FLEIBLE
DIETING

A **SCIENCE-BASED, REALITY-TESTED** METHOD FOR ACHIEVING & MAINTAINING YOUR **OPTIMAL PHYSIQUE, PERFORMANCE & HEALTH**

ALAN ARAGON

VICTORY BELT PUBLISHING INC.
LAS VEGAS

First published in 2022 by Victory Belt Publishing Inc.

ISBN-13: 978-1-628601-37-4

Cover and interior design by Elita San Juan

Illustrations by Allan Santos and Charisse Reyes

Printed in Canada

TC 0122

This book is dedicated to
Jeana, Lex, and Max—my life's
main source of pure joy.

ACKNOWLEDGMENTS

There are many people to thank. Instead of attempting a comprehensive list and still inevitably missing some dearly beloved and important individuals, I'll make this less specific, but nonetheless from the heart. I want to first thank my family for all of your love, support, patience, and wisdom. All of my real friends, you know who you are—thank you for always being there for me, especially when the chips were down. To all of my colleagues and co-authors, from the trenches to the ivory tower—thank you for helping me sharpen my skills. To all of you who have followed my career since the olden days, you have a special place in my heart. To the Victory Belt Publishing team (and my dear friend Bret Contreras for introducing us)—thank you for transforming my words and ideas into a book for the ages. To those who are new to my work, thank you for getting on the *knowledge gainz train* and trusting me to lead the way. Thank you all for providing the platform for me to have a career doing what I'm most passionate about.

TABLE OF CONTENTS

PART I

IMPORTANT INTRODUCTORY STUFF

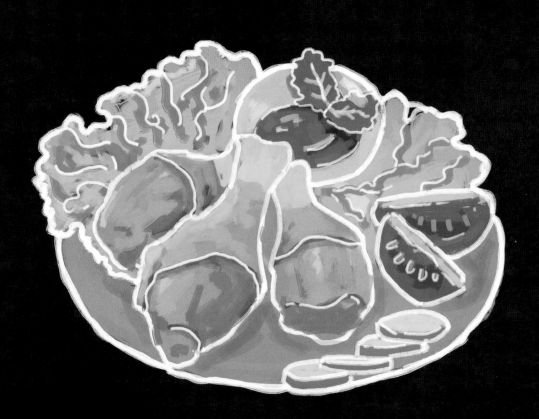

ABOUT THIS BOOK

A bit of background

The first book I ever wrote was *Girth Control*—which I self-published in 2007. By that time, I had already been in the fitness field for 15 years (I started training clients in 1992). My goal was to present the state of the science of that time, as well as my field observations.

Here we are nearly 15 years after the publication of *Girth Control*. I've accumulated a substantial amount of knowledge and experience since 2007, and I'm ready to unleash it. Over the years, I've had the honor of collaborating on various research publications that form the basis for much of the evidence-based practice guidelines for coaches, trainers, athletes, nutritionists/dietitians, and educators. Clinicians have also found utility in these publications. A special shout-out to Brad Schoenfeld is warranted here, as he has been instrumental in pulling me from the trenches into my periodic bouts in the ivory tower (the halls of academia).

The purpose of the book

Enlightenment in the area of diet and nutrition amounts to freedom from unnecessary effort, expense, health risk, and wasted time. In some cases, it can be lifesaving. But here's the colossal challenge: How do we reach the general public, who constantly walks through a minefield of diet-related misinformation? How can we teach them what we know? I suppose we can get in a pulpit and preach away, but how can we engage the public to learn? It's not as if they can just dive into the research literature and navigate their way through it. And even if they could, the in-the-trenches wisdom would still be missing. We evidence-based practitioners seem to know all the "secrets," but our efforts to effectively communicate them to the lay public have largely failed.

A frequently asked question I get is, what comprehensible yet non-quacky book do I recommend for learning what to eat to reach fitness-related goals? This book is the answer—or at least it's my answer, backed by mountains of evidence from academia and the real world. Of course I'd love for a book to go viral and change the world in a single swoop. The least I'm hoping for is to initiate the butterfly effect and perhaps inspire a handful of brilliant people with greater reach and resources than I have to continue to make the world better with evidence-based information.

Who this book is written for

I have a ton of literary space to work with here, so why not cover the needs and goals of a wide range of populations? We're in the midst of a trend toward "narrowing your niche" in the health and fitness realm. This is fine for those who want to create catchy sound bites and memorable marketing hooks, but I have the opportunity to go full-textbook in terms of breadth and depth, and I'm going to take it. Stark beginners (and those with very basic nutrition knowledge) will benefit from this book as much as high-level competitive athletes and experienced coaches. The needs and goals of the Regular Joe/Jane, all the way to folks who consider themselves "elite" on the track, field, ring, and court, are covered. This wide range of populations reflects the people I've worked with throughout my career.

With that said, I do have a soft spot for the middle-aged soccer mom/dad. I also have an affinity for the corporate desk jockey trying to recapture the glory days of early adulthood, when the idea of going to the beach or the pool didn't bring immediate pangs of anxiety. But make no mistake, my aim is to make this book life-changing (or at least genuinely useful) for everyone from couch-potato noobs to professors to professional athletes.

How to read this book

I suppose it's not common for authors to explicitly coach their audiences on how to read their books. In this case, I feel that you'll get the most out of my book by beginning with the first chapter, which details the definition of flexible dieting. It's important to know the meaning behind the title of the book. There are plenty of misconceptions about flexible dieting, perhaps the most annoying one being that flexible dieting begins and ends with tracking macro (macronutrient) grams.

So, read chapter 1 first. Then read the subsequent chapters on the *big picture of science* and, if you can stomach it, *demystifying scientific research*. These are important foundational perspectives to carry with you as you tackle the remaining chapters. In fact, these perspectives are important to have as you consume nutrition- and fitness-related media in general.

Once you've read chapters 1 and 2 (and 3 if you're brave), the next three chapters do a deep dive into how the major macronutrients—protein, carbohydrate, and fat—affect your body and its ability to function optimally during exercise. I then explore dietary supplements before finally getting into dietary programming. You are free to bounce around these chapters as you wish, but keep in mind that each one ends with an "in a nutshell" summary in case you're feeling lost.

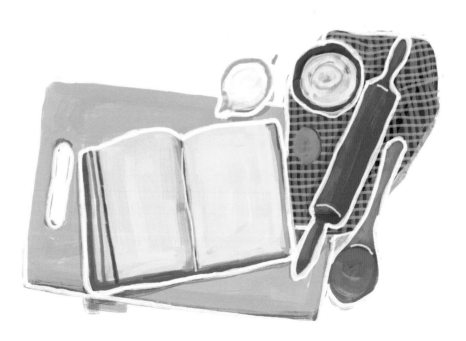

ABBREVIATION LIST

ABBREVIATION	MEANING
AA	arachidonic acid
AARR	Alan Aragon Research Review
AAS	anabolic-androgenic steroids
ACSM	American College of Sports Medicine
ADA	American Dietetic Association
ADF	alternate-day fasting
AHA	American Heart Association
ALA	alpha-linolenic acid
AMDR	acceptable macronutrient distribution range
AND	Academy of Nutrition and Dietetics
APP	Athletic Performance: Primary
APS	Athletic Performance: Secondary
ATP	adenosine triphosphate
BCAA	branched-chain amino acid
BF%	body fat percentage
BHB	ß-hydroxybutyrate
BMI	body mass index
CKD	cyclical ketogenic diet

ABBREVIATION	MEANING
CLA	conjugated linoleic acid
DHA	docosahexaenoic acid
DHT	dihydrotestosterone
DRI	Dietary Reference Intake
DSHEA	Dietary Supplement Health and Education Act
EAA	essential amino acid
EBP	evidence-based practice
EFA	essential fatty acid
EPA	eicosapentaenoic acid
eTRF	early time-restricted feeding
EVCO	extra-virgin coconut oil
FFM	fat-free mass
FFMI	fat-free mass index
GI	glycemic index
GL	glycemic load
HDL	high-density lipoprotein
HIIT	high-intensity interval training
ICAN	internal cue awareness nurturing
IF	intermittent fasting

ABBREVIATION	MEANING
IIFYM	if it fits your macros
IOC	International Olympic Committee
ISSN	International Society of Sports Nutrition
LBM	lean body mass
LDL	low-density lipoprotein
MCT	medium-chain triglyceride
MFGM	milk fat globule membrane
MPB	muscle protein breakdown
MPS	muscle protein synthesis
mTOR	mammalian target of rapamycin
MVM	multivitamin-mineral
NEAT	non-exercise activity thermogenesis
NHANES	National Health and Nutrition Examination Survey
PDH	pyruvate dehydrogenase
PICO	population, intervention, comparator, outcome
PRISMA	Preferred Reporting Items for Systematic reviews and Meta-Analyses
PUFA	polyunsaturated fatty acid

ABBREVIATION	MEANING
RCT	randomized controlled trial
RD	reduction diet
RDA	Recommended Dietary Allowance
RDI	Reference Daily Intake
REE	resting energy expenditure
RET	resistance exercise training
RMR	resting metabolic rate
SFA	saturated fatty acid
T2D	type 2 diabetes
TBW	target bodyweight
TFA	trans fatty acids
TRF	time-restricted feeding
USDA	United States Department of Agriculture

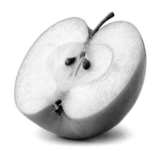

THE ORIGIN & EVOLUTION OF FLEXIBLE DIETING

1

PLEASE BE WARNED: I'm going to throw a lot of dates and citations at you in this chapter because the historical timeline is important for understanding the development and definition of flexible dieting in the research literature. This chapter might feel like reading Leviticus at times, but please bear with me as you grit through it. The following battery of findings is necessary to clear up the confusion about what flexible dieting actually is versus what the popular media and fitness culture have erroneously morphed it into.

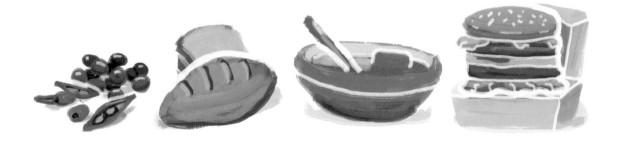

RIGID VERSUS FLEXIBLE DIETARY CONTROL

Tracing the origins of flexible dieting in the peer-reviewed literature takes us back to 1975, when Herman and Mack[1] were the first to examine high versus low levels of *restraint* (degree of self-imposed restriction for weight loss) on normal-weight individuals. They found that low-restraint individuals' food intake after a milkshake preload was inversely proportional to the preload. In other words, larger milkshakes were followed by less food intake and vice versa. This was not the case with high-restraint individuals, whose intake was directly proportional to the size of the milkshake preload. This led the authors to conclude that the low-restraint individuals showed the characteristics of folks who successfully self-regulate and maintain leanness while the high-restraint subjects shared similar eating behavior with folks who struggle with bodyweight.

FLEXIBLE VOCAB

Preload

A preload is a food or beverage consumed at a designated time before a meal in experiments that test effects on hunger, satiety, and caloric consumption in the subsequent meal. Common preloads include protein shakes, bars, and plain water.

So, what does cognitive restraint have to do with flexible dieting? Fast-forward to 1991, when Westenhoefer[2] proposed that dietary restraint (interchanged with "dietary control") can be stratified into two subcategories: flexible and rigid.

- **Rigid control** involves an inflexible, all-or-nothing approach to eating; food choices and timing are based on set, nonnegotiable rules.

- **Flexible control** utilizes more dynamic and accommodating tactics such as smaller servings instead of complete avoidance of certain foods, allowing for greater variety and flexibility. Flexible control also permits the compensation or counterbalancing of "unhealthy" food consumption with "healthy" foods in subsequent meals to limit the chances of excess intake overall.[3]

An important finding was that rigid control was associated with greater *disinhibition.* In this context, disinhibition is a tendency to overeat in the presence of palatable foods or other stimuli such as emotional stress. On the other hand, greater flexible control was associated with lower disinhibition. More concerning is that greater rigid control was associated with more problematic eating behaviors, with binging being the predominant problem. Flexible control was linked to the opposite: fewer reports of dysfunctional or disordered eating. So, the stricter the diet, the more likely the dieter was to break the rules and overeat.

Subsequent consistency of favorable outcomes from flexible dietary control

Similar findings were seen over the next decade. In 1994, Shearin and colleagues[4] found that flexible control was inversely associated with body mass index (BMI). In other words, a more flexible approach to dieting was associated with lower bodyweight.

The following year, Williamson and colleagues[5] also reported that flexible control was inversely correlated with BMI, in addition to finding that a combination of high dietary restraint and overeating was positively correlated with bulimic symptoms in normal-weight women. In 1999, Smith and colleagues[6] found that flexible dieting was associated with lower bodyweight, an absence of overeating, and lower levels of anxiety and depression. Conversely, rigid dieting was associated with overeating and increased bodyweight.

Also in 1999, Westenhoefer and colleagues[3] formally validated the concepts of flexible and rigid restraint across a range of populations. They concluded that rigid control is associated with greater disinhibition, higher bodyweight, and more frequent and severe episodes of binge eating, while flexible control is associated with the opposite outcomes, including a higher probability of long-term weight loss maintenance. In 2002, Stewart and colleagues[7] found that rigid dieting (but not flexible dieting) was associated with eating disorder symptoms, body image disturbance, and higher BMI.

Macronutrient counting makes a splash in the literature

In 2020, Conlin and colleagues[8] compared the effects of a macronutrient-tracking approach versus a meal plan–based approach using a 10-week hypocaloric phase followed by a 10-week ad libitum (unrestricted) phase in resistance-trained subjects. During the 10-week dieting phase, both groups retained lean mass and lost fat mass, with no significant differences between the groups. In the 10-week ad libitum phase, the macro-counting group gained significantly more lean mass (+1.7 kg) than the "rigid" group (–0.4 kg). Overall, with the exception of lean mass gain in the ad libitum post-diet phase in the macro-counting group, there was a lack of meaningful differences between the groups. The participant dropout rate was slightly higher in the macro-counting group. The authors speculated that the meal plan–based approach could have been easier to follow because it didn't involve any planning or calculating.

> ### FLEXIBLE VOCAB
>
> **Hypocaloric, hypercaloric, and eucaloric**
>
> A hypocaloric diet simply entails eating fewer calories than you burn, which will cause you to lose weight. Hypercaloric means the opposite—more calories and less burn equal more weight gain. Eucaloric falls in between; it's a diet designed to maintain your current weight.

The meal plan–based approach was appropriately labeled "rigid," while the macro-counting approach was labeled "flexible." This classification is at least partially justified because there were no restrictions on the food choices comprising the macronutrient targets. However, this approach carries the potential for rigidity (without flexibility of the targeted gram amounts), but also a potentially unhealthy level of micromanagement. The authors' opinion on macro-counting is worth quoting: *"When taken too far, it can pathologize into what is commonly observed with rigid dieting."*

DICHOTOMOUS THINKING: THE BACKBONE OF RIGID DIETARY CONTROL

Dichotomous thinking is the tendency to perceive events or stimuli as binary. For example, someone with dichotomous thinking might believe that specific foods are either good or bad, those being the only two possible states. In reality, every food offers different levels of nutritional value.

In 2000, Tiggemann[9] was perhaps the first to present the concept of dichotomous thinking as a factor that can influence dietary outcomes. Dichotomous perceptions of food and dieting (e.g., "good" versus "bad" or "clean" versus "dirty") were implicated as a dysfunctional cognitive style. In 2003, Byrne and colleagues[10] investigated the psychological factors associated with weight loss maintenance and found that dichotomous thinking was one of the strongest predictors of weight regain. In 2008, Ramacciotti and colleagues[11] reported that dichotomous reasoning was one of the characteristics of obese individuals with binge-eating disorder, and those without this disorder did not show dichotomous reasoning. In 2011, Lethbridge and colleagues[12] reported that dichotomous thinking was one of the factors linked to disordered eating. In 2015, Palascha et al.[13] found that failed bodyweight regulation was associated with dichotomous food and dieting beliefs rather than dietary restraint per se. In 2018, Berg and colleagues[14] found that in overweight and obese women averaging 69 years of age, increased flexible dietary restraint combined with decreased rigid restraint was associated with greater weight loss.

An overlooked result of dichotomous thinking is the attribution of moral characteristics to foods that are labeled "bad" or "dirty" instead of "good" or "clean." This black-or-white thinking paves the way for perceiving certain foods and eating behaviors as "right" or "wrong." Rigid dietary control facilitates and reinforces this view. While a dichotomous approach of right and wrong might apply to criminal law, food and dieting are more productively approached from a relativistic standpoint. This allows for nuance and shades of gray that are more reflective of reality. Importantly, a flexible approach enables individualization when it comes to programming. Figure 1a provides an overview of dietary restraint and its subcategories.

Figure 1a: Dietary Control: Subcategories & Implications

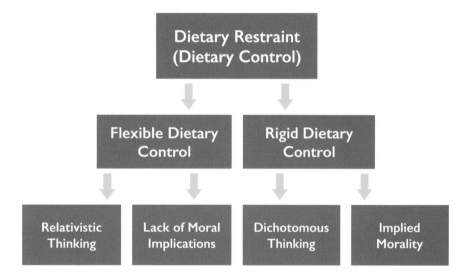

Harboring the perception of "good" and "bad" foods opens up the potential for moral judgment of oneself or others who might be eating a bad food, thus committing a bad deed, and thus being a bad person. Labeling foods in this manner gives them undeserved power. "Bad" foods become perceived as forbidden fruit. This sets the stage for overconsumption (or binging) because the dieter swears that this will be the last dance with this morally reprehensible food.

Bottom line: it's just food. Give the power to yourself, not the food. Of course, there needs to be some degree of moderation of foods that have problematic potential. This makes a good segue into the concept of *discretionary calories.*

DISCRETIONARY CALORIES: ALL FOODS CAN FIT WHEN PROPERLY MODERATED

The influence of flexible dieting principles on public health recommendations goes back to 1996, when the *ADA Courier* (the newsletter of the American Dietetic Association, or ADA, now called the Academy of Nutrition and Dietetics, or AND) designated March as National Nutrition Month. Its slogan was "All foods can fit." This simple and memorable slogan was first published in the peer-reviewed literature in the September 1997 issue of the *Journal of the Academy of Nutrition and Dietetics*.[15] In 2002, the position stand of the ADA on communicating nutrition information was that "all foods can fit into a healthful eating style."[16] The ADA's position was that labeling foods as "good" or "bad" had the potential to foster unhealthy eating behaviors. This stance was almost certainly influenced by research on the dysfunctional impact of dichotomous thinking.

FLEXIBLE VOCAB

Position stands

This term may seem a bit redundant, but a position stand serves a specific, important purpose: it's a scientific institution's most authoritative evidence-based statement on a relevant topic in its field. It is intended to represent the scientific consensus on the topic.

In 2005, the US Department of Health and Human Services and the US Department of Agriculture (USDA) coined the term *discretionary calorie allowance*,[17] defined as the margin of calories remaining when recommended nutrient intakes are met through a predominance of nutrient-dense foods. In other words, you can have your discretionary calories after you eat your vegetables.

This allows the flexibility to include added fats, added sugars, and alcohol. But here's the catch: discretionary calories amount to roughly 10 to 20 percent of total daily caloric intake. The remaining 80 to 90 percent of the diet should come from whole and minimally refined foods. This guideline has withstood the test of time due to its realistic application of moderation.

Using a 2,000-kcal diet as an example, this amounts to a "discretionary" allotment of 200 to 400 kcal per day from whatever foods an individual wants. Of course, junk foods (I prefer to call them *indulgence foods*) don't have to be forced into a diet if a person has no desire for them. The point is that a diet consisting of 100 percent stereotypically healthy foods will not necessarily constitute better health. This is especially true if long-term adherence is better when the diet allows the option to consume indulgence foods. If you feel that consuming a diet that's completely junk food–free 100 percent of the time is most sustainable for you, then that's fine—if it truly is your personal preference.

FLEXIBLE VOCAB

kcal

The abbreviation kcal is often used interchangeably with "calories." This is because kcal originally meant kilocalorie, or one large calorie equal to 1,000 small calories. This gets into the physics and chemistry of how calories convert to energy, but for the purposes of nutrition, let's just say that one kilocalorie equals one calorie worth of usable energy.

IIFYM: an inside joke that turned into a worldwide brand

Some of you reading this book already know that IIFYM stands for *if it fits your macros*. Few people know the details of the inception and transformation of this acronym, so I'll give you the scoop. I was one of the folks who inadvertently helped create this monster. I watched IIFYM go from an inside joke on the message boards to the brand name of a dietary approach of hitting daily macronutrient gram targets with minimal regard for food choices and diet quality. Let's take a short walk through a smidge beyond the past decade.

In 2009, Eric Koenreich, a fellow veteran member of bodybuilding.com's nutrition forum, thought of making an acronym out of an answer we'd give to newbies on the forum. This was due to a high volume of posts asking if various foods could be consumed during a cutting (fat loss) phase. The foods in question were everything outside of a narrow range of stereotypical bodybuilding foods traditionally used for contest prep. For example, if someone asked if whole eggs could be consumed instead of egg whites, we'd say, "If it fits your macronutrient targets, go ahead and have that food."

After an exhausting repetition of daily questions like this, Eric (out of frustration) thought of a quick, snarky way to respond by making an acronym out of the answer. Typing "IIFYM" was a lot easier than typing out the "If it fits your macronutrient targets..." answer dozens of times a day. From 2009 through 2011, we regularly responded to posts in this cheeky, not-very-helpful manner. "Can I have dark meat instead of chicken breast?"—"IIFYM." "Can I have bananas while cutting? What about white rice? What about peanut butter?"—"IIFYM." And on and on, and we chuckled among ourselves about it. Little did we know that this clumsy acronym we flippantly threw around would go viral and become an international brand of sorts.

People had no clue of its origin and intent, so IIFYM morphed into the name of a diet that gave the green light to eating like a reckless child as long as macronutrient gram targets were hit. Many folks were excited to fulfill their macronutrient targets with however much junk food they wanted and still hit their bodyweight (or body composition) goals. At the same time, many ran into the inevitable problems of predominating the diet with energy-dense, hyperpalatable foods that lacked micronutrition and satiating power. There's also an ongoing degree of opposition to and disdain for IIFYM for supposedly promoting an unhealthy lifestyle.

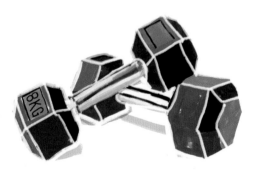

The effort to educate people about discretionary calories (10 to 20 percent) within the IIFYM framework has been a hard-fought battle, but the message seems to be making some headway. Confusion should slowly but surely dissipate once this book makes it into enough personal (and maybe even some public) libraries. On a side note, IIFYM reminds me of the ADA's 1996 National Nutrition Month slogan, "All foods can fit." However, the important stipulation is that all foods can fit into an overall healthy diet where discretionary calories comprise roughly 10 to 20 percent of total energy intake. Enjoy indulgence foods in moderation; your diet should still be composed primarily of whole, healthful foods.

Important technical note: IIFYM and flexible dieting are not synonymous

It's frustrating to see people mistakenly use the terms "IIFYM" and "flexible dieting" interchangeably. It's also been frustrating to watch this confusion unfold and persist to this day—among the lay public as well as academics. For example, Conlin and colleagues[8] put IIFYM, macro-counting, and the term "flexible dieting" in the same boat. The unintentional implication is that tracking and micromanaging grams of the macronutrients exemplifies flexible dieting when it does not. Furthermore, it was a missed opportunity for the proper origin and intent of IIFYM to be stated in the peer-reviewed literature, but alas, we can't expect Conlin and colleagues to know such underground info. Well, reader, now *you* know.

As we've reviewed during this three-decade walk down memory lane, flexible dieting is not the equivalent of checking a macro-tracking app, seeing you have an odd amount of protein, carbs, and fat left for the final stretch of the evening, and agonizing over whether you've stocked the proper foods to meet those targets. On the contrary, flexible dietary control pertains to the cognitive style of dietary restraint.

Do you control your diet in a rigid, black-or-white, dichotomous way, or do you allow flexibility of tracking/accountability style, nutrient ranges, food choices, and timing throughout the day or week? Flexible dietary control is the latter; it's not a different name for the practice of tracking macros. While setting macronutrient targets and tracking them indeed allows flexibility of food choices, it also carries the rigidity of hitting the numbers. A potential problem is that tracking your dietary intake to the gram is the very definition of micromanagement. In my observations, imposing a high degree of precision (of intake and tracking) can exacerbate people's preexisting obsessiveness.

The bombshell twist: *true* flexible dieting accommodates degrees of rigidity

Here's a concept that's important to process: flexible dieting involves individualizing the degree of dietary flexibility (or rigidity). It also individualizes the precision of tracking and accountability. Some folks can sustain the practice of gram-tracking just fine, and some even enjoy it (although, in my observations, they're in the minority). Some folks would rather track portions of each food group, as in the traditional exchange system used by dietitians. Other approaches include tracking just protein and total calories—or just protein. There's also the option to not track anything at all in the formal sense. Rather, you just maintain an awareness of your requirements for the least amount of dietary variables that still allows progress (or maintenance of progress). This option involves developing your awareness of hunger and satiety cues.

Flexible dieting encompasses all of these approaches, which are covered in this book. *Remember that flexible dieting is not a specific diet*—it's a style of dietary control. It eschews dichotomous thinking and facilitates better individualization and long-term adherence. Figure 1b outlines the continuum of dietary control and shows the true nature of flexible dieting. Other continuums related to the precision of intake and tracking will be introduced later in the book after programming has been discussed.

Figure 1b: Continuum of Dietary Control

FLEXIBLE ⟷ **RIGID**

- Protein gram or serving target, with the rest of the diet based on internal hunger and satiety cues

- Intuitive eating (all intake based on hunger and satiety cues)

- Food groups serving ranges

- Guidelines without quantitative targets (i.e., eat more versus less of certain foods or food groups)

- Any of the above with discretionary serving allotments

- Total calorie target

- Protein target with flexible carbohydrate and fat intake (as long as total kcals are met)

- Macronutrient targets with the freedom to choose food sources

- Any of the above with discretionary calorie allotments

- Any of the above with designated "cheat" meals or "cheat" days (which is not actually cheating if it's within the plan; I prefer to call them *indulgence meals* or *days off*)

- Allowed and prohibited foods

- Allowed and prohibited foods or macronutrients at certain times of day

- Specific daily menu with minimal variation or food options within meals (minimal regard to personal preference of food choice)

FLEXIBLE DIETING in its truest form is flexibility of dietary control. This means the freedom to engage in any of the approaches above, alone or in combination, depending on the individual's goal at the time. For example, during competitive phases, athletes may engage in more rigid or precise strategies and then loosen up the approach during noncompetitive phases. The more rigid the approach, the greater the risk for adverse consequences or unsustainability. Therefore, long-term solutions for the general public typically involve graduating toward more flexible dietary control and away from the extreme end of rigid dietary control.

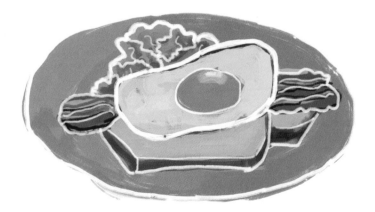

CHAPTER 1 IN A NUTSHELL

- Flexible versus rigid dietary restraint (which eventually came to be called dietary control) has been studied extensively since the early 1990s. *Flexible dietary control* has consistently been associated with favorable outcomes, while rigid dietary control has consistently been associated with symptoms of eating disorders (particularly binge-eating) and a lack of successful bodyweight regulation.

- *Rigid dietary control* is characterized by dichotomous thinking (the tendency to perceive events or stimuli as binary opposites: an all-or-nothing/black-or-white approach). This cognitive style consistently is associated with adverse outcomes, including the false attribution of morality to foods (i.e., "good" versus "bad"), consequently straining the conscience of the dieter and compromising long-term success.

- An antidote to the pitfalls of rigid dieting is *discretionary calorie allowance* (10 to 20 percent of total kcal from any food the individual wants), with the remaining 80 to 90 percent of the diet coming from whole and minimally refined foods. This predominance of nutrient-dense foods combined with a moderated allowance for indulgence foods ensures a healthy diet overall that increases the chances of long-term adherence.

- IIFYM (if it fits your macros) started as an inside joke on the bodybuilding message boards and morphed into the name of a diet that gives a green light to eating all the junk food you want as long as it fits your macronutrient targets. This was not the original intention of the acronym, and anyone who thinks otherwise is misinformed.

- Flexible dieting is not the name of a specific diet. Flexible dieting is not synonymous with IIFYM, nor is flexible dieting merely another term for tracking macronutrients (aka "macro counting").

- Flexible dieting accommodates nuances and shades of gray rather than imposing a universal approach or set of dieting rules. It operates on the basis of individual preferences, tolerances, and goals. Flexible dieting includes flexibility and individualization of macronutrient targets, food choices, meal timing, and tracking/accountability/awareness methods.

- The clincher: flexible dieting even allows the freedom to choose the degree of flexibility (or rigidity) that best suits the individual. This includes hybrids of rigid and flexible dietary control that can vary according to individual goals. So, yes, the hidden gem is that flexible dieting includes flexibility in the dietary approach itself.

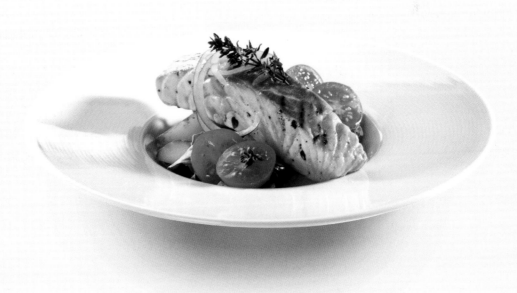

PART 2

SCIENTIFIC FOUNDATIONS

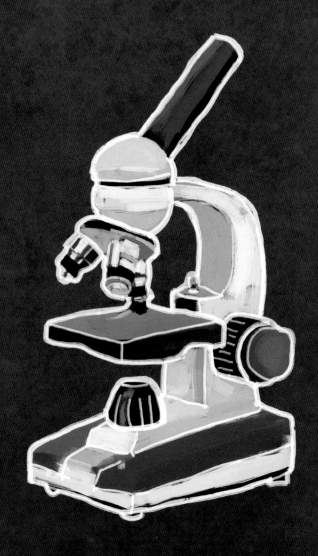

THE BIG PICTURE OF SCIENCE

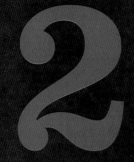

WHY IS THE GENERAL PUBLIC SO CONFUSED ABOUT WHAT TO EAT?

As I see it, there are three main interacting factors driving the public's confusion about diet and nutrition:

- Everybody eats.

- Misinformation is rampant.

- Scientific literacy is scarce.

First of all, everyone must eat as a matter of survival. Since everybody eats, there's a tendency for people to develop a sense of authority about what works—especially if their personal eating habits have been working well for them. Many feel that they have automatic dominion or expertise in this area, so the teaching, preaching, and bold claims proceed from there.

Of course, many of these claims have no evidence basis other than personal testimony or mere opinion tainted by confirmation bias, among other things. This is a unique problem within the field of nutrition. For example, you don't see people pervasively offering legal advice at social gatherings; there's no obligatory link between lawyering and human survival. But alas...everybody eats, so everyone is an "expert" at it.

Misinformation: anyone can write a diet book

The second factor driving the widespread confusion is that unqualified people (and outright quacks) have a knack for writing diet books that become quite popular. As a group, the science-minded people qualified to write books or dish out nutrition advice to the public are a) too busy counseling clients or treating patients, b) lacking in marketing savvy, or c) unwilling to bend the truth into something that hits all the right emotional hot-buttons. As a result, the people succeeding at reaching the masses are serving up a lot of misinformation.

Marton and colleagues[18] examined the current top 100 bestselling diet book authors' credentials and occupations as well as the claims made in those books. Their results are shown in Figure 2a.

Figure 2a: Author Occupations for the Top 100 Bestselling Diet Books

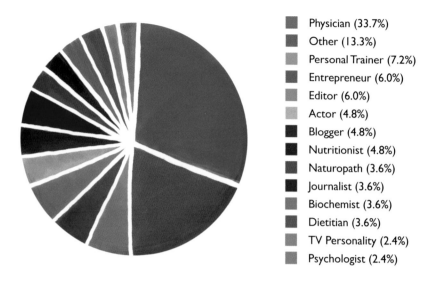

- Physician (33.7%)
- Other (13.3%)
- Personal Trainer (7.2%)
- Entrepreneur (6.0%)
- Editor (6.0%)
- Actor (4.8%)
- Blogger (4.8%)
- Nutritionist (4.8%)
- Naturopath (3.6%)
- Journalist (3.6%)
- Biochemist (3.6%)
- Dietitian (3.6%)
- TV Personality (2.4%)
- Psychologist (2.4%)

Perhaps unsurprisingly, physicians comprised the largest proportion (33.7 percent) of the 14 occupations in the sample. The general public is unaware of how woefully inadequate the nutrition course requirements are for physicians.[19] In contrast, dietitians (who have undergone rigorously extensive training in nutrition) comprised only 3.6 percent of the occupations, making them third to last, in front of TV personalities and psychologists, who were tied for last place at 2.4 percent. It was also found that most of the authors of these books were not active in the peer-reviewed literature. The following excerpts from the paper illustrate my point perfectly:

> "In all, our assessment of the summaries of bestselling books on nutrition shows that they may provide information or misinformation about very important matters... [...] it is likely that many, probably the large majority, contain substantial misinformation and claims that have no scientific foundation.

> "The information spread in these books may eventually have more impact on the public than the peer-reviewed scientific literature, as more consumers reported using nutritional information from friends and family members or from news articles or headlines or news on TV..."

A third factor underpinning the general public's confusion about nutrition is a lack of scientific literacy.

SCIENTIFIC LITERACY: NECESSARY FOR NAVIGATING THE MINEFIELD OF MISINFORMATION

The National Research Council has defined scientific literacy as the ability to *"use evidence and data to evaluate the quality of science information and arguments put forth by scientists and in the media."*[20] The general public's lack of scientific literacy leaves them vulnerable to everything from well-meaning spreaders of misinformation to individuals and companies who purposely lie to consumers to extract cash. While many people will read this book for direct answers to their nutrition- and fitness-related questions, I'm going to insist on taking some time to teach you how to fish instead of handing you a fish (although plenty of fish are served throughout the book). New information will always be surfacing through multiple sources, and it's important to have a basic skill set for discerning the quality of the information fed to you or people you care about.

The discussion of scientific literacy must begin with defining what science is. The National Academy of Sciences defines science as *"the use of evidence to construct testable explanation and prediction of natural phenomena, as well as the knowledge generated through this process."*[21] Science functions as a system of inquiry and discovery that maximizes objectivity and minimizes bias. Thus, here's my personal definition of science:

> *Science is the set of principles that guide research toward uncovering the truth without kidding anyone—or yourself.*

Science and research, though used interchangeably, are more accurately seen as two separate but related entities. Science is a "flawless" set of principles, while research is the vehicle that attempts to carry out those principles. Since research is done by humans, it's inevitably flawed. It's messy, and it's subject to varying degrees of error and bias. Nevertheless, scientific research is the best tool we have for investigating the way things in the material world actually work. The alternative to scientific research is baseless speculation, imagination, opinion, and personal testimony.

The forward march of research is virtually endless because of the vast expanse of the unknown—especially when it comes to the complexity of human physiology. The goal of research is to bring more definitive answers and understanding to the broad swaths of gray area in our knowledge. Concrete, measurable skills of scientific literacy include the ability to identify a valid scientific argument, evaluate the validity of sources, identify the misuse of scientific information, understand the elements of research design, interpret quantitative data generated by research, and evaluate conclusions based on these data.[22] A basic understanding of statistics and methodology is important, but not as important as the ability to use sound logic and reason in order to ask the right questions.

FLEXIBLE VOCAB

Qualitative versus quantitative

Qualitative and quantitative studies differ in both the data collected and the methods of collection. Whereas qualitative studies collect non-numerical data such as personal accounts, quantitative studies rely on data that is numerical or measurable.

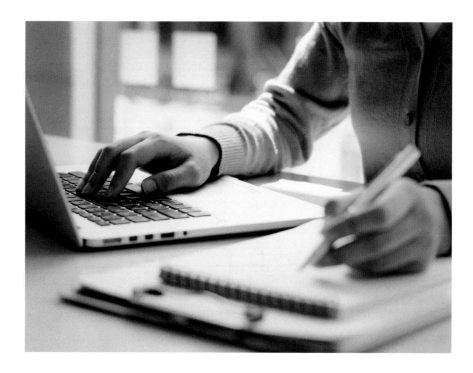

THE SCIENTIFIC METHOD

The scientific method is something many of us learned in grade school but have rarely (if ever) revisited. Please bear with the flashback; it is crucial to the discussion of scientific literacy. While there's no singular, universally accepted version of the scientific method, its variations share the same fundamental progression:

1. Observation and description of the phenomenon (or phenomena) that cannot immediately be explained; generation of the problem/purpose.

2. Formulation of a hypothesis to explain the observed phenomena and predict quantifiable outcomes.

3. Testing of the hypothesis and its predictions through experimental design that appropriately addresses the question being investigated.

4. Analysis of the results/data; evaluation of the potential applicability of new insights to the field.

5. Repetition of the process—with improved methodology, when possible. Replication of results from independent labs strengthens the likelihood that the findings were not erroneous.

These steps will further crystallize when we discuss randomized controlled trials (RCTs), the type of research considered highest on the evidence hierarchy due to its ability to demonstrate cause and effect.

In a nutshell, the process is to observe, make an educated guess, and then test that guess. If your guess doesn't pass the test, it needs to be scrapped, and then the process can continue with alternative hypotheses. If your hunch was correct, then that's the beginning of an evidence basis, which gets strengthened if others can replicate the results.

A prime example of the scientific method at work is the discovery and confirmation of the effectiveness of creatine supplementation for increasing muscle size and strength. Let's break down the process using an example.

OBSERVATION: The observation in the case of creatine begins with the long-standing knowledge that adenosine triphosphate (ATP) is required to fuel all biological processes in the body, hence ATP's description as the body's energy currency. The phosphagen system (also called the ATP-creatine phosphate system) provides a limited amount of ATP, which can supply energy for skeletal muscle to perform short-term, maximal-effort work. Within the muscle cells, phosphocreatine functions as an energy buffer, prolonging the availability of ATP.

HYPOTHESIS: The educated guess, based on observation and existing knowledge, was that supplementing with creatine could increase intramuscular creatine levels. This in turn could form phosphocreatine, which could serve as a buffer to resynthesize ATP, which would increase the capacity to perform maximal-effort anaerobic exercise.

FLEXIBLE VOCAB

Anaerobic exercise

Anaerobic exercise differs from aerobic exercise in that it's higher in intensity, burning more calories per unit of time. You've no doubt done an anaerobic workout at some point and not even realized it. Basically, it's any short, high-intensity activity that uses glucose for energy while making your oxygen demand surpass your supply. This can be accomplished with high-effort resistance training, sprinting, and other intense exercise.

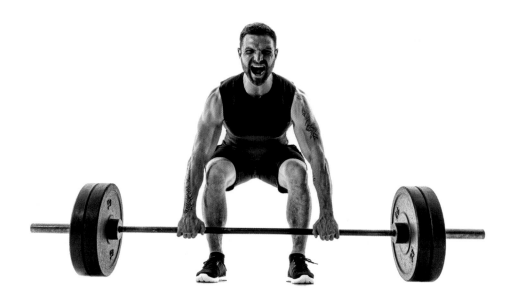

EXPERIMENTATION: Intervention trials compared the effects of creatine supplementation with a placebo (inert substance) in order to see whether it works. If you are familiar with the way creatine works, you know that it's a matter of saturating intramuscular stores; this is discussed in Chapter 7.

ANALYSIS OF THE RESULTS: Creatine's effects on high-intensity, strength/power-oriented activities are significantly greater than a placebo, and these results are not likely due to bias or confounding variables. Therefore, the hypothesis is accepted as viable.

REPLICATION: The majority of studies—several hundred since the 1990s across a wide range of populations and circumstances—have shown the effectiveness of creatine for enhancing muscular size, strength, and power.[23]

The big point here is that creatine's legitimacy is based on consistent support from research that properly carries out the scientific method. Creatine's evidence base is not merely speculation, hype, and celebrity endorsements.

In contrast to creatine, a compound called conjugated linoleic acid (CLA) is touted as a weight loss supplement. It worked great in rodents, and initial research in humans showed promise. However, a systematic review and meta-analysis by Onakpoya and colleagues[24] found that CLA's long-term effects are too negligible to be considered clinically relevant. As I'll discuss in the next section (point #4), a scientific perspective of CLA would not conclude with 100 percent certainty that it's useless for fat loss; it's just unlikely to have meaningful effects, as far as the current body of evidence stands.

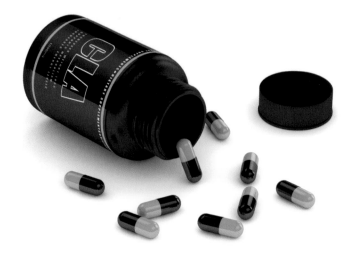

THE NATURE OF SCIENCE (CORE PRINCIPLES)

In addition to having a basic grasp of the scientific method, it's equally important to be familiar with the fundamental nature of science and how this familiarity assists in scientific reasoning and knowing the right questions to ask. A collaboration headed by the National Academies of Sciences, Engineering, and Medicine outlines the five core principles and assumptions of scientific inquiry:[25]

1. **Nature is not capricious.** In other words, science operates under the presumption that nature follows rules that are consistent. So, if a new experiment is performed under the conditions with the same variables as another experiment, the results should be replicated.

2. **Knowledge grows through exploration of the limits of existing rules and mutually reinforcing evidence.** The discovery of new relationships among the variables in question allows for the expansion of the evidence base of any given topic. When different types of studies (i.e., observational and interventional designs) arrive at similar conclusions, it's called a convergence of evidence, or consilience. The greater the consilience of results on a given topic, the more confidence we have in the phenomena being true, and not merely due to error or bias. Rules that hold true beyond the context in which they're discovered are steps toward discovering the limits of their generalizability. However, finding the limits of how far we can generalize or apply these results/rules is important for the progress of science. For example, if a particular result of a given diet or protocol is seen in untrained but not trained individuals, this suggests that the relationship may be affected by training status or other characteristics that may lead to further investigation. Basically, science thrives by finding and testing the boundaries of our knowledge.

3. **Science is a communal enterprise.** In other words, science is an ongoing, shared endeavor among researchers who build upon their own work and the work of their peers. In addition to studying previous findings and learning novel ones, researchers critically appraise one another's work as a means of quality control. Each properly conducted study is a piece that contributes meaningfully to the larger puzzle. The collective body of research is also crucial for educating practitioners, clinicians, and the public.

4. **Science aims for refined degrees of confidence rather than certainty.** Scientific findings have an inherent degree of uncertainty. The tentative nature of science is actually one of its strengths, since an openness to improving existing models and systems of knowledge is impossible when operating under the presumption of certainty. Researchers should understand and disclose the uncertainties and limitations of their work. Individuals or entities seeking to use a given study's results should also be aware of its limitations.

5. **Scientific knowledge is durable and mutable.** The state of scientific knowledge on any given topic evolves as existing models are tested in new contexts or with improved technology. The scientific process allows a consistency of new (credible) evidence to modify and in some cases overturn previous positions or opinions, even if they were deemed to be well established. The fact that scientific knowledge is subject to change shouldn't be seen as a weakness. It's actually the progression toward a deeper, clearer understanding of how nature works.

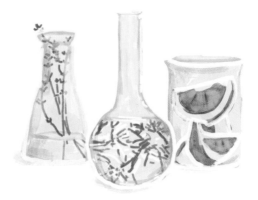

Pseudoscience: how not to do it

Pseudoscience is an important term that refers to any concept or practice that claims to be scientific (or appears scientific to the untrained eye) but is not actually rooted in the scientific method. The research evidence base of pseudoscientific claims is weak to nonexistent. Pseudoscience often relies on misused (or made-up) technical jargon and the misapplication of legitimate research in order to fabricate a scientific aura.

Classic examples of pseudoscience are astrology and homeopathy. Basing diets on body type or blood type are examples of pseudoscience in the nutrition realm. Characteristics of pseudoscience include an over-reliance on anecdotes/testimonials, an avoidance of peer review, a lack of biological plausibility, and a lack of research evidence. Understanding the nature of unscientific approaches to knowledge can help us understand scientific approaches to knowledge by a simple contrasting comparison (Table 2a).[26]

Table 2a: Approaches to Knowledge

	SCIENTIFIC	UNSCIENTIFIC
General approach	Empirical	Intuitive
Observation	Controlled	Uncontrolled
Reporting	Unbiased	Biased
Definitions of concepts	Clear	Ambiguous
Instruments	Accurate/precise	Inaccurate/imprecise
Measurement	Reliable/repeatable	Unreliable
Hypotheses	Testable (falsifiable)	Untestable (unfalsifiable)
Attitude	Critical	Uncritical

Evidence-based practice: bridging the gap between the lab and the trenches

Evidence-based practice (EBP) in the fitness context is an offshoot of evidence-based medicine, which originated from the need to raise the scientific standard of patient care.[27] Thanks to bickering matches on social media (typically won by whoever has the most PubMed links ready for inundating the opposition), EBP is commonly misunderstood. EBP has three main components: the current body of scientific literature, field experience, and individualization of client/patient needs.

The peer-reviewed literature is crucial to EBP and functions as a starting point from which to individualize programs. Relying on the scientific literature can often save people time, energy, and money because they can go straight to the agents and protocols that have the greatest probability of being effective. However, it's only a fraction of the empirical body of knowledge. Gray areas or knowledge gaps in the literature must be bridged by experience and observations in the field. EBP is where science and practice converge. Thus, having the most PubMed links is not enough. Furthermore, protocols must be tailored to individual needs and preferences, regardless of what has been published (or not). Figure 2b illustrates the misconception versus the actual components of EBP.

Figure 2b: Evidence-Based Practice (EBP)

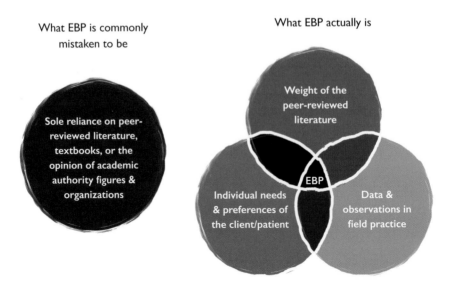

What EBP is commonly mistaken to be

Sole reliance on peer-reviewed literature, textbooks, or the opinion of academic authority figures & organizations

What EBP actually is

Weight of the peer-reviewed literature

Individual needs & preferences of the client/patient

Data & observations in field practice

EBP

CHAPTER 2 IN A NUTSHELL

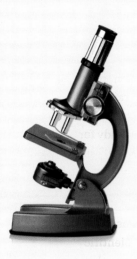

- The general public is utterly confused about what to eat for three main reasons: 1) Everybody eats (and thus feels a sense of authority over this domain). 2) Dietary misinformation abounds in the mass media due to highly biased and/or unqualified people with large audiences. 3) The public lacks scientific literacy.

- Scientific literacy, which is the ability to discern scientifically valid information from hype and speculation, is important for navigating your way through the minefield of misinformation.

- A collaboration headed by the National Academies of Sciences, Engineering, and Medicine outlines the five core principles and assumptions of scientific inquiry as follows: 1) Nature is not capricious. 2) Knowledge grows through exploration of the limits of existing rules and mutually reinforcing evidence. 3) Science is a communal enterprise. 4) Science aims for refined degrees of confidence rather than complete certainty. 5) Science is durable and mutable.

- Pseudoscience is non-science disguised as science, thanks to the clever use of jargon and misapplication of research. Pseudoscience profits from taking advantage of the general public's interest in and lack of understanding of science.

- Evidence-based practice (EBP) bridges the gap between theoretical and practical knowledge. There will always be gray areas of knowledge yet to be definitively covered by scientific research. Although the peer-reviewed literature is a crucial component of EBP, field experience and observations combined with individual client/patient needs complete the evidence-based approach.

DEMYSTIFYING SCIENTIFIC RESEARCH

3

TYPES OF RESEARCH

A big part of winning the battle to understand scientific research is knowing how it's categorized and knowing the purpose, strengths, and limitations of each type. That is, you should know which types of research have the most validity, how much weight to give them, and how to tell them apart. Figure 3a depicts the various types of research, existing on a continuum from research that can convey observations to research that's capable of establishing causation.

Descriptive research

Descriptive research includes case studies, surveys, and historical research. The objective is self-explanatory: to describe what is observed. The strength of descriptive research is that it's relatively straightforward and less prone to rogue variables (called *confounders*) that can introduce error or bias. It merely describes observable phenomena at face value and does not attempt to determine what agent causes a given effect.

Despite a lack of intervention (control of the variables), descriptive research can be quite valuable. For example, case studies of successful bodybuilders' contest preparation strategies have provided clues regarding what might work for individuals beyond the person being studied in the publication.

Figure 3a: The Research Continuum

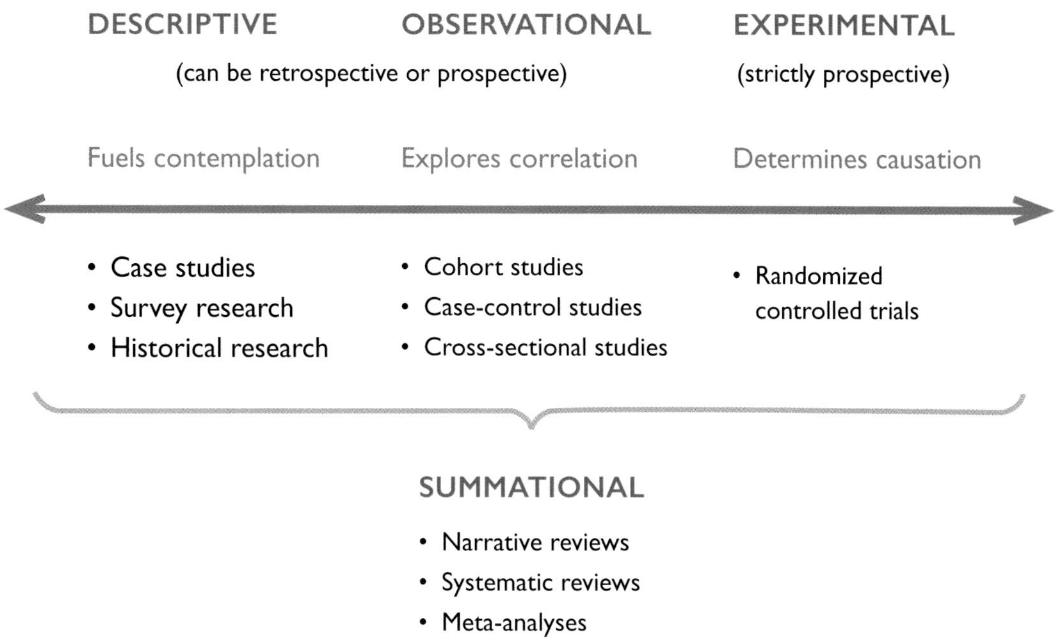

DESCRIPTIVE   OBSERVATIONAL   EXPERIMENTAL

(can be retrospective or prospective)   (strictly prospective)

Fuels contemplation   Explores correlation   Determines causation

- Case studies
- Survey research
- Historical research

- Cohort studies
- Case-control studies
- Cross-sectional studies

- Randomized controlled trials

SUMMATIONAL

- Narrative reviews
- Systematic reviews
- Meta-analyses

With several case studies published, patterns and commonalities can be detected and put to trial in the real world.

The main limitation of descriptive research is that it's incapable of indicating the nature of the relationships between the things being observed. This question of "what" sets the groundwork for progressing toward the question of "how."

Observational research

As we move along the continuum, observational research (cohort studies, case-control studies, and cross-sectional studies) has a greater capability to identify the nature of how things, events, or phenomena are related to one another. Observational research is capable of finding associations or correlations between variables.

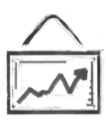

Under the umbrella of observational research is a more common term, *epidemiology*, which is the study of disease at the population level. The majority of headlines (usually health scares involving various foods and risk for chronic diseases or death) are generated by epidemiology. The main strength of epidemiology is its capacity to study large populations over long periods. Researchers can study the associations of various lifestyle factors and disease outcomes (including mortality), which can take several years or decades to manifest. This would be nearly impossible to examine via controlled interventions due to logistical and ethical constraints as well as financial expense.

In terms of limitations, observational research is largely considered to be hypothesis-generating rather than confirmative of fact. In other words, observational research is useful for raising questions but not for providing definitive answers. Barring certain theoretical technicalities such as meeting the Bradford Hill criteria,[28] observational research cannot determine cause and effect. The saying that "correlation does not imply causation" applies perfectly in the case of observational research.

FLEXIBLE VOCAB

Correlation does not imply causation

This saying, which is popular in pro-science circles, describes the inability to determine a cause-and-effect relationship based solely on correlation. To think otherwise—that correlation does imply causation—is a logical fallacy. In other words, just because two things happen at the same time or under the same circumstances does not mean they are related or that one caused the other.

Randomized controlled trials

At the far right of the research continuum are randomized controlled trials (RCTs), considered to be true experimental research (as opposed to quasi-experimental research, which omits the process of randomization). Thanks to the rigorous control and manipulation of the variables, RCTs can establish cause and effect.

A prime example of the value of RCTs is the study of artificial sweeteners and bodyweight. Observational studies have suggested an association between diet/artificially sweetened food and beverage consumption and overweight/obesity,[29] leading some folks to blame things like diet soda for causing weight gain. In contrast, RCTs consistently show that replacing sugar with artificial sweeteners supports weight loss.[30] Therefore, the indictment of artificial sweeteners by observational data is an error of *reverse causality*. In other words, overweight and obese individuals tend to seek out artificially sweetened "diet" products rather than the other way around. And we know this thanks to the ability of RCTs to investigate cause and effect.

While RCTs have merits beyond other types of research on the continuum, they're not free of shortcomings. Common limitations of RCTs include short trial duration and small sample sizes. The tight control and isolation of the variables in question can sometimes compromise *external validity* (the real-world relevance of the effects seen in the sterile environment of the lab).

FLEXIBLE VOCAB

Sample size

The sample size in a study refers to the number of participants. This must be calculated when the study is proposed because too large a sample is infeasible and too small a sample is unscientific. Getting the sample size right is a critical part of research.

Summational research

Summational research is necessary to provide a synthesis or aerial view of the state of the evidence as a whole. Given the vast and ever-growing body of nutrition and exercise studies, we can get a big-picture perspective of what is known and unknown from narrative reviews, systematic reviews, and meta-analyses, all of which help provide a clearer path for future investigation. Narrative reviews offer qualitative assessments and speculations while also relaying experiences from the field. They strive to surpass mere editorials by avoiding selective reporting or glorification of protocols that suit the authors' personal preferences. Narrative reviews are particularly useful for addressing areas of controversy born from equivocal data or widespread misunderstanding.

A narrative review that's special to me (because it's my first peer-reviewed publication) is titled "Nutrient timing revisited: is there a post-exercise anabolic window?"[31] This paper discusses the misconceptions surrounding a narrow, rapidly disappearing post-exercise window to consume rapidly absorbed protein and carbohydrate for the goal of muscle gain.

In contrast to the more fluid and untethered format of narrative reviews, systematic reviews adhere to specific reporting systems such as the PRISMA (Preferred Reporting Items for Systematic reviews and Meta-Analyses) that maximize the transparency, thoroughness, and quality of both the review itself and the studies included in the review.[32]

Meta-analyses involve pooling the data of several studies addressing a similar question and quantitatively analyzing the magnitude of the effects.

THE (NEW AND IMPROVED) HIERARCHY OF EVIDENCE

In addition to knowing the purpose, strengths, and limitations of the various types of research, it's important to have the proper perspective of their rank on the hierarchy of evidence (Figure 3b). There are multiple versions of this hierarchy floating around the lay media as well as the peer-reviewed literature. They have subtle differences but are fundamentally similar, with the two common threads being that RCTs are ranked higher than observational studies (i.e., cohort, case-control, and cross-sectional studies), with systematic reviews and meta-analyses sitting at the top of the hierarchy. What's pictured in Figure 3b is my updated and nuanced version of the traditional schematic.

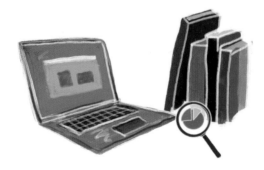

Figure 3b: Hierarchy of Evidence

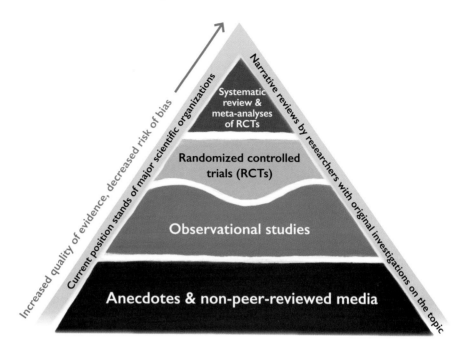

Anecdotes and non-peer-reviewed media

Going from the weakest to the strongest evidence, we begin at the bottom with anecdotes and non-peer-reviewed media. Anecdotes are stories relaying individuals' personal experiences or observations. Imagine someone raving over a new diet, supplement, or exercise device: "I tried Product X, and it works great!"

The problem with anecdotes is that they're subject to the biases of the individual (not to mention their level of knowledge or reasoning capability pertaining to the anecdote). An important caveat about anecdotes, aside from commercial bias if some sort of endorsement deal is at play, is the possibility of confirmation bias. If the marketing or persuasion tactics behind Product X (or Training Protocol X, or Diet Protocol X) led someone to believe in the product, this could lead to false fulfillment of preexistent expectations, and then confirmation of preexistent belief occurs.

Another example is if someone watches a documentary on a particular diet that paints the diet in an overwhelmingly positive light. When the person adopts this diet, confirmation bias can facilitate the selective perception or acknowledgment of the favorable effects of the diet while actively ignoring (or denying) the downsides.

Non-peer-reviewed media include magazine articles, blog posts, popular diet books, and documentaries (or, more accurately, *docudramas*). All of these sources of information are subject to multiple biases—not to mention agendas. In most cases, their main goal is to generate views and revenue, so scientific diligence takes a backseat to good storytelling.

Observational studies and RCTs

Observational studies (cohort, case-control, and cross-sectional studies) are the next tier up. Now, we've entered the realm of original investigations, also called primary research. As mentioned earlier, observational studies have the limitation of being incapable of demonstrating causation. They can give strong hints, though, and provide hypotheses for further testing in RCTs when feasible. It's important to note the wavy line separating observational research and RCTs, indicating that the quality of these studies needs to be assessed on an individual basis. Study design alone is insufficient grounds to assign validity rankings. A more flexible/fluid perspective is warranted here.

FLEXIBLE VOCAB

Primary and secondary research

Primary research refers to any type of research performed firsthand, such as surveys, interviews, and experiments. Secondary research encompasses editorials, narrative reviews, and systematic reviews—basically, interpretations or evaluations of primary research.

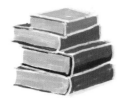

This brings us to the next tier up, RCTs, often called the "gold standard" of research design due to their ability to demonstrate causation rather than mere correlation. Although this label has been reasonably well earned, RCTs vary widely in quality and relevance. An RCT can have strong internal validity—in other words, it properly controls the variables in question and accurately tests and measures the targeted end points. However, high internal validity does not automatically equal external validity (relevance to humans in the real world).

So, despite their purported gold standard status, RCTs are far from exempt from critical scrutiny. I've already discussed the main limitations of RCTs, but a pervasive one that bears repeating is that they often involve small numbers of subjects (participants). The problem with small subject numbers is that they compromise the ability to extrapolate or generalize the findings to the overall population in question.

Systematic reviews and meta-analyses

The aforementioned problem is alleviated to a certain degree in systematic reviews and meta-analyses of RCTs, which sit near the top of the evidence hierarchy. The aim of these types of research is to quantitatively investigate the weight of the evidence on a given topic. This is done by calculating effect sizes and pooling the data of multiple studies to determine which direction the evidence leans.

Meta-analyses can alleviate the problem of small subject numbers in individual studies. However, meta-analyses are only as good as the studies they contain. Even then, heterogeneity remains a persistent issue that challenges attempts to draw firm conclusions. Nevertheless, meta-analyses are a useful and far more diligent alternative to cherry-picking the studies whose results align with one's personal beliefs.

In most incarnations of the evidence hierarchy, systematic reviews and meta-analyses are at the very top. However, meta-analyses are still plagued by considerable limitations. Not the least of these are the recurrent methodological shortcomings of individual studies, whose flaws are merely baked into the meta-analyses that include them. Systematic reviews and meta-analyses tend to cover narrow slices of the state of the evidence; they typically concentrate on single questions or facets of a given topic.

Heterogeneity and homogeneity

These opposing concepts are often used in the sciences to relate the uniformity of a study or collection of studies. Something that is heterogeneous is distinctly nonuniform in composition or character (e.g., size, distribution, or design), while something that is homogeneous is marked by the uniformity of those qualities. In other words, homogeneity in a collection of studies refers to methodological sameness, while heterogeneity calls out methodological differences.

In the model I'm proposing (refer to Figure 3b on page 47), notice the top layer of the pyramid in light blue, spanning the length of its sides. This depicts position stands and narrative reviews as having the potential to surpass the tip of the pyramid, which traditionally is reserved for systematic reviews and meta-analyses.

Position stands and narrative reviews

Position stands aim to convey the state of the evidence on a given topic, and they're authored by several researchers who are typically among the most prolific or accomplished researchers in the given area of interest. Furthermore, they rely on data from current systematic reviews and meta-analyses. They therefore represent the scientific consensus.

Unlike most systematic reviews and meta-analyses, position stands include applications that can be useful for personal and professional practice. When seeking answers to nutrition- or training-related questions, the position stands of the major organizations in these areas of study are a good place to start:

- American College of Sports Medicine (ACSM): www.acsm.org/acsm-positions-policy/official-positions/ACSM-position-stands

- Academy of Nutrition and Dietetics (AND): www.eatrightpro.org/practice/position-and-practice-papers/position-papers

- International Society of Sports Nutrition (ISSN): www.biomedcentral.com/collections/ISSNPosP

- National Strength and Conditioning Association (NSCA): www.nsca.com/about-us/position-statements/

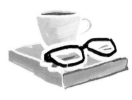

The main drawback of position stands is their low frequency of updates, which happen every several years to roughly a decade, if at all, due to the enormous amount of work that goes into evaluating and summing up vast multitudes of studies and cohesively conveying the state of knowledge. This is why I allowed for a more flexible ranking of them on the evidence hierarchy. It's possible for position stands to be significantly out of date, but it's also possible for current position stands to represent the scientific consensus more comprehensively and with more applicability than systematic reviews and meta-analyses. The problem of evolving evidence in the face of infrequently updated position statements can be alleviated with "living" practice guidelines that are continually updated as the evidence trickles in. An example of this is the American Diabetes Association's Standards of Medical Care in Diabetes, which now receive *living updates*.

If there are no current position stands on a topic you're investigating, then I suggest searching for systematic reviews first and then meta-analyses on the topic in question. A quick-and-dirty Google search hack is to type the topic along with "systematic review." You can do the same with your chosen topic and the term "meta-analysis." Note that systematic reviews are often combined with meta-analyses. Another trick that cuts through a lot of noise is to add the term "PubMed" to any topic you want to seek out. PubMed is a free search engine maintained by the US National Library of Medicine that provides access to the MEDLINE database on life sciences and biomedical topics.

Also missing from published evidence hierarchies are narrative reviews. As in the case of position stands, I convey narrative reviews as having a fluid ranking—anywhere from at the top to near the bottom, depending on their quality. It's possible for narrative reviews to be good for not much more than food for thought (or food for face-palming, in some cases).

Editorials are a type of narrative review, but they're essentially opinion pieces. Editorials often express a point of view that has equally vigorous counterpoints. If editorials were converted to video form, you'd see a certain amount of emotion and theatrics. Editorials are valuable when the author has a lot of experience and knowledge of the topic and/or is diligent about assessing the totality of the evidence fairly. However, this isn't always the case, since editorials considerably lacking in scientific rigor have been published even in high-profile journals.[33,34]

In contrast, there are narrative reviews that are collaborations by active, extensively published researchers in a given area, which do a very thorough and diligent job of evaluating the state of the evidence.[35-37]

RESOLVING THE CONUNDRUM OF CONFLICTING STUDY RESULTS

It's common to dismiss scientific research as a pointless mishmash of conflicting findings. People often claim that for every study showing a given product or protocol is effective, there's another study showing it isn't.

It's important to maintain the perspective that a single study with contrary results cannot overturn an existing body of evidence. It might add new insight and challenge the existing research by using better instrumentation or a more relevant protocol. If a new study has across-the-board better methodological aspects than previous research, including a longer trial period, a larger number of subjects with a more relevant profile relative to the research question, better/more rigorous control measures, or better technology for measuring the targeted changes, then it's worthy of consideration as something that can upset the apple cart. But again, this is a long shot. As we proceed through this discussion, you'll see that there are many possible methodological differences that can result in divergent outcomes between studies asking similar questions.

When two studies examining the same question yield conflicting results, the first question you should ask is whether you're comparing studies of the same design. Are they both RCTs, or are you pitting an RCT against an observational study? In the latter scenario, the RCT has the advantage of being a notch above observational research on the evidence hierarchy. Just remember the important nuance: studies are not automatically stronger or more valid based on their design; there are poorly done studies of all types. Nevertheless, RCTs have the advantage of being capable of demonstrating causation since they test an experimental treatment against a control condition while equating all other variables.

The PICO framework

If you're comparing two RCTs on the same topic with different results, running each of them through the PICO framework can reveal the reasons for the discrepancy. PICO originated as a method to formulate well-focused research questions in evidence-based medicine.[38] There are subtle variations, but for our purposes, PICO is an acronym for population, intervention, comparator, and outcome.

The PICO framework is used as a guide for literature searches, and it's also a practical guide to determine which piece of research is more relevant to your interests. A less commonly used version of PICO adds an "S" to the end of the acronym to signify *study design*, to narrow down and filter out irrelevant studies for the given literature search.[39] Let's examine the components of PICO, along with the questions you should ask when weighing the validity of two conflicting RCTs.

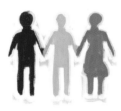

Population

What were the characteristics of the subjects? Healthy or diseased? Young or old? Male or female? Lean/normal-weight or overweight/obese? Trained or untrained? If they were trained, were they merely nonsedentary or recreationally trained, or were they competitive athletes, and at what level?

All of these characteristics can impact results in different ways. For example, a nutritional intervention's lack of effect in untrained subjects is still subject to further research in trained subjects, who are less prone to the masking effect of substantial "newbie gains" in muscle size and strength. When the positive effects of a given intervention are seen in trained subjects, the intervention is more noteworthy since eliciting changes in folks who are closer to their potential requires considerably more potency/effectiveness.

FLEXIBLE VOCAB

Newbie gains

This term refers to how women and especially men with little to no previous experience tend to enjoy rapid increases in muscle mass when they start weightlifting. In their first year, most men can gain 20 to 25 pounds of muscle, while women can gain about half that. After that point, progress tends to slow dramatically.

A classic example in the nutritional realm is the age-related difference in muscle protein synthesis (MPS) in response to protein feeding. Subjects in their seventies require nearly double the protein dose in a single meal to maximally stimulate MPS compared to subjects in their twenties.[40] There's a lot to unpack on the topic of age-related anabolic resistance, but we'll get to that in a later chapter.

Another point of consideration is animal research, which has its place but also has distinct limitations. At best, animal research is hypothesis-generating when there's a lack of human studies on the topic. At worst, it's either meaningless or misleading in the presence of available human studies. A prime example is mice, in whom ketogenic diets have caused severe hepatic insulin resistance,[41] impaired cardiac function,[42] and substantial accumulation of visceral fat.[43] These adverse effects in mice are not reflective of (and are in large part antithetical to) the effects of ketogenic diets in human trials.

Finally, I'll reiterate that the most important question to ask about the population is, how relevant is this population to the topic or question at hand? How reflective or relevant is this population to you and your circumstances?

Intervention

This refers to what agent, product, or protocol is being tested. It's also called the experimental treatment, the treatment condition, or just the treatment.

Several questions should be asked. Are the dose and dosing scheme appropriate? If it's a training program, are the programming variables (set volume, loading, progression, level of effort) appropriate for the population? What compliance measures were imposed? How frequent and in-depth was the interaction between the subjects and the research personnel? What was the level of surveillance or accountability of meal consumption or supervision of the training sessions? If a supplement is being tested, what chemical form was it? Is it an acute (short-term) response study, or is it longitudinal (also called a chronic study, lasting several weeks or months)?

Acute studies have the advantage of being conducive to tight control measures and exploring potential mechanisms, but the disadvantage of questionable generalizability to the long term. Longitudinal studies shine in the latter department, but control of the variables is often a lot looser for the trial to be feasible.

The most important question to ask about the intervention is, how relevant is this agent or protocol to the topic or question at hand? How reflective or relevant is this intervention to you and your circumstances?

Comparator

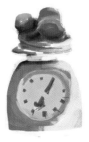

This component is also called the control treatment, the control condition, or just the control. It refers to what the intervention was compared to. In some studies, it's a placebo, which is an inert substance. Some studies do not involve a placebo when they directly compare different diet types.

A prime example is the comparison of diets differing in carbohydrate content. When the aim is to examine the effects of carbohydrate restriction, then total daily protein and energy intake needs to be equated between the carb-restricted diet (the treatment) and the higher-carbohydrate/conventional diet (the control).

It's amusing that a failure to equate protein and calories in studies that investigate low-carbohydrate diets has been a regular occurrence in the research over the past few decades. When the research involves exercise performance, a common lack of control is the failure to standardize/equate dietary intake in the days leading up to the testing period, or the evening meal before testing in the morning, or the pre-testing meal if exercise testing occurs in the middle of the day or at some point significantly after waking. Differences in these aspects of control can yield varying results. Pay attention to how these controls reflect your own situation.

Outcome

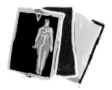

This is the anticipated effect of the potential cause (the intervention/ treatment) being tested. In short, the outcome is what you would hypothesize to happen—or not happen. Examples of outcomes are fat loss, muscle gain, exercise performance, and various health parameters, states of disease, and death.

In clinical jargon, *intermediate outcomes* are used as proxies or surrogate markers for disease; they can't be felt or observed symptomatically.[44] Intermediate outcomes attempt to track disease progression. Examples include changes in biomarkers such as blood lipids and glucose levels.

In contrast, *health outcomes* (also called *hard outcomes*) are changes in quality of life or functional status. Examples are actual states of disease and of course death. In the fitness realm, acute/short-term anabolic response (measured by markers such as MPS) can be considered an intermediate outcome, while changes in lean mass and fat mass can be viewed as hard outcomes or concrete end points.

FLEXIBLE VOCAB

Muscle protein synthesis (MPS)

Muscle protein synthesis is an anabolic (growth-oriented) process by which the body responds and adapts to nutrition and exercise. Net gains in muscle protein eventually result in increased muscle mass. I'll explain more about this process in the next chapter, which is all about protein.

Although both types of outcomes provide useful data, hard outcomes typically carry more evidential weight. In addition to evaluating how appropriate the outcomes are to the research question, an important consideration is the instrumentation used to measure them. Differences in the method of measuring body composition can explain the differences in the outcomes between studies.

On the note of results, when an outcome (for example, bodyweight change) is deemed "statistically significant," zoom in on the data and ask whether this difference is practically meaningful. Often, it is not, and honest researchers will point this out when discussing their work. Once again, when weighing the validity of one study versus another, you want to determine how reflective or relevant the outcomes are to you and your circumstances. It's rare for two studies to use identical methodology to measure identical outcomes. In other words, what do these outcomes (and the way they were reached) mean for you and your unique lifestyle factors?

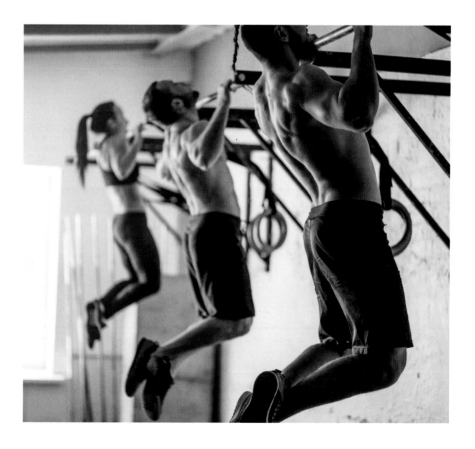

FURTHER STUDY AND RESOURCES FOR SHARPENING YOUR RESEARCH SKILLS

The journey of gaining knowledge is not solely contained within this book. It helps to have some fundamental research skills to continue that journey beyond these pages. You might be an avid secondary researcher whether you realize it or not. If you regularly search for answers through the scholarly literature, you're in the club. As mentioned previously, some of the best answers to health- and fitness-related questions are contained in position stands of the major science-based organizations. But, due to the potential for some position stands to be outdated, searching for systematic reviews in addition to checking out the position stands can keep you more current. Now that you've got the research continuum, evidence hierarchy, and PICO in your toolbox, you can scan the literature with a better understanding of what you're seeing.

One of the most practical resources on conducting a literature search is a paper by Ecker and Skelly[45] titled "Conducting a winning literature search." It's an open-access publication, so the full text is free.

For those who'd rather watch a tutorial than read one, I highly recommend a video called "Conducting a literature search using PubMed," put together by the Medical College of Wisconsin Libraries. It's freely accessible on their YouTube channel, and it's thorough yet concise (21 minutes)—they really nailed the perfect balance of simplicity and comprehensiveness.

Box 3c lists my personal favorite tutorials and resources for those interested in sharpening their research skills and scientific literacy.

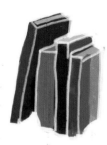

BOX 3C: RESOURCES FOR IMPROVING RESEARCH SKILLS AND SCIENTIFIC LITERACY

Literature search tutorials

- Conducting a winning literature search (Ecker and Skelly): www.ncbi.nlm.nih.gov/pmc/articles/PMC3609008

- Conducting a literature search using PubMed (Medical College of Wisconsin Libraries): www.youtube.com/watch?v=0lill6yUmk8

Research methodology tutorials

- Designing a research project: randomised controlled trials and their principles (Kendall): https://emj.bmj.com/content/20/2/164.full

- Publishing nutrition research: a review of study design, statistical analyses, and other key elements of manuscript preparation, part 1 (Boushey et al.): https://jandonline.org/article/S0002-8223(05)02036-5/fulltext

- Publishing nutrition research: a review of study design, statistical analyses, and other key elements of manuscript preparation, part 2 (Boushey et al.): https://jandonline.org/article/S0002-8223(08)00003-5/fulltext

- Research methodology series (multiple papers, various authors) in the *Journal of the Academy of Nutrition and Dietetics*: https://jandonline.org/content/researchDesign

- Estimating the size of treatment effects (McGough and Faraone): www.ncbi.nlm.nih.gov/pmc/articles/PMC2791668/

- Progressive statistics for studies in sports medicine and exercise science (Hopkins et al.): https://journals.lww.com/acsm-msse/Fulltext/2009/01000/Progressive_Statistics_for_Studies_in_Sports.2.aspx

- Understanding the basics of meta-analysis and how to read a forest plot: as simple as it gets (Andrade): https://pubmed.ncbi.nlm.nih.gov/33027562/

Databases

- PubMed (not all open-access): https://pubmed.gov

- PubMed Central (all open-access): www.ncbi.nlm.nih.gov/pmc

- Cochrane Library (not all open-access): www.cochranelibrary.com

CHAPTER 3 IN A NUTSHELL

- The main types of research are observational, experimental, and summational. Each type serves important purposes; observational research is incapable of demonstrating causation but can help us draw correlation-based inferences in large populations and, in some cases, over long periods. Experimental research (RCTs in particular) has the advantage of being able to establish causation, but its common limitations are short trial durations, small numbers of participants, and a lack of real-world relevance due to the sterility of the lab environment. Summational research is important for providing an aerial (and practical) view of the big picture, since it's easy to get lost in a mix of studies differing in designs and results.

- There are many incarnations of the hierarchy of evidence. The version I created (Figure 3b) attempts to provide more completeness, clarity, and nuance than the traditional models. At the bottom of the hierarchy are anecdotes and non-peer-reviewed data; in the middle are RCTs and observational studies; and at the top are systematic reviews and meta-analyses of RCTs.

- Of more widely variable status in this hierarchy are position stands/scientific consensus statements of major organizations. The rank of these articles in the hierarchy can diminish in the face of newer, higher-quality evidence. Narrative reviews, though subject to various biases when not done according to predetermined systematic standards (such as PRISMA), can nonetheless accurately represent the current state of the evidence when authored by the most active/prolific researchers in the topic area.

- Conflicting study results are the inevitable consequence of differences in study design/methodology, instrumentation, and subject profile. A useful tool for evaluating RCTs is the PICO framework, which is an acronym for population, intervention, comparator, and outcome.

- The art and science of improving research skills and scientific literacy can be a long and winding journey. To minimize the roadblocks in this process, I have provided a collection of research resources that I personally have found to be very helpful (Box 3c).

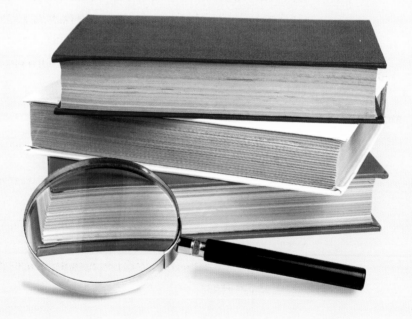

PART 3

EXAMINING THE COMPONENTS

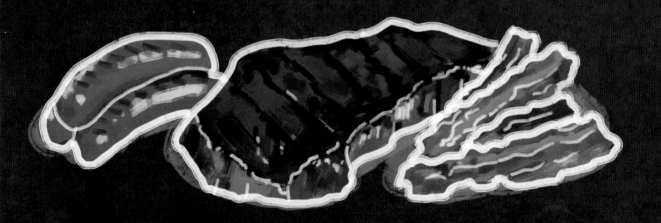

PROTEIN

Here we are at the meat of things (literally and figuratively) as we tackle the topic of protein. First things first, though—let's give credit to a Dutch chemist named Gerardus Johannes Mulder for coming up with the name *protein* in 1838.[46] He based it on the Greek word *proteus*—which carries implications of being first in rank or importance.

This name is fitting given protein's necessity for sustaining life, as well as the multitude of crucial roles protein plays in the body. All cellular processes involve protein in some way. Proteins function as structural components, enzymes, hormones, immune factors, transporters, acid-base regulators, and neurotransmitters. The single largest tissue store of bodily protein is skeletal muscle.[47] The importance of maintaining the health and functionality of muscle tissue cannot be overstated.

Protein is known to most of the readers of this book as one of the macronutrients, with the other two being carbohydrate and fat. Macronutrients have also been called energy nutrients since they provide calories (4 kcal per gram of carbohydrate or protein, 9 kcal per gram of fat) to fuel the myriad bodily processes. There's controversy over whether alcohol can rightly be classified as a macronutrient, but it technically does provide metabolizable energy (7 kcal per gram).

Protein is considered an essential nutrient because the body cannot biosynthesize enough of it to maintain health and survival. Protein therefore must be obtained from the diet. Proteins are large molecules consisting of amino acids. Of the 20 amino acids that comprise proteins, nine are considered essential amino acids (EAA—also called indispensable amino acids/IAA) and thus must be obtained from food.

A perpetual narrative in dietetics curriculums is that the general population overconsumes protein to a degree that's detrimental to health. This claim is unfounded, and the concern is overblown. The latest National Health and Nutrition Examination Survey (NHANES) data shows that the protein intake of US adults averages 88.2 grams per day (1.1 g/kg), which amounts to 14 to 16 percent of total daily calories.[48] This is within the Institute of Medicine's acceptable macronutrient distribution range (AMDR) of 10 to 35 percent of total daily calories.[49] Furthermore, the intake of 1.1 g/kg is not excessive by any scientifically sound standard. In fact, it's suboptimal for older and dieting populations who are physically active (more discussion about this ahead). With the exception of preexistent kidney disease, there does not appear to be any imminent risk with higher protein consumption than the aforementioned upper thresholds.

Regarding concerns for kidney health, a recent 28-study meta-analysis by Devries and colleagues[50] compared high protein intakes (≥1.5 g/kg bodyweight or ≥20 percent energy intake or ≥100 grams of protein per day) with normal/lower protein intakes (≥5 percent less energy intake from protein per day compared with the high-protein group) on kidney function. It was concluded that higher protein intakes have a trivial to nonexistent effect on kidney function. Furthermore, a series of studies by Antonio and colleagues[51-53] with protein intakes ranging from 2.5 to 3.4 g/kg and trial durations ranging from two to six months found no adverse effects on kidney function or any other health parameter. In addition, a high protein intake (averaging 2.8 g/kg) over a six-month period in trained women had no harmful effects on bone mineral content or density.[54] Subsequently, a meta-analysis by Groenendijk and colleagues[55] showed that higher protein intake (above the RDA of 0.8 g/kg) resulted in a significant *decrease* in hip fractures compared to lower protein intake.

In other words, the average American's protein intake is far from problematically high. If anything, it may be a little low.

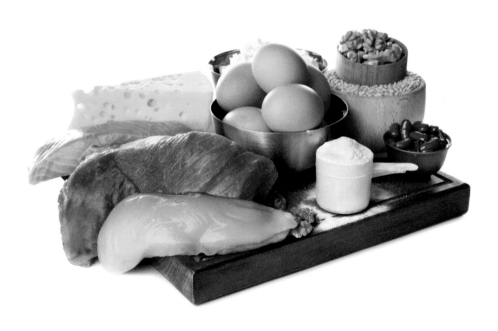

INTAKE HIERARCHY OF IMPORTANCE

There's an underlying order of importance when it comes to protein intake (and diet design for various goals). Maintaining this perspective will enable you to better assess the claims you hear, or the magnitude of the programming moves you make when manipulating the king of the macros. From most to least important, the hierarchy is as follows:

1. **Total daily protein amount.** This is the most influential factor for all goals as far as protein is concerned. Although it's theoretically possible to get total daily intake right but lack quality to a critical degree, it's somewhat far-fetched. Hevia-Larraín and colleagues[56] saw no significant differences in muscular size and strength gains between vegans and omnivores, and this presumably was due to sufficient total daily protein intake (~1.6 g/kg). I'd still reiterate that the use of untrained subjects leaves open questions. Nevertheless, in the big picture, total daily intake is the weightiest factor.

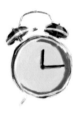

2. **Distribution of protein throughout the day.** This refers to the spread or pattern of intake (dosing, spacing, and positioning) of protein over the course of a day. For example, there is ongoing research comparing the impact of evenly spread versus skewed feeding patterns, higher versus lower feeding frequencies, and broad versus time-restricted feeding windows. While all of these are potentially important lines of inquiry, they take a distant backseat to total daily protein intake.

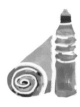

3. **Timing of protein relative to the training bout.** This factor has the least impact, especially in programs with typical (multiple) protein feedings per day, amounting to an adequate total. A case can be made for the utility of specific timing of protein in cases of exceptionally low meal frequency (one or two meals per day). In that case, the positioning/timing of protein can potentially influence training performance or muscle growth, but even then, it's rare that individuals consuming one or two meals per day have pressing concerns of optimizing either of those goals. The nuances will be addressed in subsequent chapters.

Keep in mind that this hierarchy applies mainly to protein. A similar hierarchy applies to dietary fat, with distribution and timing being virtual nonconcerns. An exception is that the consumption of large amounts of fat prior to competition can potentially cause gastrointestinal distress and impair endurance performance—but this is uncommon and unlikely. In contrast to protein and fat, strategic timing of carbohydrate can be a critical factor for endurance-oriented exercise performance.

With that bit of nuance out of the way, let's have a look at protein requirements for the goal of muscle gain, followed by the goals of fat loss and then athletic performance.

ROLE IN MUSCLE GAIN

First, it's important to discuss the broader context of how muscle growth (also called *muscle anabolism* or *muscle hypertrophy*) occurs and how this process is optimized. In addition to total daily protein intake, overall caloric intake is an integral factor influencing muscle gain. While muscle growth is possible regardless of energy balance, surplus conditions facilitate maximal rates of growth. More protein equals more muscle.

There are two main mechanisms underlying this process: greater MPS and greater resistance training capacity. Muscle protein is in a constant state of *turnover;* MPS and muscle protein breakdown (MPB) are cyclical and ongoing throughout the day. Muscle growth is the result of net gains in MPS over the long term. So, MPS must consistently exceed MPB in order to achieve net gains in muscle protein balance and thus net gains in muscle growth. In contrast, hypocaloric conditions (caloric deficit) have consistently been shown to impair MPS and anabolic signaling.[57] Furthermore, hypocaloric conditions are unable to accommodate increasing training demands (load and volume of work).

To reiterate, although muscle growth has been seen in hypocaloric conditions, this phenomenon is limited mostly to overweight/obese untrained subjects. Therefore, hypercaloric conditions should be employed if the goal is to maximize rates of muscle gain.

Muscle protein turnover

Human muscle is in a constant cycle of breakdown and synthesis—a phenomenon known as muscle protein turnover. As we get older, MPS can diminish, especially with a lack of physical activity and muscular work. This leaves us vulnerable to age-related muscle losses and a range of adverse metabolic consequences. The other major contributor to age-related muscle loss is low protein intake. To optimize muscle protein balance, both resistance training and adequate protein intake are necessary.

The next question becomes, how much of a caloric surplus is required? Put simply, the more advanced your training status—the closer you are to your potential for muscular development—the smaller the caloric surplus can be without gaining excessive amounts of fat.[57]

Total daily protein requirements (muscle gain)

Total daily protein intake is the top tier of importance, regardless of goal (not just for muscle gain). The general population without specific athletic or body composition–oriented goals aside from general health should consume protein at a minimal range of 1.2 to 1.6 g/kg per day.[58] This is 50 to 100 percent greater than the Recommended Dietary Allowance (RDA) of 0.8 g/kg.

It's important to realize that the RDA was derived from studies on sedentary individuals using nitrogen balance, which is a crude and archaic method of estimating changes in muscle protein status. Therefore, the RDA—now over 40 years out of date—does not apply to physically active and/or dieting populations[59] or the elderly.[60]

Frailty and sarcopenia are among the greatest health threats to the aging population. These conditions are often referred to interchangeably due to their common ground of unintended, progressive weight loss. However, frailty is a state of increased vulnerability due to age-related decline and dysfunction across multiple physiologic systems,[61] while sarcopenia refers more specifically to the loss of skeletal muscle mass.[62] Prevalence of both conditions increases with advancing age.

Age-related anabolic resistance is characterized by a diminished MPS response to an anabolic stimulus (e.g., protein, amino acids, and/or resistance exercise).[63] Anabolic resistance is typically seen in older adults, but it is also instrumental to skeletal muscle atrophy that occurs during periods of disuse from inactivity and bed rest, regardless of age.[64] Nevertheless, due to decreasing levels of physical activity with advancing age, the resultant anabolic resistance is considered to be a key driver of age-associated skeletal muscle atrophy. The ESPEN Expert Group[65] recommends at least 1 to 1.2 g/kg per day for healthy older people, 1.2 to 1.5 g/kg per day for older people who are malnourished or have acute or chronic illness, and higher intakes for individuals with severe illness or injury. The PROT-AGE Study Group[65] recommends an average daily intake of 1 to 1.2 g/kg per day for healthy people, 1.2 to 1.5 g/kg per day for those with acute or chronic disease, and up to 2 g/kg for those with malnutrition, severe illness, or injury.

In addition to hitting the targeted daily total, overcoming the blunted MPS response characteristic of anabolic resistance involves consuming enough high-quality protein per meal. The PROT-AGE Study Group recommends 25 to 30 grams of protein per meal containing ~2.5 to 2.8 grams of leucine.[65] However, more recent data show that this dosing range is on the low end, so I would consider this a minimum—especially if your goal is to maximize adaptations to resistance training. An optimal approach to total protein intake and distribution is discussed next, and the recommendations apply to older adults as well.

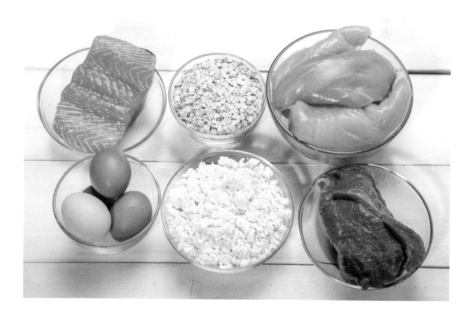

I was fortunate enough to be one of the collaborators of the most comprehensive systematic review and meta-analysis of its kind on protein intake and resistance training adaptations.[66] The analysis involved data from 49 studies containing a total of 1,863 subjects. We concluded that maximizing muscle growth can be achieved with 1.6 to 2.2 g/kg (0.7 to 1 g/lb). Keep in mind that we excluded hypocaloric studies from our analysis, so our conclusion is potentially limited to eucaloric (maintenance) and hypercaloric conditions. I'll quote the manuscript directly since these figures have been highly influential, shaping the current field practice guidelines (note that FFM stands for fat-free mass and RET stands for resistance exercise training):

> *"Here we provide significant insight by reporting an unadjusted plateau in RET-induced gains in FFM at 1.62 g protein/kg/day (95% CI: 1.03 to 2.20). [...] Given that the confidence interval of this estimate spanned from 1.03 to 2.20, it may be prudent to recommend ~2.2 g protein/kg/d for those seeking to maximise resistance training–induced gains in FFM."*

Protein quality: the plant versus animal debate

Protein quality is defined by a given source's ability to provide the amino acids needed to fulfill a person's physiological needs, which is determined by its digestibility and amino acid profile.[67] High-quality proteins are characterized by high digestibility and high proportion of EAAs.[68] Protein quality ranking systems include the Protein Digestibility Corrected Amino Acid Score and its successor, the Digestible Indispensable Amino Acid Score.

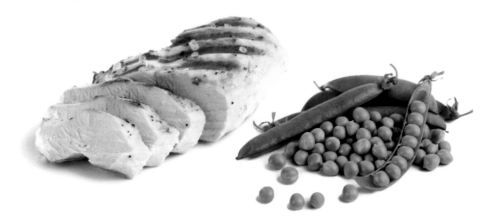

Animal-derived proteins (e.g., meat, fish, poultry, eggs, and dairy) tend to be higher quality than plant-derived proteins. Furthermore, animal proteins have shown greater anabolic responses in head-to-head comparisons examining MPS.[69-72] Animal proteins generally have higher EAA and branched-chain amino acid (BCAA) content. Among the BCAAs, leucine acts as an anabolic signaling molecule and plays a key role in stimulating MPS and suppressing MPB.[73]

FLEXIBLE VOCAB

Leucine and BCAAs

Leucine is an EAA used in protein biosynthesis—one of three branched-chain amino acids (BCAAs), which are purported to have a unique ability to stimulate muscle growth. Leucine is sometimes considered the "main" BCAA thanks to its special role in boosting MPS and reducing MPB. As a result, many people in rigorous training programs use BCAA supplementation. As I'll discuss in Chapter 7, this is superfluous in the context of adequate total daily protein intake, which already delivers sufficient BCAAs.

Traditionally, plant proteins have been considered inferior to animal proteins due to their lesser proportion of EAAs. Combine this with lower digestibility, and you end up with a seemingly obvious conclusion about where plant proteins stand in the pecking order.[74-76]

But of course, it's not that simple. It's noteworthy that current protein quality ranking systems don't account for functional or morphological outcomes. One strength of acute anabolic response studies is that a high degree of control and precision can be imposed upon the variables being manipulated. The main limitation of these studies is that an acute MPS response does not guarantee the same superiority in terms of muscle growth over the longer term. Indeed, recent longitudinal studies showed a lack of obviously consistent/unanimous animal protein superiority.

FLEXIBLE VOCAB

Anabolic response

Anabolism is the aspect of your metabolism involved in "building up." In other words, your anabolic response is your body's metabolic reaction to the muscle protein synthesis (MPS) I've been talking so much about.

The sole plant protein supplementation study showing superior effects to whey is by Babault and colleagues,[77] who found that pea protein supplementation (25 grams twice daily) increased biceps muscle thickness to a slightly greater degree than whey protein. However, subsequent comparisons cast doubt upon the reproducibility of the latter findings. An eight-week trial by Banaszek and colleagues[78] found no significant difference between the effects of pea versus whey protein (24 grams before and after training) on muscle thickness, body composition, and strength. A subsequent study by Nieman and colleagues[79] reported that whey (0.3 g/kg) outperformed pea protein for mitigating muscle damage after five days of intensive eccentric exercise.

Mixed results across several studies created the perfect opportunity to conduct a meta-analysis to see which treatment (if any) has the stronger effect when the data from all of the relevant studies are pooled together. This is exactly what Messina and colleagues[80] did in 2018, attempting to determine how animal versus plant protein supplementation (soy, specifically) affects muscle size and strength gains in subjects undergoing resistance training.

Soy protein was reported to be similarly effective for increasing muscle size and strength compared to the animal protein comparators (in most studies, whey was used; other sources included milk and beef). While vegans and plant-based diet proponents might be quick to conclude that this finding puts plant and animal proteins on a level playing field, there are some important caveats here.

Of the nine studies in the meta-analysis, three favored dairy protein, and six showed no significant advantage of either protein type. None of the studies found soy to be the superior performer; either animal protein won, or it was a wash. Only two of the studies involved "optimal" total daily protein intakes at or above 1.6 g/kg. Only one of the nine studies involved resistance-trained subjects. A more recent, larger meta-analysis by Lim and colleagues[81] concluded that younger adults (<50 years) had greater absolute and proportional lean mass gains with animal versus plant protein supplementation. Still, this meta-analysis suffered many of the same limitations of Messina's meta-analysis.

Importantly, none of the studies in the aforementioned meta-analysis compared a completely plant-based/animal-free diet with an omnivorous one. All of the diets were omnivorous, varying only in the type of protein supplement employed. So, if only a minority of total daily protein intake varies between the comparators, it's somewhat predictable that the performance of the diets overall would not differ much.

A plant-based diet versus an omnivorous diet

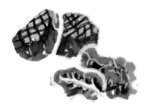

A recent 12-week study by Hevia-Larraín and colleagues[56] challenged long-standing presumptions of superiority based on protein quality rankings. For the first time, plant protein supplementation (soy) versus animal protein supplementation (whey) was compared in the context of a completely plant-based diet versus an omnivorous diet, and no between-group differences were seen in gains of lean mass and strength.[56]

A strength of this study (aside from the unprecedented comparison of a vegan diet with an omnivorous one in this context) was the assignment of adequate total daily protein (at least 1.6 g/kg). The main limitation was the use of untrained individuals. In novices, potential differences in the effects of the treatments are often masked by large responses (hence the term "newbie gains"). Replication of this study—particularly in trained subjects—is warranted before settling on the conclusion that vegan diets are on par with omnivorous diets for maximizing muscular adaptations to resistance training.

In sum, animal proteins produce a greater anabolic response than plant proteins on a gram-for-gram basis; they are more efficient than plant proteins for the purpose of growth. This is due to higher EAA content—particularly leucine—and potentially due to other constituents such as taurine, carnosine, creatine,[82,83] collagen,[84-86] and even cholesterol,[87,88] none of which are present in plant foods. Furthermore, vegan diets tend to lack sufficient essential nutrients without supplementation and/or careful dietary construction. The most commonly cited population-wide nutritional shortcomings among vegans are vitamin B12, omega-3 fatty acids (EPA/DHA), vitamin D, calcium, iodine, iron, and zinc.[89-91] However, those who avoid consuming animal products are not necessarily doomed to lesser muscle gains. A recent review by Pinckaers and colleagues[92] proposed the following tactics to correct the inferior anabolic effect of plant proteins:

1. Consume more protein to compensate for the lesser quality.

2. Use specific blends of plant-based proteins to create a more balanced amino acid profile.

3. Fortify the plant-based protein with the free amino acid(s) that are lacking.

Of the aforementioned tactics, total protein amount is arguably the simplest to implement. My rough estimate is that a 15 to 30 percent greater total daily protein intake from a variety of high-quality plant-based sources could at least match leucine content and potentially level the anabolic playing field with animal-based protein.

Let's imagine an omnivorous individual weighing 80 kg whose protein intake is 1.6 g/kg, or 128 grams per day. The target in a completely plant-based diet would be increased by 15 to 30 percent, amounting to 147 to 166 grams. This amounts to an additional 19 to 38 grams beyond an omnivore's intake if the goal is to maximize growth. Accomplishing this with whole foods can be done using legumes, which contain high-quality proteins and provide roughly 0.5 gram of leucine per 100-gram (3.5-ounce) serving of cooked weight.[93]

On a related note, the isoflavone content of soy foods has been a long-standing topic of controversy due to its estrogenic potential. This concern is not completely unfounded, since testosterone decreases have been reported with soy protein isolate supplementation dosed as low as 20 grams per day in resistance-trained men[94] and 56 grams per day in untrained men.[95] However, the evidence on the whole does not support concerns about soy isoflavone consumption having feminizing effects in men.

A recent meta-analysis by Reed and colleagues[96] involving 41 studies reported that soy protein or isoflavone intake had no significant effects on sex hormones. A sub-analysis of isoflavone dose (<75 mg versus >75 mg per day) found no effect. While 75 mg is a reasonable cutoff point to represent a high intake (intake among older adults in Japan is 25 to 50 mg per day),[97] it's not implausible to presume that folks with a heavy reliance on soy to meet protein targets could be overdoing it. A classic example is a case study by Siepmann and colleagues,[98] who described a 19-year-old male with erectile dysfunction and hypogonadism, whose blood parameters normalized and sexual function returned within one year of abandoning a vegan diet that contained large amounts of soy products with an isoflavone content of 360 mg per day.

Keep in mind that case studies lack the control to demonstrate causality. Nevertheless, sole reliance on large amounts of soy protein supplementation and soy products to hit daily protein targets poses a certain degree of risk for adverse hormonal effects.

Current bodyweight versus target bodyweight versus lean mass

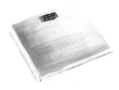

With rare exceptions, protein recommendations in the peer-reviewed literature are based on total bodyweight rather than lean mass. This is mainly due to the complexity and error potential involved with estimating body composition. Although it's simpler to base protein recommendations on total bodyweight, this carries the built-in presumption that we're talking about normal-weight individuals. The pitfall is that it's possible to over- or underestimate protein intake targets if someone is highly over- or underweight. For example, if an individual weighs 300 pounds and has 50 percent body fat, a protein intake of 300 grams per day would be excessive.

FLEXIBLE VOCAB

Body composition

Believe it or not, the makeup of your body is much more important and accurate for assessing your health than your weight. That's the whole idea behind body composition: to improve the overall makeup by focusing on factors such as body fat, body water, lean mass, bone mass, and daily caloric intake. Usually, it refers to losing fat while gaining muscle.

A relatively simple solution is to base protein intake on goal bodyweight or *target bodyweight* (TBW). Current bodyweight can be used to estimate protein needs if you're seeking to maintain your current weight. This method is an effective way of approximating lean mass with a built-in margin of safety.

For those who are hell-bent on basing protein intake on lean mass or FFM, a reasonable range for maximizing muscle growth is 1.8 to 2.6 g/kg of FFM. This range is derived from IAAO data in recent studies I discussed in the October 2019 issue of AARR (my monthly research review at alanaragon.com/aarr). To simplify things, a target of 2.2 g/kg of FFM (1 g/lb of FFM) shoots right in the middle of the "optimal" range. This is a safe baseline target for the goal of muscle gain.

Sex-based differences in protein metabolism

The collective evidence does not warrant different protein intake levels between the sexes. This lack of meaningful difference is reflected in the absence of separate recommendations for men and women by the position stands and consensus statements of major scientific organizations.

A classic review by Tipton[99] relayed the findings of several studies showing a lack of sex-based differences in whole-body protein turnover (the cycle of synthesis and breakdown) and no difference in net muscle protein balance. Furthermore, there's no human evidence that ovarian hormones inhibit MPS. Subsequent research by Smith and colleagues[100] found no meaningful differences in MPS during either the fasted or fed state between young adult and middle-aged men and women.

Continuing along these lines, Dreyer and colleagues[101] found no differences in post-exercise increases in MPS and mTOR between men and women. Adding a small wrinkle here, a recent review by Witard and colleagues[35] reported that greater basal MPS rates have been shown in women over 65 years old. This can at least partially explain the slower age-related loss of muscle in older women compared to older men.[102] Another interesting detail is that during endurance training, men oxidize more protein and leucine than women.[103-105] Whether these differences have any meaningful/ functional consequences is open for debate, but they're unlikely to matter in the context of protein intake within the ranges recommended here.

The main sex-based difference relevant to setting protein intake targets is the higher proportion of body fat in women. Since women have a lower proportion of lean mass, total bodyweight-based protein recommendations can potentially be skewed toward overestimating women's needs. However, this dilemma can be solved relatively simply by starting at the lower end of the "optimal" range (1.6 to 2.2 g/kg). Men and women can use 1.6 g/kg as a baseline from which to adjust upward. It's reasonable to assume that women require less protein per unit of total body mass since they tend to carry a higher proportion of body fat than men. Therefore, women's needs will likely hover around the lower end of the 1.6 to 2.2 g/kg range.

FFM-based protein targets are more complicated and not necessarily more accurate, but they can satisfy some people's desire for precision. As such, 2 g/kg of FFM (0.9 g/lb of FFM) is a reasonable baseline target for general purposes. Individuals specifically aiming for muscle gain (as well as dieters running a caloric deficit) can start at 2.2 g/kg of FFM (1 g/lb of FFM) and adjust according to individual response.

Distribution of protein throughout the day (muscle gain)

The goal of *maximizing* muscle gain warrants special attention to distribution—which is the pattern, frequency, or spread of protein doses over the course of the day. I emphasize "maximizing" because muscle growth is still possible without paying much attention to anything other than hitting the total daily protein target. However, exhausting all theoretical avenues toward maximal growth is accomplished by consuming MPS-maximizing doses throughout the day,[37] from waking to pre-bed.[106]

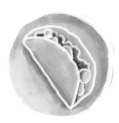

A succession of recent research has refuted the long-standing presumption that 20 to 25 grams of high-quality protein elicits a maximal anabolic response. Macnaughton and colleagues[107] reported greater MPS with 40 versus 20 grams of whey after a high-volume resistance training session, and Park and colleagues[108] reported greater MPS with 70 versus 35 grams of beef protein within a mixed macronutrient meal.

These and similar findings have served to challenge the *leucine trigger hypothesis* (also called the leucine threshold hypothesis), which proposes that a certain dose of leucine (~2 to 3 grams contained within 20 to 25 grams of protein) needs to be reached to maximize MPS.

The basis of this idea is largely rooted in research examining the effects of isolated protein doses rather than protein within solid food matrixes or mixed meals, which are likely to increase the anabolic ceiling of protein dosing.[109] Considering the collective evidence from short-term and longitudinal research, it appears that a minimum of four feedings dosed at ~0.4 to 0.55 g/kg per meal is ideal for maximizing muscle growth.[37]

Whether or not muscle growth can be maximized with just three protein feedings per day is one of the gray areas of research ripe for investigation. I would speculate that the difference between three protein feedings per day and four (or more) is not likely to be meaningful outside of competitive conditions where very small differences can determine placings. However, in some individuals, fewer than three protein feedings per day can present practical challenges such as the gastrointestinal issues associated with huge meals.

I'll reiterate that a wider (waking to pre-bed) and more even spread (similarly sized protein doses within the main meals) is ideal. I would also caution that what you can sustain in the long term is more important than what is supposedly ideal. In any case, protein feeding frequency and distribution will remain an area of controversy as long as there's a lack of direct comparisons of different meal frequencies in resistance trainees in trials that measure body composition changes over time. The research simply isn't there yet, so I recommend doing what feels right for you. In the meantime, Table 4a provides total and per-meal dosing specifics.

Table 4a: Protein Distribution for Maximizing Muscle Growth

BODYWEIGHT	TOTAL DAILY PROTEIN	DOSE PER MEAL (3 MEALS)	DOSE PER MEAL (4 MEALS)
50 kg (110 lbs)	80–110 g	27–37 g	20–27 g
55 kg (121 lbs)	88–121 g	29-40 g	22–30 g
60 kg (132 lbs)	96–132 g	32-44 g	24–33 g
65 kg (143 lbs)	104–143 g	35-48 g	26–36 g
70 kg (154 lbs)	112–154 g	37–51 g	28–38 g
75 kg (165 lbs)	120–165 g	40–55 g	30-41 g
80 kg (176 lbs)	128–176 g	43–59 g	32-44 g
85 kg (187 lbs)	136–187 g	45–62 g	34-47 g
90 kg (198 lbs)	144–198 g	48–66 g	36–50 g
95 kg (209 lbs)	152–209 g	51–70 g	38–52 g
100 kg (220 lbs)	160–220 g	53–73 g	40–55 g
110 kg (242 lbs)	176–242 g	59–81 g	44–60 g
120 kg (264 lbs)	192–264 g	64–88 g	48–66 g
130 kg (286 lbs)	208–286 g	69–95 g	52–71 g

Fasting is not your friend if your main goal is muscle growth

Various forms of fasting have been gaining momentum in mainstream popularity over the past decade or so. Fasting confers an array of speculative and objectively demonstrated health benefits, but the prime mechanism underpinning these benefits is the reduction or control of total caloric intake.[110] Specifically, you're eating less, so you lose weight.

Of specific relevance to the present topic—there's nothing anabolic about not eating. I'm not saying that to be cheeky or sardonic. There's actually a faction of intermittent fasting fans who believe that fasting benefits muscle growth because of growth hormone elevations. Well, the transient rise in growth hormone as a result of fasting is *not* a net anabolic event. It's a compensatory phenomenon, a homeostatic stress response. It's merely the body's attempt to mitigate what it perceives as a threat to survival. Think of growth hormone elevations during fasting as the emergency lights of a building popping on when the main power goes out.

FLEXIBLE VOCAB

Transient fluctuations

Transient means "passing through quickly," so it stands to reason that a transient rise or fall in hormones is a temporary phenomenon at best—not the best way to realistically identify beneficial changes in the human body.

As a general principle, transient hormonal fluctuations at the physiological (as opposed to pharmacological) level are not reliable indicators of muscle growth. A much better short-term indicator of the trajectory of muscle growth is MPS, which is suppressed during fasting. This doesn't mean that fasting will cause rapid declines in muscle mass (the body is smarter than that), but fasting sure as heck does not optimize muscle growth. Is heavy resistance training bad for muscle growth because it causes transient elevations in cortisol? Of course not. Sleep deprivation can cause transient elevations in growth hormone. Is this good for muscle growth? Of course not. These are just a few examples of many. If fasting were a superior way to grow muscle, we'd see it in the peer-reviewed literature, but the opposite is apparent. Quoting a recent paper by Williamson and Moore:[111]

"Thus, based on the acute research to date, we argue that the lost opportunity for amino acid-induced MPS with more feedings may not be compensated for with fewer feedings at higher doses, as what is likely to occur with intermittent fasting. [...] It is our position that intermittent fasting likely represents a suboptimal dietary approach to remodel skeletal muscle, which could impact the ability to maintain or enhance muscle mass and quality, especially during periods of reduced energy availability."

Timing of protein relative to the training session (muscle gain)

In the ISSN's position stand on diets and body composition,[59] I call total daily nutrient and calorie intake the "cake," while the specific timing of its constituent doses is the "icing." Again, protein timing is of distant secondary importance to total daily intake. It's common for folks to fall prey to marketing hype that puts timing on a pedestal, claiming that timing relative to training trumps all. This is false—particularly in the case of protein. Get the cake right first, and then you can apply the icing.

Pre-exercise

Pre-exercise protein intake—on its own—has received minimal attention as a tactic for the goal of muscle growth. My colleagues and I ran a 10-week comparison of pre-exercise versus post-exercise protein intake (25 grams of whey) in resistance-trained subjects.[112] There was no meaningful muscle strength or hypertrophy advantage to either timing protocol. Our findings echoed that of previous work by Candow and colleagues,[113] who conducted a similar comparison in resistance-trained subjects involving a placebo either before or after exercise—with the opposite treatment being protein dosed at 0.3 g/kg. No effect on muscle mass and strength was observed. There appears to be a lack of difference in the anabolic effects of immediate pre- versus post-exercise protein consumption. The effect of timing protein intake closely to both sides of the training bout has yielded mixed results; we'll get to that shortly when discussing the "anabolic window" concept.

During exercise

Protein (or amino acid) intake during training is another potential opportunity to promote net gains in muscle. But how inherently effective is it in the fed-state, typical-length training?

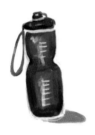

Bird and colleagues[114] reported that MPB was suppressed by a 6 percent liquid carbohydrate solution with essential amino acids (Gatorade plus 6 grams of EAA) consumed during full-body resistance training. This protection against MPB was greater than that from carbohydrate alone or a non-nutritive placebo. This finding is interesting, but the threat of resistance training–induced MPB is likely to be limited to fasted sessions. (In Bird's study, the pre-exercise fasting period was four hours.)

Similarly, Beelen and colleagues[115] found that a combination of carbohydrate and hydrolyzed casein (each dosed at 0.15 g/kg per hour during a two-hour resistance training session) outperformed carbohydrate alone. Net muscle protein balance was positive in the combination treatment, whereas it was negative in the carb-only treatment. These results were seen despite the testing in this trial being done in the evening rather than fasted in the morning. Still, we're looking at a two-hour resistance training session, which understandably might benefit from special attention to "intraworkout" support.

Nevertheless, the body is smarter than we give it credit for. Deldicque and colleagues[116] reported a greater anabolic signaling response to a post-exercise meal after overnight fasted exercise compared to exercise in fed conditions. A potential explanation for this is that the body amplifies its utilization of the post-exercise nutrients in response to what it perceives to be an energy crisis. This doesn't mean fasted training is optimal for growth; it just means the body has its ways of evening things out to preserve homeostasis. But, for individuals who train immediately after waking and have no time for pre-exercise protein, intraworkout protein might be justified if the goal is to pull out all theoretical stops to mitigating MPB. In the latter conditions, protein during your workout might help and couldn't hurt.

Post-exercise

The post-exercise period is a hotbed of claims and lore. The "post-exercise anabolic window" concept was brought to the general fitness audience in the early 2000s thanks to Ivy and Portman's research and their popular paperback *Nutrient Timing: The Future of Sports Nutrition*.[117] The premise is that the timing of specific nutrients immediately post-exercise (quickly absorbed protein and carbs within an hour of finishing the exercise bout) could make or break muscular gains. Essentially, it put the icing before the cake in terms of importance.

This principle grew deeply ingrained in the mantra of trainees and coaches and eventually became accepted as a matter of fact. However, Ivy and Portman's ideas were based on short-term anabolic response studies that measured MPS and/or glycogen resynthesis. At the time their book was published, there were few to no longer-term trials putting those ideas to the test.

However, several studies published over the decade following the release of Ivy and Portman's book yielded equivocal results. The post-exercise anabolic window concept thus amassed considerable doubt from my colleagues and me. So, we conducted a meta-analysis of the relevant research.[118]

Protein-timed conditions were defined as protein ingestion within an hour of either side of the resistance training bout, while non-timed conditions involved a minimum of two hours of protein neglect on both sides of the training bout. A basic analysis (not accounting for covariates such as total daily protein) showed a slight advantage of protein-timed conditions on muscle hypertrophy.

FLEXIBLE VOCAB

Covariates

In statistics, a covariate is any variable that can affect a response variable (also called the dependent variable, which reacts to the independent variable in a study) but is not of specific interest in a study. Basically, it is a variable that isn't the focus of the study but must be accounted for to ensure accurate results.

However, when accounting for covariates, we found that the advantage was due to greater total daily protein intake in protein-timed conditions compared to the non-timed conditions (1.66 versus 1.33 g/kg, on average). A sub-analysis of the studies that *did* equate total daily protein between the groups still failed to show an advantage of protein timing within an hour of training. We therefore concluded that if an anabolic window of opportunity exists for protein intake, it's likely a longer time frame than the fabled one-hour period surrounding the training bout.

So, post-exercise timing seems to have the best evidence to support it. That said, instead of focusing on a narrow post-exercise "anabolic window," the period between the pre- and post-workout meal (the *periworkout* period) should be the focus. The anabolic effect of a protein-rich meal is roughly three to five hours, potentially longer, depending on the size and composition of the meal.[31] According to personal preference and tolerance, liquid or solid meals can be consumed at any point within the three- to five-hour periworkout period. Protein dosing in both the pre- and post-workout meals should maximize the anabolic response (0.4 to 0.55 g/kg).[37] For most individuals, this amounts to a minimum dose of roughly 30 to 50 grams. Figure 4a illustrates the current strategy of periworkout protein timing relative to training.

Figure 4a: Periworkout Protein Timing

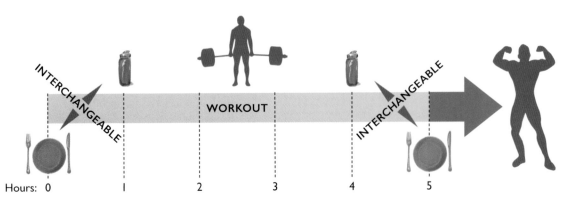

ROLE IN FAT LOSS

Total daily protein requirements (fat loss)

Protein requirements for individuals in hypocaloric (dieting) conditions are higher due to the greater threat to lean mass loss from bodily protein being used to battle the energy deficit. The increased protein needs depend on the severity of the deficit and the dieter's degree of leanness.[59] The more aggressively you're dieting, the more protein functions as a layer of protection.

In hypocaloric conditions, untrained individuals with moderate to high body fat lose a greater proportion of their bodyweight from fat mass. The leaner you get, the greater the threat of lean mass loss. With that said, low protein intakes in sustained eucaloric (weight maintenance) conditions,[119] and even in hypercaloric (weight gain) conditions,[120] can still jeopardize muscle mass. Based on the collective evidence, 1.6 g/kg per day is an optimal baseline protein intake from which dieters in general can adjust upward according to individual response.

Athletes' requirements

The inherent threat to muscle preservation by inadequate protein intake is amplified in hypocaloric conditions. A 2019 review by Hector and Phillips examined the needs of elite athletes in hypocaloric conditions.[121] The reasons for dietary caloric restriction in this population includes "making weight" for sports separated by weight classes, improving power-to-weight ratio, improving overall athletic performance, and improving body composition in aesthetic sports or physique competition. The authors concluded that an appropriate range of protein intake for athletes in hypocaloric conditions is 1.6 to 2.4 g/kg.

Pushing the envelope

In the only systematic review of its kind, Helms et al.[122] examined the needs of resistance-trained subjects in hypocaloric conditions and reported that 2.3 to 3.1 g/kg of fat-free mass was appropriate, with the dose escalating according to the severity of the deficit and leanness level. However, the limitations of this paper are important to elucidate.

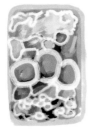

Of the six studies included in the review, only three examined highly trained competitive athletes. Only one study (Mäestu and colleagues[123]) examined the intakes of competitive bodybuilders, and it reported that the pre-contest protein intake of drug-free world-class bodybuilders ranged from 2.48 to 2.68 g/kg. Based on a mean body fat level of roughly 18 percent among the subjects in the treatment groups of Helms et al.'s systematic review (which included men and women),[37] this translates to 1.9 to 2.5 g/kg (0.86 to 1.14 g/lb) of total bodyweight. Chappell and colleagues[124] reported that elite-level drug-free bodybuilding men and women who placed in the top five had pre-contest protein intakes of 3.3 and 2.8 g/kg, respectively.

An important caveat is that these findings are observational. Therefore, they are incapable of establishing cause and effect. Nevertheless, these observations are valuable and provide strong hints about what might be optimal for this population. The late Jim Rohn wisely said, "Success leaves clues," and this statement applies here. Collectively, we can distill the envelope-pushing protein range to 2.2 to 3.3 g/kg (1 to 1.5 g/lb) of TBW.

Recomposition

Recomposition (nicknamed "recomp" by the fitness community) is simultaneous fat loss and muscle gain. The capacity to recomp diminishes alongside the progression of an individual's training status.[125] In other words, recomp happens more dramatically in untrained (or previously trained) folks with excess body fat. The closer you are to your potential, the less margin is available for recomp.

With advancing proximity to your potential, recomp eventually becomes an impractical target. Advanced trainees and most later-stage intermediates are better off focusing on one goal at a time—fat loss or muscle gain, not both simultaneously.

The hierarchy of recomp capacity, from greatest to least, is

1. Formerly fit/trained folks with excess body fat

2. Overweight novices

3. Intermediates

4. Advanced trainees who are relatively lean

Formerly fit folks typically make the most dramatic before-and-after transformations, especially if they overate while remaining sedentary for several years. There are at least two potential mechanisms underlying this ability of the formerly fit to dramatically rebound back into shape.

First, training increases the number of myonuclei within the muscle fibers.[126] This allows strength and size gains to rebound faster via increased mitochondrial remodeling. Training-induced myonuclear increases are resistant to apoptosis (cell death). These cellular components can remain intact despite extended time off from training.[127]

FLEXIBLE VOCAB

Myonuclei and mitochondrial remodeling

Myonuclei are commonly thought of as the "control centers" of muscle fibers, and when you work out and grow muscle, more get added. But here's the cool part: they don't completely go away when muscle fibers shrink; instead, they facilitate muscle regrowth. Hence the term "muscle memory." They accomplish this through mitochondrial remodeling, which describes the ability of mitochondria to adapt to environmental cues.

Another potential mechanism is the persistence of training-induced increases in capillarization (increased vascular networks within the muscle).[128] When you combine these mechanisms with greater neural efficiency reducing the learning curve of the exercises, it's clear that the recomp advantages of previously trained folks (who have gained body fat) put them at the top of the hierarchy due to rapid "rebound gains."

A consistent finding across multiple studies (including studies on trained subjects) is that higher protein intakes are more conducive to recomp. A recent paper by Barakat and colleagues[125] is the first of its kind in the peer-reviewed literature to specifically examine the recomp phenomenon. They concluded that consuming 2.6 to 3.5 g/kg of FFM may increase the likelihood or magnitude of recomposition. This turns out to be very similar to the envelope-pushing range of 2.2 to 3.3 g/kg (1 to 1.5 g/lb) of TBW.

A note about gluconeogenesis and ketosis

Gluconeogenesis is the process of generating glucose from glucogenic amino acids. There's a widespread belief that dietary protein is easily converted to glucose. This is one of the reasons many ketogenic dieters are afraid of high protein intakes; they fear that gluconeogenesis might kick them out of ketosis.

FLEXIBLE VOCAB

Ketosis

Commonly abbreviated "keto," ketosis forms the foundation of a popular low-carb diet. Ketosis occurs when the body lacks sufficient carbohydrates to burn for energy and, as a result, burns an increased proportion of fat (now in greater supply, thanks to the diet) while producing energy-supplying by-products called ketones.

A classic study by Khan and colleagues[129] used tracer methodology to estimate the gluconeogenesis of 50 grams of protein from cottage cheese, which put 9.68 grams of glucose into circulation. More recent work by Fromentin and colleagues[130] used a more sophisticated tracer method and reported that ingesting 23 grams of egg protein produced 3.9 grams of glucose, which they described as a small amount, despite optimal conditions for gluconeogenesis to occur (after an overnight fast and in the absence of dietary carbohydrates).

The moral of the story is that while protein ingestion can result in glucose production, the amount is inconsequential in normal circumstances in healthy individuals. In extreme conditions such as prolonged fasting and starvation, the body can ramp up gluconeogenesis as a survival measure, where it can catabolize bodily protein for the production of glucose to fuel vital cellular functions.

Under normal conditions in typical diets, blood ketone levels are low (<3 mmol/L). Ketosis is attained either by fasting or by restricting carbohydrate to a maximum of about 50 grams or 10 percent of total daily calories, with the predominance of energy intake from fat (60 to 80 percent).[59] This brings circulating ketone levels to 0.5 to 3 mmol/L. The primary ketone in circulation is ß-hydroxybutyrate (BHB).

FLEXIBLE VOCAB

mmol/L

For our purposes, this unit of measurement stands for millimoles of glucose per liter of blood, where a millimole is one-thousandth of a mole, which measures the mass of molecules. To put it simply, it's a way to measure glucose levels in your blood.

In their book *The Art and Science of Low Carbohydrate Performance*,[131] ketogenic diet research pioneers Jeff Volek and Stephen Phinney recommend blood BHB levels ranging from 0.5 to 3 mmol/L to achieve *"optimal fuel flow during keto-adaptation."* They define nutritional ketosis as a BHB level ranging from 1 to 3 mmol/L. Of relevance to the present discussion, they recommend a relatively low protein intake (0.6 to 1 g/kg of lean mass).

Many took this as gospel and avoided high protein intakes for fear of getting kicked out of ketosis. This apprehension is based on the potential for a fraction of dietary protein to be converted to glucose during gluconeogenesis. However, there's enough evidence from controlled intervention trials to confidently say that protein intakes beyond traditional recommendations still result in BHB levels that would satisfy keto proponents.

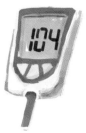

Table 4b lists studies showing that high protein intakes can allow blood ketone levels within the range of 0.5 to 3 mmol/L.[132-134] Note that two of the three studies showed blood ketone levels promoted by keto connoisseurs (1 to 3 mmol/L).

Table 4b: Studies Showing Ketosis Despite High Protein Intakes

PUBLICATION	POPULATION	PROTEIN INTAKE	CARB INTAKE	BLOOD KETONE LEVEL
Wilson JM, et al. *J Strength Cond Res.* 2020 Dec;34(12):3463-74.	25 college-aged resistance-trained men	1.7 g/kg	31 g/day	1 mmol/L
Burke LM, et al. *J Physiol.* 2017 May 1; 595(9):2785-807.	21 elite race walkers	2.2 g/kg	33 g/day	1.8 mmol/L
Volek JS, et al. *Metabolism.* 2016 Mar;65(3):100-10.	20 elite ultra-marathoners and Ironman distance triathletes	2.1 g/kg	82 g/day	0.7 mmol/L

Distribution of protein throughout the day (fat loss)

This subsection represents a developing area of research with a few twists and turns. It's possible that the body may have an asymmetric control system regarding muscle retention (in a caloric deficit) versus growth in maintenance or hypercaloric conditions. The body appears to be more lenient/flexible with protein distribution for retaining muscle mass under caloric deficit conditions, as long as total daily protein is optimized and resistance training is engaged. Protein distribution involves the number, evenness, and placement of protein doses throughout the day. As you'll see, all of these variables have lacked consistency in influencing fat loss. So, protein can help you maintain muscle mass, but will it help you lose fat?

In 2015, colleagues and I conducted the only meta-analysis of its kind to date, examining the effect of meal frequency on weight loss and body composition.[135] Fifteen studies were included in the analysis. Meal frequency did not affect total bodyweight change, but higher meal frequencies were associated with greater losses of fat mass and greater retention of lean mass.

However, we ran a sensitivity analysis that tested the influence of individual studies on the overall analysis. The removal of a single study (Iwao and colleagues[136]) eliminated the effect of meal frequency on changes in body composition. We thus concluded that, since adherence is a prime concern, the number of daily meals should come down to personal preference for the goal of fat loss.

The main limitation of our meta-analysis was a lack of studies with structured exercise protocols (let alone progressive resistance training programs). Protein intakes sufficient for maximizing muscle retention were also lacking among the studies in our analysis. These shortcomings have since been addressed in more recent research, which I'll get to in a moment.

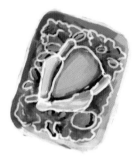

Skewed intake

Even skewed intake patterns fall under the umbrella of protein distribution. In a skewed pattern, the bulk of the day's protein intake is concentrated toward one meal (or one section) of the day.

Earlier work by Arnal and colleagues[137] showed a lack of difference in nitrogen balance between an even protein distribution over four meals versus a skewed pattern providing 80 percent of daily protein at lunch in young subjects (average age of 26 years) consuming total daily protein dosed at 1.7 g/kg of lean mass. Another study by Arnal and colleagues of the same design,[138] this time on older subjects (average age of 68 years), actually found *better* nitrogen retention in the skewed pattern.

FLEXIBLE VOCAB

Nitrogen balance

Maintaining positive nitrogen balance is a rough indication that lean body mass is in an anabolic state; in other words, a state of growth. All the macronutrients contain carbon, hydrogen, and oxygen, but only protein contains a nitrogen molecule as well. Thus, tracking nitrogen balance can, in theory, tell us whether the body has sufficient protein for muscle growth. However, given that skeletal muscle is only one of several nitrogen sources in the body, this is not always the most reliable metric.

Both studies were short (two weeks); nitrogen balance is a relatively crude measure of bodily protein status; and body composition (lean mass and fat mass) was not assessed. Nevertheless, these findings indicate a lack of threat to lean mass with skewed protein intakes compared to evenly distributed intakes when total protein is adequate (≥1.6 g/kg). I'll reiterate that consistent fat loss advantages to any particular protein distribution have thus far been elusive.

Time-restricted feeding

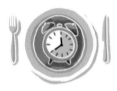

Also relevant to the context of protein distribution is time-restricted feeding (TRF, also called time-restricted eating), which is a type of intermittent fasting. TRF involves shortening feeding windows to about eight hours or less, typically compared with at least a 12-hour feeding window in the control condition.

TRF is the functional equivalent of a skewed distribution, with the control conditions representing more even distributions. TRF studies involving resistance training and adequate protein (≥1.6 g/kg) have revealed similar effects on lean mass in the TRF and control (evenly distributed) conditions.[139-141]

A fat loss advantage of TRF versus the control diet was evident in one study.[139] One study saw the potential for a fat loss advantage in TRF, which was no longer present with an *intention-to-treat* analysis, which estimates outcomes based on data from all subjects regardless of whether they complied with the intervention protocol or dropped out. The most recent study in this line of research[141] saw no body composition advantage to either the TRF or the control diet. Importantly, a comprehensive and sophisticated four-compartment model was used to assess body composition. In addition, muscle morphology (cross-sectional area, thickness, quality) was assessed via ultrasound.

Findings, or the lack thereof

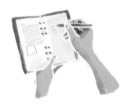

Collectively, these equivocal and mostly unremarkable differences lead us to conclude that the influence of protein distribution on fat loss is somewhere between questionable and negligible. In the quest to optimize body composition outcomes, the protein intake pattern that you prefer and can best stick to in the long term is the one that you should implement. For the goal of fat loss, it's evident that a wide range of possible distributions (including number of feedings and skewed versus even feedings throughout the day) produce similar results, as long as the appropriate daily total is hit.

A simple, pragmatic approach would be to maintain the same protein feeding pattern in a fat loss program as you would for muscle gain. What supports muscle growth in maintenance or surplus conditions (a *minimum* of three to four protein feedings that maximize the acute anabolic response) is likely to support muscle retention in hypocaloric conditions. However, I'd point out that those who choose to push the boundaries of low meal frequency can do so with minimal concern for muscle loss—once again, as long as the total daily protein target is hit.

Timing of protein relative to the training session (fat loss)

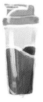

Fasted cardio has traditionally been claimed to enhance the fat loss process. This is due to the greater rate of fat oxidation (fat "burning") that occurs during exercise done in an overnight fasted state. However, an important principle I'd like to get across is that what happens in a snapshot of time (i.e., during a training bout) does not necessarily translate to changes in body composition over longer periods. What ultimately matters is *net fat balance* (the difference between fat oxidation and fat storage) by the end of the day, week, month, etc.

FLEXIBLE VOCAB

Oxidation

In science, oxidation is the result of a chemical reaction where an atom or molecule loses one or more electrons. In our context, what athletes refer to as "burning" fat is more accurately described as the consumption of a bodily fuel source (stored as any of the three macros, not just fat) combined with the delivery of oxygen to create energy.

My colleagues and I investigated this topic in a direct comparison of fed versus fasted aerobic exercise over a four-week period in controlled, hypocaloric conditions.[142] The treatment we employed was a 250-kcal meal replacement shake consisting of whey protein (20 grams), maltodextrin (40 grams), and trace amounts of fat (0.5 gram).

This was the first—and thus far, the only—study of its kind to assess body composition changes in these conditions. Both the fasted cardio and the fed cardio groups lost body fat and retained lean mass, with no significant differences between the groups. Importantly, all of the dietary variables (total daily calories and macronutrient intake) were the same for both groups; the only difference was the placement of the first meal before versus after exercise. No fat loss advantage was seen with fasted cardio.

Our findings were echoed in a subsequent systematic review and meta-analysis by Hackett and Hagstrom[143] containing five studies and 96 subjects in total. The overall lack of difference in fed versus fasted training on body composition led them to conclude that programming in this vein can be flexible and based on individual preference, since no particular approach appears to be superior for fat loss.

Finally, there's an interesting line of research showing that protein taken prior to exercise causes greater increases in post-exercise energy expenditure compared to carbohydrate.[144,145] However, short-term differences in energy expenditure don't guarantee differences in body composition over the longer term. It's premature to assume that "protein-enhanced" exercise bouts impart a fat loss advantage. So, at least in terms of fat loss, go with the protein intake program that suits your unique needs.

ROLE IN ATHLETIC PERFORMANCE

Total daily protein requirements (athletic performance)

Again, we begin with the highest tier of importance—total daily amount. The increase and preservation of muscle mass is crucial to increasing and preserving its strength and functional capacity. Therefore, it's not surprising that protein requirements for athletic performance closely resemble protein requirements for maximizing muscle growth.

No distinction is established between the needs of strength-oriented versus endurance-oriented athletes. Their similar needs make sense since the increased needs of strength athletes are generally directed toward increasing muscle mass, while the increased needs of endurance-oriented athletes are directed toward preventing muscle loss. The safest bet for protein intake guidelines for athletic populations are the position stands of the major scientific organizations in this area of specialization.

Table 4c outlines the latest position stands of the major nutrition (and exercise) organizations on protein requirements for athletic populations. The protein recommendation of the ISSN[146] has been the same since its initial position stand on this topic in 2007. The Academy of Nutrition and Dietetics, Dietitians of Canada, and American College of Sports Medicine[147] have increased the upper end of their previous 2009 position stand from 1.7 to 2 g/kg in light of new research. In retrospect, the ISSN was ahead of the game.

Table 4c: Position Stands on Protein Requirements for Athletic Goals

PUBLICATION	POPULATION	RECOMMENDATION
International Society of Sports Nutrition Position Stand: Protein and Exercise, 2017	Physically active individuals, including competitive and recreational athletes aiming to enhance muscular strength, endurance, or size	1.4–2 g/kg *"Higher protein intakes (2.3–3.1 g/kg FFM/d) may be needed to maximize the retention of lean body mass in resistance-trained subjects during hypocaloric periods."*
Position of the AND, DC, and ACSM: Nutrition and Athletic Performance, 2016	Competitive athletes in a range of sports spanning the strength-endurance continuum	1.2–2 g/kg *"Higher intakes may be indicated for short periods during intensified training or when reducing energy intake."*

Although the position stands of these organizations represent the scientific consensus, this doesn't mean they are indisputable. The indicator amino acid oxidation (IAAO) technique is a validated method used for determining indispensable amino acids in humans.[148] Recent studies using the IAAO technique have shown protein requirements greater than the low end of the protein ranges listed in the position stands.

Kato and colleagues[149] reported that endurance athletes on a training day had an estimated average requirement of 1.65 g/kg, with an upper 95 percent confidence limit of 1.83 g/kg. More recently, Bandegan and colleagues[150] found that the estimated average protein requirement in endurance-trained subjects in the 24-hour post-trained period was 2.1 g/kg, with an upper 95 percent confidence limit of 2.6 g/kg. The latter findings call into question the lower end of the recommendations of the current position stands on protein intakes for athletes, which range from 1.2 to 1.4 g/kg. Based on the current evidence, I would not recommend dipping below 1.6 g/kg for competitive athletes, or recreational athletes who take winning seriously.

FLEXIBLE VOCAB

Confidence limits

In statistics, a confidence limit is the number at the upper or lower end of a confidence interval, which is a range of estimates for an unknown parameter. Basically, confidence limits are the estimated upper and lower lower boundaries that would contain the true value we're testing for, in the theoretical absence of bias.

Timing of protein relative to the training session (athletic performance)

Pre-exercise

To date, only one study has directly compared protein with other macronutrients on endurance performance. Rowlands and Hopkins[151] compared the effects of a high-fat, high-carbohydrate, or high-protein meal 90 minutes prior to a test involving sprinting and 50-km performance in competitive cyclists. No significant differences were observed between the treatments compared.

This study asked an interesting question and unfortunately has not been replicated. To my knowledge, there is no study specifically comparing pre-exercise protein with other macronutrients on strength performance.

During exercise

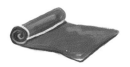 A commonly overlooked factor that can greatly influence the ergogenic potential of intraworkout nutrition is the presence versus absence of preworkout nutrition. From a bioavailability standpoint, preworkout nutrient ingestion can function as intraworkout nutrition since digestion and absorption can last several hours.

FLEXIBLE VOCAB

Ergogenic

Ergogenic means "enhancing physical performance." But it's a bit more nuanced than that. It can mean anything from boosting energy levels to bolstering post-workout recovery, and aids are usually classified as nutritional, pharmacological, physiological, or psychological. Remember to use caution with ergogenic aids. Not all are legal or allowed in competition.

In the most recent meta-analysis to examine the effect of protein and carbohydrate co-ingestion versus carbohydrate only on endurance performance, Kloby Nielsen and colleagues[152] reported that the protein-containing conditions enhanced endurance. However, this was seen in trials that equated carbohydrate intake, and the addition of protein led to greater intake of total calories, which explained the advantage. In comparisons that equated total calories, there was no endurance performance advantage of a carb-protein mix versus carbs alone. So, the addition of protein is beneficial for performance only when insufficient carbohydrate is consumed during exercise.

A wrinkle I would add is that Saunders and colleagues[153,154] found that carb-protein beverages at a 4:1 ratio consumed during and after endurance exercise are superior for suppressing muscle damage compared to carbohydrate-only solutions. In these combination beverages, protein and carbohydrate were dosed at 0.038 and 0.15 g/kg for every 15 minutes (0.15 and 0.6 g/kg/hour, respectively) of exercise. This amounts to roughly 8 to 15 grams of protein per hour of training. But, once again, the big confounder here is a lack of protein-containing pre-exercise nutrition, hence a lack of real-world validity for endurance competition.

It's worth reiterating that preworkout nutrition can function as intraworkout nutrition. A perfect example in the protein context is by Power and colleagues,[155] who found that after ingesting 45 grams of whey, it takes about 45 minutes for amino acid levels to peak in the blood and another two hours for them to return to baseline levels.

Keep in mind that this was an isolated dose of quickly digested protein. Within a mixed-macronutrient meal containing this protein dose, it would take even longer for circulating nutrient levels to peak and longer for them to return to baseline. Therefore, the question of intraworkout protein intake only potentially applies to fasted training—and even in this case, intraworkout protein would not be an efficient fuel for athletic performance. I'll discuss more of that in the next chapter, which covers carbohydrate.

Post-exercise

Protein combined with carbohydrate can generate more insulin output, which in turn has been shown to enhance glucose uptake in the post-exercise period. However, in a recent meta-analysis, Craven and colleagues[156] reported that protein co-ingested with carbohydrate does not expedite post-exercise glycogen resynthesis (or subsequent exercise performance) compared to carbohydrate alone, especially when carbohydrate dosing is at or near 1 g/kg/hr. This finding reflects recent position stands on post-exercise carbohydrate dosing (1 to 1.2 g/kg/hr) for maximizing glycogen replenishment under time-constrained conditions where exhaustive endurance bouts are separated by less than eight hours.[147,157]

FLEXIBLE VOCAB

Glycogen resynthesis

Glycogen is a polysaccharide that acts as energy storage, so synthesis of glycogen from glucose—also called glycogenesis—is a major player in energy creation for exercise. Therefore, glycogen resynthesis refers to methods for replenishing these energy reserves and enhancing performance.

Given this finding, the addition of protein may be viewed as a tool to expedite glycogen resynthesis when carbohydrate dosing—for whatever reason— is restricted to levels below 1 g/kg. It's worth mentioning that although post-exercise protein isn't directly ergogenic in the presence of optimal carbohydrate dosing (>1.2 g/kg), it's still an opportunity to feed, and that opportunity should be taken since there's no downside. It's an opportunity to stimulate MPS and partially fulfill the daily protein requirement (and help fulfill the protein feeding frequency target). Purposely neglecting protein in the post-exercise period is not conducive to minimizing muscle damage or expediting recovery and growth.

In sum, protein timing is a relative non-factor in athletic performance; carbs are king in this domain. Although there's the potential benefit of intraworkout protein intake for the purpose of mitigating MPB to indirectly preserve strength, this only applies to a complete absence of preworkout (and/or post-workout) protein intake.

CHAPTER 4 IN A NUTSHELL

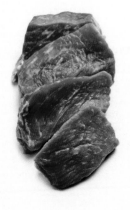

- Proteins are large molecules consisting of amino acids. Of the 20 amino acids that comprise proteins, nine are considered essential and thus must be obtained from the diet. Proteins function as structural components, enzymes, hormones, immune factors, transporters, acid-base regulators, and neurotransmitters.

- Animal-derived proteins (e.g., meat, fish, poultry, eggs, and dairy) tend to be higher quality than plant-derived proteins, showing more efficient stimulation of muscle protein synthesis (MPS). Nevertheless, there is recent evidence showing that a vegan diet can yield similar gains in muscle size and strength when total daily protein intake is 1.6 g/kg, at least in untrained subjects.[56]

- From the most to least important considerations of protein intake, the hierarchy is as follows: 1) total daily protein amount, 2) distribution of protein throughout the day, and 3) timing of protein relative to the training bout.

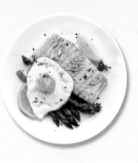

- The general population without specific athletic or body composition goals aside from general health should consume protein at a minimal range of 1.2 to 1.6 g/kg per day. Maximizing muscle growth can be achieved with 1.6 to 2.2 g/kg (0.7 to 1 g/lb). An appropriate range of protein intake for athletes in hypocaloric conditions is 1.6 to 2.4 g/kg. Per the current position stands of the major scientific organizations, maximizing athletic performance requires 1.4 to 2 g/kg. On the note of pushing the envelope, the protein needs of lean, resistance-trained subjects in hypocaloric conditions are 2.3 to 3.1 g/kg of fat-free mass (FFM). Athletes "pushing the envelope" physiologically under stressful conditions such as prolonged caloric deficits can use the guideline of 2.2 to 3.3 g/kg (1 to 1.5 g/lb) of target bodyweight (TBW). Recomposition (the simultaneous loss of fat mass and gain of lean mass) has been seen with protein intakes ranging from 2.6 to 3.5 g/kg of FFM.

- FFM-based protein targets are more complicated and not necessarily more accurate, but they can satisfy some people's need for precision. For general purposes, 2 g/kg of FFM (0.9 g/lb of FFM) is a reasonable baseline target. Individuals specifically aiming for muscle gain (as well as dieters running a caloric deficit) can start at 2.2 g/kg of FFM (1 g/lb of FFM) and adjust according to individual response.

- A simple solution to the complexity of basing protein on FFM is to base protein intake on goal bodyweight or TBW. Current bodyweight can be used to estimate protein needs if you're seeking to maintain your current weight. This is an effective way to approximate lean mass with a built-in margin of safety.

- While muscle growth is possible regardless of energy balance, surplus conditions facilitate maximal rates of growth. A caloric surplus of 20 to 40 percent above maintenance in novices and 10 to 20 percent in more advanced trainees is needed (alongside optimized protein dosing) for maximizing muscle growth.

- The goal of *maximizing* muscle gain may warrant special attention to distribution—which is the pattern, frequency, or spread of protein doses throughout the day (a minimum of four feedings dosed at ~0.4 to 0.55 g/kg per meal). Refer to Table 4a for specific protein doses and corresponding bodyweights.

- Instead of focusing on a narrow post-exercise "anabolic window," the period between the pre- and post-workout meal (the periworkout period) should be the focus. The anabolic effect of a protein-rich meal is roughly three to five hours, potentially longer, depending on the size and composition of the meal.

- Although there's the potential benefit of intraworkout protein intake for the purpose of mitigating muscle protein breakdown (MPB), this applies only to an absence of preworkout (and/or post-workout) protein intake—or if the training session approaches or exceeds two hours of continuous/exhaustive work. Pre- and post-exercise protein doses that max out MPS (~0.4 to 0.6 g/kg) ideally would frame the periworkout period. This means protein should be consumed within two hours prior to training and again within two hours after training. Refer to Figure 4a.

- Unlike with carbohydrate, which has specific applications for sport, protein timing is a relative non-factor in athletic performance.

- Although post-exercise protein isn't ergogenic in the presence of sufficient carbs, it's still an opportunity to stimulate MPS in addition to contributing to the daily protein total.

- Due to an overall lack of differences in anabolic response, there's insufficient evidence to program different protein targets, either in total or per meal, based on sex.

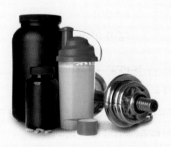

CARBOHYDRATE

5

Carbohydrate is a perpetually newsworthy nutrient. It's a lightning rod for controversy and vilification. But here's the rub: culpability belongs to the combination of refined carbohydrate and fat in highly processed foods, yet carbs are selectively blamed. Many popular diet books are based on the manipulation, careful selection, or avoidance of carbohydrate. Unfortunately for the general public, where carbs go, misinformation follows.

Well, as the saying goes, the buck stops here. As you proceed through this book, you'll be severely disappointed if you're looking for magic food sources, dose manipulations, or intake levels of carbohydrate that can be universally prescribed to end humanity's ills and create superheroes. That simply is not reality.

Individual preferences, tolerances, and goals determine carbohydrate intakes to suit various needs. The promises and claims made in the majority of popular diet books are rooted in speculation rather than science. Here, we will stick to the science, unless I specify that we're treading on hypothetical ground or personal observations.

From a nutritional standpoint, carbohydrate is one of three macronutrients, with the others being protein and fat. Carbohydrates function primarily as an energy source. They also play key roles in glucose and insulin action, as well as cholesterol and triglyceride metabolism and fermentation.[158]

Carbohydrate can further be classified in terms of its structure:

- **Simple carbohydrates (monosaccharides and disaccharides)** consist of single and double monosaccharide units, respectively. Examples of monosaccharides include glucose, fructose, and galactose. Examples of disaccharides include sucrose, maltose, and lactose.

- **Complex carbohydrates (oligosaccharides and polysaccharides)** consist of short and long chains of monosaccharide units. Of these, polysaccharides are more abundant and relevant to the human diet. Common examples of polysaccharides include amylose, amylopectin, and glycogen (the body's stored form of polysaccharide).

FLEXIBLE VOCAB

Polysaccharides

What do you get when you put together *poly*, which means "many," and *saccharide*, which refers to a compound with sugar as a base? The most abundant carbohydrate found in nature! Polysaccharides are large molecules made up of many smaller monosaccharides that can store energy, send cellular messages, and even support cells and tissues.

FIBER: A COMPLEX CARBOHYDRATE

Dietary fiber falls under the complex carbohydrate umbrella. Fiber is a plant-based compound that includes a wide range of non-starch polysaccharides that are not fully digested in the human gut. Types of dietary fiber include beta-glucan, cellulose, hemi-cellulose, gums, lignin, pectin, mucilage, and resistant starch.

The current evidence collectively supports a minimum fiber intake of 25 to 29 grams per day for lowering the risk of all-cause and cardiovascular related mortality and incidence of coronary heart disease, stroke, type 2 diabetes (T2D), and colorectal cancer.[159] These findings are in line with the recommended dietary fiber intakes for both children and adults: 14 grams per 1,000 kcal.[160,161]

However, insufficient data are available for drawing definitive recommendations of fiber sources and fiber subtypes. Traditional classification of fiber is based on solubility, but a more recent focus has been on gel-forming capability. Insoluble fiber has benefits on colonic health (i.e., the bulking of stool), while viscous soluble fiber has shown benefits that include improved glycemic control, blood pressure, and lipid profile.

Fiber is technically not calorie-free; its metabolizable energy is ~2 kcal/g on average.[162] Interestingly, higher fiber intakes have been found to promote greater weight loss and dietary adherence independently of macronutrient and caloric intake.[163] Further supporting the weight-regulating impact of fiber, Jovanovski and colleagues[164] conducted a meta-analysis of RCTs and found that supplementation with viscous soluble fiber to an ad libitum (unrestricted) diet reduced bodyweight and waist circumference. The moral of the story is that fiber may technically provide calories, but it tends to favor weight loss—through mechanisms that are not entirely clear. Potential explanations are increased satiety that decreases energy intake overall, along with increased energy expenditure via the greater thermic effect of higher-fiber foods.[165]

Resistant starch

There's a considerable amount of hype behind resistant starch, particularly for the goal of weight loss. As the name implies, this type of starch is resistant to digestion and absorption. In a similar manner to fiber, resistant starch is shielded from digestion in the upper gastrointestinal tract, undergoes fermentation in the large bowel, produces short-chain fatty acids, and imparts the potential to improve gut health.[166]

The health news media perpetually recycles research showing that rice that's been cooled after cooking has a significantly higher resistant starch content.[167] Normally cooked rice has a low resistant starch content, typically less than 3 percent.[168] This increase in resistant starch is purported to reduce the metabolizable energy (usable calories) of the food, which is supported by the observation of a lower glycemic response to consuming the specially cooked/cooled rice.[167]

What proceeded from that point was a leap of faith that resistant starch is the answer to the obesity problem, which is essentially a problem of overeating. Well, that hypothesis has not panned out as hoped. A recent systematic review by White and colleagues[169] reported that resistant starch does not increase satiety or reduce appetite and food intake in subjects with prediabetes. A subsequent systematic review by Guo and colleagues[170] included 11 studies, six of which specifically assessed body composition (resistant starch doses ranged from 13 to 40 grams per day). Compared to regular (digestible) starch, resistant starch showed beneficial effects on glucose control and insulin sensitivity but had no effect on bodyweight or body composition.

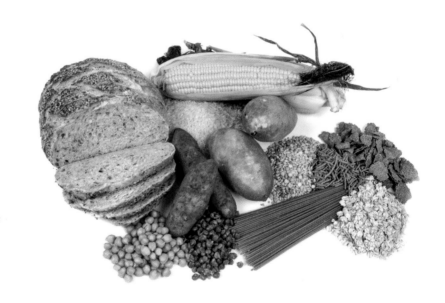

GLYCOGEN: STORED CARBOHYDRATE

Glycogen levels (levels of stored carbohydrate) can vary considerably depending on lean body mass (LBM), diet composition, and training demands. Adults store ~350 to 700 grams of glycogen in skeletal muscle and 100 grams in the liver.[171]

Carbohydrate intake directly influences glycogen levels, which can significantly influence muscle mass since every gram of glycogen is chemically bound to 2.7 to 4 grams of water.[172] At ~4 kcal/g, carbohydrate and protein have similar energy yields, while fat has 9 kcal/g. Despite fat having nearly double the energy content of carbohydrate, the oxidation ("burning") of fat is an inefficient way to produce ATP (the body's energy currency). ATP production via glucose oxidation is two to five times faster than from fat oxidation.[173,174] The latter carries implications for carbohydrate dosing to optimize performance at various exercise intensities, with carbohydrate dependency increasing alongside increasing intensity. At greater than 60 percent of maximal oxygen consumption (high-moderate intensity and beyond), the primary fuels to produce ATP are blood glucose and muscle glycogen due to progressively greater recruitment of fast-twitch motor units.[175]

FLEXIBLE VOCAB

ATP

Adenosine triphosphate isn't called the body's energy currency for nothing. Found in every known form of life, this remarkable compound provides the energy behind many processes in living cells, from muscle contraction to chemical synthesis. The body has several systems for making ATP, which work together in phases to respond to the demands you put on your body.

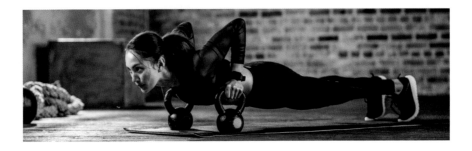

Glycemic index: missing the forest for the trees

Much ado has been made about the glycemic index (GI) of foods since its inception in 1981.[176] GI is a ranking of a food's ability to raise blood glucose levels. Specifically, GI is the glycemic response from a fixed amount of carbohydrate (50 grams) in a given food within a fixed time frame (two hours). This value is indexed against a reference food (pure glucose or white bread, which is assigned a GI of 100).

Arbitrary categories of GI have been designated as low (GI ≤ 55), medium (GI 56–69), and high (GI ≥ 70). Glycemic load (GL) is a parameter that accounts for total carbohydrate in addition to GI and was meant to be an improvement upon merely using GI to judge carbs. These classification systems are not only arbitrary, but fail to account for nutrient density and food quality.[177]

Most importantly, the majority of the research on the various effects of GI fails to equate macronutrition between the diets compared. Protein, fat, and fiber content consistently lower a given food's GI. The common research design flaw is the failure to match macronutrition (and fiber) in comparisons of foods differing in GI. This imparts an unfair advantage to the lower-GI treatment.

In dietary comparisons that equate macronutrition and fiber between the groups, differences in GI do not impact body composition or markers of cardiovascular risk.[178-180] For these reasons, GI is a problematic metric for judging carbohydrate quality. I'd go as far as to say that GI is an irrelevant distraction. GL is just as meaningless once macronutrition and fiber are equated in diet comparisons.

A sound, science-based approach would place the focus on consuming a predominance of whole and minimally refined carbohydrates instead of judging foods by their GI ranking. An example of the folly of a GI focus would put Snickers candy bars and full-fat ice cream in a superior position to fresh fruit such as pineapple and watermelon. Of course, that's absurd. And yes, one could argue that ice cream and Snickers bars have a greater GL than fruits. Well, congratulations, you're one step closer to focusing on what matters more than GI or GL: total amount of carbohydrate within a diet of predominantly unrefined carbohydrate sources.

SUGAR: REALITY VERSUS ALARMISM

Given the interlocking crises of obesity, diabetes, and heart disease, a ton of research has been done on the impact of dietary sugars. Keep in mind we're talking about added sugars (also called extrinsic sugars), not sugars intrinsic to foods such as milk/milk products and fruits.

One of the most notable papers in recent years is by Khan and Sievenpiper,[181] and it summarizes the evidence on this topic from the highest level (systematic reviews and meta-analyses). Their focus was fructose-containing sugars, since fructose is the most commonly vilified monosaccharide. Their conclusion strongly challenges the pop-diet/sugar-scaremongering narrative: fructose-containing sugars can only increase bodyweight and cardiometabolic disease risk in the context of an overconsumption of total daily calories. Quoting the paper directly:

> "When the calories are matched, fructose-containing sugars do not appear to cause weight gain compared to other forms of macronutrients including complex carbohydrates, fats and protein, and in low doses fructose might even show benefit."

A subsequent meta-analysis by Khan and colleagues[182] determined that the threshold of harm for cardiovascular disease mortality via added sugars was 65 grams, or 13 percent of total energy. In practical terms, 65 grams of added sugar is the equivalent of 13 teaspoons (4.33 tablespoons) of sugar or syrup. Mean dietary intake of added sugars among US adults is estimated to be 14.9 percent of total energy intake,[183] an amount that breaches the aforementioned threshold of harm.

A caveat to consider is that these findings were based on the general population, not performance athletes (who can benefit from added sugar intakes beyond the norm). Added sugar recommendations by the major health organizations are inconsistent (ranging from 5 to 25 percent of total energy). Furthermore, these figures are based on low-quality evidence lacking a scientific basis.[184] A practical solution hearkens back to Chapter 1, and that is to set a discretionary calorie allotment of 10 to 20 percent of total intake from essentially whatever your heart desires; added sugar would fall within that allotment.[17]

THE RELATIVITY OF ESSENTIALITY

Carbohydrate is often labeled the "nonessential" macronutrient because the body can biosynthesize all the glucose it needs for survival by drawing on noncarbohydrate tissues and their metabolites. However, the question that needs to be asked is…*essential for what?*

The traditional, clinical definition of *essentiality* refers to survival, but within the context of maximizing athletic performance (especially at higher intensities) or muscle mass, it can be argued that carbohydrate is indeed essential. The combination of carbohydrate and fluid has been called *"the largest single determinant of ensuring optimal performance during prolonged endurance events"* aside from genetic capacity and training.[185]

The ergogenic benefit of carbohydrate was published in the scientific literature as far back as 1920.[186] Subsequent milestones in the timeline of carbohydrate research include the 1960s showing a clear relationship between glycogen availability and endurance capacity and the 1980s showing that performance was increased via carbohydrate consumption during exercise.[187]

The early 2000s began a new era of research investigating the finer details of carbohydrate amount and type consumed during exercise to optimize performance at various durations. Novel strides were made in the understanding of the role of multiple transportable carbohydrate intake. The most recent decade spawned larger investigative strides in carbohydrate periodization, the strategic manipulation of carbohydrate availability for enhancing endurance performance. On the note that nutritional essentiality is goal-specific (rather than merely required for survival), the goal of optimal health/maximal prevention of chronic disease would simply not be possible on a zero-carbohydrate diet. A major shortfall would be the absence of dietary fiber, the health benefits of which were discussed previously. So, carbs are essential for optimal health.

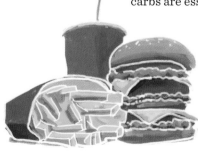

Periodization

Periodization refers to strategically varying a training program over time to improve results. When it comes to carbohydrate periodization, this means manipulating carb availability by consuming low, moderate, or high amounts depending on the day or meal. Doing so can alter carbohydrate availability (or glycogen content) for your next training session.

Sex-based differences in carbohydrate metabolism

As in the case of protein, the collective evidence does not warrant different carbohydrate intake levels between the sexes. The broader range of variation in carbohydrate needs across individuals further reinforces the lack of utility in generalizing different requirements for men and women. Once again, this lack of meaningful difference is reflected in the absence of separate recommendations for men and women by the position stands of major scientific organizations.

With that said, classic work by Tarnopolsky and colleagues[104] found that in the context of endurance exercise, women use 25 percent less glycogen than men (who also oxidize more protein/aminos). This is due to women's higher intramuscular triglyceride stores, which facilitate a higher rate of fat mobilization and use as fuel during exercise.[188]

However, this doesn't mean that women in competitive athletics should downplay carbohydrate intake in favor of fat intake. This difference in substrate utilization does not change the objective to maximize carbohydrate availability for athletic performance goals. Furthermore, when carbohydrate dosing is optimized, post-exercise glycogen resynthesis rates,[189] as well as glycogen loading capacity (relative to lean mass),[190] are similar between men and women.

ROLE IN MUSCLE GAIN

Total daily carbohydrate requirements (muscle gain)

Progressive resistance training is well established as the most effective type of exercise for maximizing muscle growth.[191] Each macronutrient plays an important role in this process. The primary role of dietary carbohydrate in muscle growth is to provide energy to support progressive resistance training. Carbohydrate serves as fuel for high-intensity muscle contraction when available from endogenous sources (from inside the body; glycogen and circulating glucose) or exogenous sources (from the diet; carbohydrate-containing foods or beverages).

It's worth reiterating that although fat is a more concentrated energy source than carbohydrate, it's a far less efficient energy substrate than carbohydrate due to its lower rate of ATP production. Given that rates of muscle hypertrophy are optimized in a sustained caloric surplus, carbohydrate's role in rapid energy production, as well as its lesser tendency toward adipose (fatty tissue) storage compared to dietary fat, carbohydrate has prime utility for programming a caloric surplus.[57]

High-load/high-effort resistance training is a largely glycolytic (glucose-dependent) activity. Resistance training bouts, which vary in volume and effort, can reduce muscle glycogen stores by 24 to 40 percent.[171] While typical resistance training bouts are not completely glycogen-depleting, this suggests the importance of maintaining a certain minimum of carbohydrate intake to support lifting performance at higher volumes of training.

In several recent studies,[192-196] ketogenic dieting conditions in resistance trainees caused either lean mass reduction or compromised gains in lean mass. Furthermore, a recent (massive) review by Ashtary-Larky and colleagues[197] examined the ketogenic diet literature spanning from 1921 to the present day. Among their conclusions was that in resistance-trained individuals, lean mass loss tends to be greater with ketogenic diets versus higher-carb/lower-fat control diets. A 13-study systematic review and meta-analysis led by the same authors[198] reinforces the finding that restricting carbohydrate to ketogenic levels (<10 percent of total energy, or less than ~50 grams per day) is counterproductive to the goal of maximizing rates of muscle hypertrophy or retention. Ketogenic diets are not a deal breaker for muscle growth, but the collective evidence shows that they can antagonize or at least suboptimize the process.

It's plausible that the daily dose for maximizing muscle growth would be similar to amounts that would maximize strength performance. In perhaps the first paper to specifically address the macronutrient needs of bodybuilders, Lambert and colleagues[199] recommend 5 to 6 g/kg. A more recent review by Slater and Phillips[200] relays survey data where competitive lifters and throwers reported carbohydrate intakes of 3 to 5 g/kg per day, while bodybuilders reported 4 to 7 g/kg per day. A systematic review by Spendlove and colleagues[201] reports that the average intake of competitive bodybuilders in the off-season is 5.3 g/kg per day. A recent position stand of the ISSN[83] maintains its recommendation of 5 to 8 g/kg per day for moderate volumes of intense training typical of lifters and strength athletes. Although this area is largely observational (thus lacking in causational data), it's safe to say that a carbohydrate intake range of 3 to 8 g/kg reflects the evidence at-large for the goal of maximizing muscle growth.

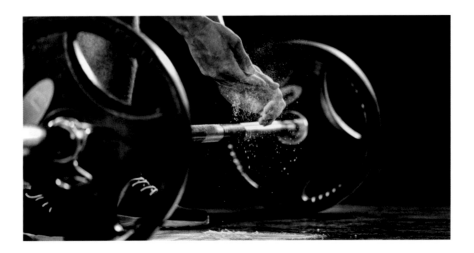

Timing of carbohydrate relative to the training session (muscle gain)

Pre-exercise

The goal of muscle hypertrophy is inseparable from the performance-based objective of progressive overload. In other words, muscle growth typically follows increases in volume load (sets × reps × load). Compromised lifting performance is not a critical issue for the goal of fat loss, whereas for muscle growth, it is. While it's possible to *maintain* lifting performance while lowballing total daily carbohydrate, the push toward continual improvement would inevitably be compromised—thereby suboptimizing rates of growth.

FLEXIBLE VOCAB

Progressive overload

Progressive overload is one of the key tenets behind the effectiveness of strength training. It advocates for gradually increasing the stress on the musculoskeletal system, which increases the body's ability to adapt over time. In other words, progressively increasing the weight (in terms of load, reps, and/or sets) helps you get stronger.

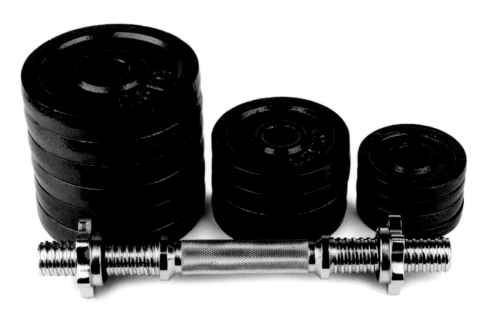

Carbohydrate consumption immediately prior to resistance training has the potential to increase work output, but the research in this area has yielded mixed results. Studies showing an ergogenic effect involved training sessions lasting 50 minutes or longer, while the majority of studies showing a lack of effect on training performance lasted no longer than 40 minutes.[202]

However, a major limitation of this research is the use of fasted subjects. When training is done in a fed state, ergogenic effects of immediate pre-exercise carbohydrate are questionable—especially in the context of resistance training, where glycogen reductions per muscle group do not normally reach critical levels. Resistance training bouts of typical length and volume deplete glycogen by roughly 24 to 40 percent.[171]

A recent study by Bin Naharudin and colleagues[203] compared a non-nutritive placebo beverage with a large breakfast having a carb dose of 1.5 g/kg (116 grams on average). Exercise commenced two hours after the meal. Significantly more repetitions were performed in upper- and lower-body exercises in the breakfast versus the fasted group.

This trial improved on previous designs by using higher-volume resistance training, as well as a typical solid-food high-carb breakfast. (Previous designs used a beverage.) Another design strength was the use of resistance-trained subjects, historically averaging four sessions per week. A notable limitation of this study is that all the subjects were habitual breakfast eaters; the results could have been different in habitual breakfast skippers. Nevertheless, these findings provide grounds for caution against fasted resistance training with the goal of growth (and, therefore, lifting performance).

The amount of carbohydrate consumed in the preworkout period for maximizing resistance training performance depends on individual circumstances. It can range from being a non-issue to a serious consideration, depending on the degree of total daily carbohydrate restriction and the nature of the training bout. For individuals seeking a cautious approach to protecting performance, training within two hours after a moderate mixed-macronutrient meal with a carbohydrate content of 0.5 to 1 g/kg is a range that accommodates the needs of most. The relatively massive dose of 1.5 g/kg used in the recent trial by Bin Naharudin and colleagues[203] is certainly an option (and it worked), but it can limit the flexibility for carbohydrate intake at other points in the day for a large segment of the noncompetitive population with lower total energy requirements.

During exercise

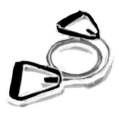

The benefit of carbohydrate intake during exercise largely depends upon glycogen availability through the course of the training bout. A hypothetical resistance training bout that would benefit from intraworkout carbohydrate ingestion is a lengthy one with a high volume of sets per muscle group—commenced immediately after an overnight fast, minus a preworkout meal that contains carbs.

In this scenario, carbohydrate ingested during training would provide fuel for high-intensity muscular work that would otherwise be waning toward the end of the session. But also notice how these circumstances (a long, exhaustive session performed after an overnight fast, minus preworkout nutrition) would reflect a very limited segment of the training population.

As anticlimactic as it is, carbohydrate intake during fed-state resistance training has limited benefit for maximizing muscle growth. A possible exception is resistance training in an overnight-fasted state for longer than roughly an hour. Another exception is training in a fed state (having eaten two to four hours pre-exercise) for 90 minutes or longer in an exhaustive, endurance-type fashion. However, both of these are far-fetched scenarios in programs specifically designed to maximize muscle growth.

For individuals engaged in particularly high-volume resistance training sessions that approach or exceed 90 minutes, a range of ~30 to 60 grams of carbohydrate per hour could offset the risk of decreased glycogen availability later in the session, especially when training in a fasted or semi-fasted state.[157]

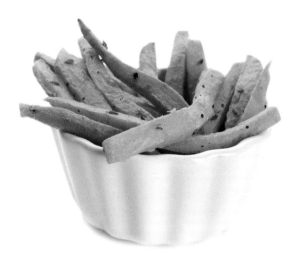

Post-exercise

Post-exercise carbohydrate always enters the discussion as a traditional component of the "anabolic window" concept, rooted in findings from earlier research on rates of glycogen resynthesis after depletion via exhaustive endurance exercise.[31] This is a separate goal from muscle hypertrophy.

MPS data from acute (short-term) studies using low protein or amino acid doses generated the presumption that the co-ingestion of carbohydrate with protein was necessary to maximize the anabolic response. It was speculated that carbohydrate's insulin stimulation beyond that of protein alone augmented anabolism. However, this idea was eventually refuted by several acute studies using higher protein doses (20 to 25 grams or more) co-ingested with or without rapidly absorbed/highly insulinogenic carbohydrate, showing no difference in MPS.[204]

Post-exercise carbohydrate is touted to play a major role in *anticatabolism* through its ability to raise insulin. However, the evidence shows that MPS plays a greater role than the suppression of MPB in net gains in muscle protein. Morton and colleagues[205] report that in healthy humans, changes in MPS are four to five times greater than MPB in response to exercise and feeding. Illustrating this, Glynn and colleagues[206] compared the post-exercise anabolic response via 20 grams of EAA plus 30 grams of carbs versus 20 grams of EAA plus 90 grams of carbs. They found only minor changes in MPB and concluded that MPS was the main driver of anabolism regardless of carbohydrate dose or insulin level. These findings are in line with research by Greenhaff and colleagues[207] showing that during sustained elevations of blood amino acid levels, muscle protein balance plateaus at insulin concentrations raised to 15 to 30 mU/L. This level of insulinemia is achievable by typical protein doses within meals, even without the co-ingestion of carbohydrate.

Corroborating these acute findings, a 12-week trial by Hulmi and colleagues[208] found no difference in muscle size and strength gains via post-exercise 30 grams of protein alone, versus protein co-ingested with 34.5 grams of maltodextrin in subjects undergoing a progressive resistance training program.

So, while the post-exercise period presents a feeding opportunity for those struggling to consume enough of any given macronutrient, the precise timing of quickly absorbed carbohydrates in the immediate post-exercise period has limited relevance to the goal of muscle hypertrophy. Exceptions exist in programs that involve training a muscle exhaustively more than once per day (which are rare in the context of programs designed to maximize muscle growth).

ROLE IN FAT LOSS

Total daily carbohydrate requirements (fat loss)

While the goal of muscle gain is compromised by underconsuming carbohydrate, the goal of fat loss is more flexible. Every level of carb intake can work as long as a net caloric deficit is sustained over the course of the day/week/month. *Sustained* is the key word here. If an individual's chosen degree of carb restriction is too difficult to sustain in the long term, then the purpose is defeated. Thus, the amount of carbohydrate required for fat loss effectively ends up being whatever the individual can best adhere to. This will vary with individual preferences, tolerances, and goals.

Contrary to popular lore, there truly is no magic threshold of carbohydrate intake below which fat loss is optimized, nor is there a magic threshold above which fat loss is inhibited.[59] Ketogenic dieting (less than 10 percent of total kcals from carbs, or a maximum of 50 grams of carbs per day) remains a popular approach to weight/fat loss due to rapid initial weight drops—largely due to decreased glycogen, which is mostly water. The "keto" diet has legions of die-hard followers, some successful with it, others yo-yoing their way through perpetual dieting frustration. The best we can say about keto is that it's a viable option—but one that is not universally sustainable.

Keto's questionable sustainability has been consistently demonstrated in subjects with T2D. This doesn't speak too well of keto, since those with T2D have a more urgent need to comply with therapeutic intervention diets. Still, long-term adherence largely fails.

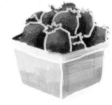

A relatively recent review of low-carbohydrate diets and T2D by van Wyk and colleagues[209] arrives at a skeptical conclusion about the emphasis on carbohydrate restriction per se. A common thread among the studies was a lack of adherence to carbohydrate restriction. Wyk's review includes nine meta-analyses and an additional 12 studies. They conclude that, overall, there were no significant differences in clinical outcomes (including glycemic control) between low-carb diets and control diets, particularly in studies exceeding six months in duration.

Once again, this is likely due to a breakdown of adherence, characterized by an up-creep in carbohydrate intake over time. Carbohydrate intake at one year in very-low-carbohydrate diets (less than 50 grams per day) ranged from 132 to 162 grams. The latter point bears repeating: subjects' carbohydrate intakes after a year of dieting ended up being about triple their keto-level carbohydrate intakes assigned at baseline.

A subsequent meta-analysis by Huntriss and colleagues[210] found that in T2D, very-low-carbohydrate diets (less than 50 grams per day) were difficult to adhere to, whereas a more moderately low-carbohydrate diet (less than 130 grams per day) was more sustainable. In a more recent meta-analysis, Goldenberg and colleagues[211] report that in T2D, low-carbohydrate diets (less than 130 grams per day) actually outperformed very-low-carbohydrate/ketogenic diets (less than 10 percent of total kcal from carbohydrate) for weight loss at six months. However, this difference was negated in subjects who were highly adherent to ketogenic diets. The recurrent implication here is that ketogenic diets appear to lack long-term sustainability compared to less restrictive low-carbohydrate diets with a limit of 130 grams per day.

The good news is that keto, high-carb/low-fat, and everything in between are viable options for fat loss. Across the multitude of studies that rigorously equate protein and total calories between ketogenic and non-ketogenic diets of varying degrees, no fat loss advantage is seen for keto.[59,197,212-214] Rather, a wide range of carbohydrate-fat proportions are similarly effective for fat loss when protein and total calories are equated. Although it might be disappointing that no magic bullet (a universally superior dietary model) exists, the bright side is that this leaves room for flexibly programming diets to suit the inevitable variability of individual needs.

Recent research involving resistance-trained subjects has shown a potential fat loss advantage to ketogenic diets amid their lack of benefit to muscle growth and retention.[198] However, one of the challenges to the presumed superiority of carbohydrate restriction for fat loss is the current data on competitors whose aim is to achieve the limits of human leanness. Chappell and colleagues[124] examined the dietary strategies of elite natural bodybuilders (placing in the top five in national-level competition). At the start of contest preparation, carbohydrate intake was reported to be 5.1 and 3.7 g/kg per day (431.1 and 340.6 grams per day) in men and women, respectively. At the end of prep, carbohydrate intakes were 4.6 and 3.5 g/kg per day (340.6 and 196.7 grams per day) in men and women, respectively. These carbohydrate intakes range from ~3.9 to 8.6 times the amount that would qualify as ketogenic.

Distribution of carbohydrate throughout the day (fat loss)

As in the case of protein, total daily intake of carbohydrate occupies the top tier of importance, with the distribution and timing of its constituent doses being a distantly secondary concern. I would go so far as to say that the distribution of carbohydrate is actually a non-concern beyond specific athletic performance applications.

For the goal of fat loss, what matters most is sustaining a net caloric deficit by the end of the day, week, month, etc. There is no special daily pattern of carbohydrate intake (meal frequency, dose per meal, length and positioning of the feeding window) beyond what maximizes adherence in the long term. This inevitably varies across individuals.

There is a wealth of speculation and mythology surrounding the topic of ideal carbohydrate placement throughout the day for fat loss. Fortunately, there is also an abundance of research refuting these glorifications and vilifications of various carbohydrate eating patterns. Perhaps the oldest tenet in this area is that breakfast (a carb-heavy one) is the most important meal of the day.

A noteworthy review by Brown and colleagues[215] discusses the false nature of the pervasive claim that skipping breakfast causes obesity, which is rooted in observational data but not supported by interventional data. A recent systematic review and meta-analysis by Sievert and colleagues[216] includes 13 RCTs and finds that breakfast consumption resulted in higher total daily energy intakes. Contrary to popular belief, the addition of breakfast showed a tendency to hinder weight loss. The authors thus conclude, *"Currently, the available evidence does not support modification of diets in adults to include the consumption of breakfast as a good strategy to lose weight."* This is not to say that breakfast is a global threat to weight/fat loss—it's just another avenue for individualizing programs based on a person's preference for maximizing sustainability.

Another widespread belief is that carbs consumed later versus earlier in the day lead to fat gain or prevent fat loss—which is nonsense. If that were true, then Sievert and colleagues' meta-analysis of breakfast studies[216] would have arrived at a different conclusion.

A tightly controlled study by Keim and colleagues[217] compared the six-week effects of eating 70 percent of daily calories in the morning versus in the evening. Subjects lived in the research center's metabolic suite throughout the study. Physical activity (including resistance and aerobic training) was standardized. The larger evening intake condition retained more lean mass without any remarkable difference in fat mass reduction; there was actually a slight advantage to the larger evening intake at one of the time points.

Another significant blow to the "no carbs at night" dogma is the longest study of its kind, a six-month trial by Sofer and colleagues.[218] Consuming the majority of carbohydrates at dinner (thus making it the highest-calorie meal of the day) was compared with spreading carbs more evenly throughout the day. The late-shifted carb intake was superior for body fat loss, glycemic control, hunger control, reducing markers of inflammation, and improving blood lipids. Although these results are compelling, the research in this area has been mixed. There indeed are studies showing bodyweight regulation benefits of earlier versus later carbohydrate intake,[219,220] but these studies have lower methodological rigor than the ones I discussed earlier.

Time-restricted feeding (TRF) is one of the intermittent fasting variants that I'll discuss further in the nonlinear dieting chapter. Briefly, the main rationale for early time-restricted feeding (eTRF, limiting caloric consumption to a time frame early in the day) is to take advantage of higher glucose tolerance at the beginning of the day.

However, eTRF research fails to consider the influence of exercise and its interaction with nutrients. I would confidently speculate that the far-reaching metabolic effects of the exercise bout would override the already modest advantages seen in eTRF. A recent trial by Savikj et al.[221] on people with type 2 diabetes found that afternoon (4 p.m.) high-intensity interval training (HIIT) was superior to morning (8 a.m.) HIIT for improving 24-hour blood glucose levels. It's reasonable to hypothesize that consuming a substantial proportion of the day's intake post-exercise would potentially augment improvements in glycemic control by leveraging the increased state of insulin sensitivity.[222,223]

FLEXIBLE VOCAB

High-intensity interval training (HIIT)

As you can guess by the name, HIIT is a kind of interval training, which means it uses rounds of exercise at varying intensity levels that include short bursts of effort that exceed 90 percent of maximal oxygen consumption or 75 percent of maximal power. HIIT is a more efficient alternative to moderate-intensity steady-state (MISS) training. However, your goals, personal preferences, and tolerances should dictate the use of HIIT and/or MISS.

Again, what ultimately matters is sustainability. The theoretical differences between carbohydrate distribution patterns are small and essentially meaningless in the big picture. The most effective approach is to honor personal preference. Whether it's a breakfast, lunch, or dinner carb bomb or a more even distribution of carbs throughout the day—all of those options are fine. An earlier versus later feeding window will not make or break health or body composition outcomes in physically active individuals making progress toward their body composition goals in the context of otherwise healthy lifestyle factors. Same goes with a narrow versus broad feeding window. The simple truth is that the best carbohydrate distribution pattern is whatever the individual can best adhere to.

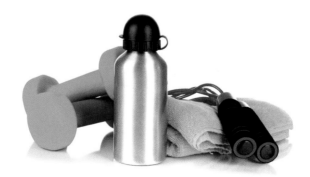

ROLE IN ATHLETIC PERFORMANCE

Total daily carbohydrate requirements (athletic performance)

Strength/power-oriented sports

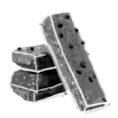

The mechanisms and requirements of carbohydrate intake for pursuit of strength gains have inevitable overlap with the goal of muscle hypertrophy. Strength/power athletes and physique/bodybuilding athletes both employ progressive overload to attain their primary goals. Athletes focused on strength/power-oriented sports performance employ periodization models that cover the continuum of metabolic and morphological adaptations (i.e., muscle hypertrophy) to functional adaptations (i.e., maximal strength and power). Within this framework, hypertrophy is typically a side effect or accessory consequence of strength adaptations. Periodization phases traditionally progress from more hypertrophy-oriented programming (higher set volume and effort, lower loads, shorter rest intervals) toward more strength-oriented programming (lower set volume, higher loads, longer rest intervals).

Compared to strength/power athletes, bodybuilders tend to take more sets to failure. In comparisons with equal work, sets to failure cause greater increases in glycogenolysis and phosphocreatine demands than sets that keep repetitions in reserve.[200] Given this, it has been speculated that rates of glycogen use as well as energy expenditure are higher during hypertrophy-focused training sessions compared to strength-focused training sessions.[202] In some cases, this would mean lower carbohydrate requirements in weight class–based sports, where maximal strength and power–to-weight ratio is sought.

Although low glycogen levels can theoretically compromise muscular force production and thus resistance training performance, the body of literature to date has not consistently demonstrated this effect.[202] The majority of studies examining the effect of ketogenic diets on resistance training have shown performance on par with control/non-ketogenic conditions.[224] Similar lifting strength on ketogenic diets compared to conventional control diets has been demonstrated in resistance-trained subjects at moderate[225] and near-maximal to maximal loading.[132,193,194] Thus, while ketogenic diets might be suboptimal for maximizing muscle gain and preservation, this disadvantage is not apparent for strength goals.

Nevertheless, the position stands of the major scientific organizations in the athletic realm have not delineated carbohydrate intake targets for the goals of maximizing gains in muscular strength versus gains in muscular size, collectively recommending a range of 5 to 8 g/kg per day.[83,147] The current body of evidence showing the effectiveness of very-low-carbohydrate/ketogenic diets on strength performance challenges these recommendations.[226,227] The recommended carbohydrate intake range in the collective literature for maximizing muscle hypertrophy is 3 to 8 g/kg per day—a broader range encompassing lower dosing.

It's reasonable to speculate that the safe minimum carbohydrate intake for maximizing strength gains is the low end of the "hypertrophy" range (3 g/kg/day). In support of this point, a recent study by Vargas-Molina and colleagues[195] involving lean resistance-trained women showed a failure to increase bench press strength on the keto diet, while the non-keto control diet caused significant strength gains.

So, for the time being, it's safe to consider under-carbing a risk for suboptimizing maximal strength development, especially in programs with a high volume of sets. In high-stakes competition, utilizing every legal ergogenic advantage (including optimal carbohydrate intake) is important. A low-end daily carbohydrate intake that won't compromise this goal remains a gray area in our knowledge, but individuals are welcome to take their chances.

Endurance-oriented sports

Of the macronutrients, carbohydrate is the one most intimately tied to total daily energy demands as well as the energy demands of specific bouts of training or competition. The scientific consensus on total daily carbohydrate intake for athletic performance is best reflected in the position stands of the major scientific organizations. Given that these organizations are looking at essentially the same body of literature, similarity of recommendations is inevitable.

The ISSN delineates carbohydrate requirements as follows: general fitness with no particular performance goals requires typical intakes, ~3 to 5 g/kg per day. I would interject that in the absence of performance goals, setting a minimum intake of carbohydrate is unnecessary. Moderate amounts of intense training (e.g., two to three hours per day of intense exercise, five or six times a week) typically require 5 to 8 g/kg per day. The latter reflects the intermediate dosing zone between strength/power-oriented sports and endurance sports. High-volume (e.g., three to six hours per day of intense training in one or two daily workouts five or six days a week) may require 8 to 10 g/kg per day of carbohydrate. The latter recommendation reflects the needs of sports that are more purely endurance-oriented.

The joint position of the Academy of Nutrition and Dietetics, Dietitians of Canada, and the American College of Sports Medicine is that carbohydrate recommendations are stratified into four levels:

- **Light** (low-intensity or skill-based activities): 3 to 5 g/kg per day

- **Moderate** (~one hour per day): 5 to 7 g/kg per day

- **High** (one to three hours per day of moderate to high-intensity exercise): 6 to 10 g/kg per day

- **Very high** (more than four to five hours per day of moderate to high-intensity exercise): 8 to 12 g/kg per day

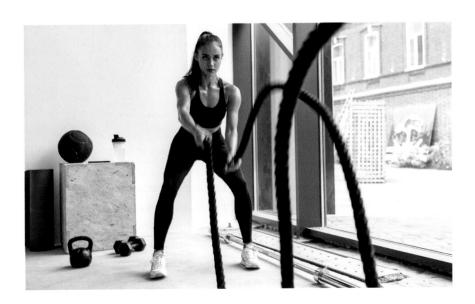

Wait a minute; doesn't keto-adaptation offer endurance benefits?

In a word, no. But first, a little background. Carbohydrate restriction and replacement with fat to become "fat-adapted" (also called *keto-adapted*) results in increased oxidation of fat and decreased glycogen utilization. This increased reliance on fat as fuel is touted to improve endurance performance due to the abundance of energy within body fat (as opposed to reliance on the body's limited store of glycogen).

FLEXIBLE VOCAB

Keto-adapted

Keto- or fat-adaptation is used to describe the process the body undergoes when it switches from using glucose to fat as its primary energy source on a keto diet. As a result, the body produces ketones, water-soluble molecules that can serve as energy in the absence of carbohydrates. It's important to note that the increased oxidation of fat is largely due to higher levels of free fatty acids in circulation and higher levels of intramuscular fat.

However, keto-adaptation has been shown to impair high-intensity exercise performance.[228-230] This is a big problem since endurance events are typically a mix of intensities, not a constant, linear pace. Dr. Jose Areta, faculty of Sport and Exercise Sciences, Liverpool John Moores University, has astutely illuminated the importance of carbohydrate availability for what he calls *race-winning moves*—sprints, climbs, lead-outs, and breakaways. The ability to best execute these moves separates the winners from the other competitors. All race-winning moves occur at high intensities and are dependent upon carbohydrate.

Perhaps the biggest knocks against keto-adaptation are three recent, well-controlled studies by Burke and colleagues.[133,231,232] They stand out because, unlike studies showing a lack of viability when using surrogate measures such as time to exhaustion,[233] Burke and colleagues went the extra mile and measured the time to complete an actual race. Impaired performance was consistently seen in keto-adapted athletes compared to the high-carb control conditions when testing most closely reflected real-world competition. Given that these effects were observed in elite-level race walkers, it's apparent that keto-adaptation can decrease exercise performance at a wide range of intensities, not just high intensities.[133,228-231,234]

Timing of carbohydrate relative to the exercise bout

Of the macronutrients, carbohydrate is the most time-sensitive, especially in the context of prolonged endurance bouts and scenarios where there is minimal recovery time between glycogen-depleting bouts. The goal of maximizing endurance performance is unique in that carbohydrate timing relative to training can be as important as total daily amount.

The combination of carbohydrate and fluid has been called *"the largest single determinant of ensuring optimal performance during prolonged endurance events"* aside from genetic capacity and training.[185] The ergogenic benefit of carbohydrate was published in the scientific literature as far back as 1920.[186] As mentioned previously, subsequent milestones in the timeline of carbohydrate research include the 1960s and 1980s,[187] with the early 2000s marking a new era of research. Advances were made in the understanding of the role of multiple transportable carbohydrates (in simpler terms, the consumption of glucose and fructose combinations for more efficient absorption and delivery). Again, the most recent decade spawned larger investigative strides in carbohydrate periodization.

Pre-exercise

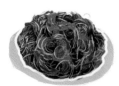

Given the crucial importance of glycogen availability for endurance performance, the main objective of pre-exercise carbohydrate intake is to "top off" or maximize glycogen stores. Pre-competition intake can be viewed as three separate phases: the days preceding the competition, within approximately four hours prior to competition, and within one hour of competition.

In the days preceding competition, *carbohydrate-loading* is a technique for attaining supernormal glycogen levels. (It is also referred to as glycogen supercompensation.) The classic carbohydrate-loading model developed by Bergström and colleagues[235] involves three to four days of glycogen depletion (low carbohydrate intake of 10 to 100 grams per day; roughly 5 to 15 percent of total kcal, combined with exhaustive exercise) followed by three to four days of carb-loading (500 to 600 grams per day; roughly 70 percent of total kcal or more) combined with reduced training volume—also called tapering.

Although carbohydrate-loading does cause glycogen supercompensation, performance advantages compared to control conditions are unlikely to occur in events that do not exceed 90 minutes.[236] Subsequent carb-loading models aimed to minimize the adverse effects on mood seen by depletion phases by focusing more on tapering and a more linear increase in carbohydrate intake. Contemporary carbohydrate-loading recommendations omit the depletion phase and institute a loading phase ranging from 7 to 12 grams of carbohydrate per day for one to three days prior to competition, while training volume is tapered.[147,157]

In the final four hours preceding competition, the objective is to maximize muscle and liver glycogen levels. After an overnight fast, liver glycogen stores can be reduced by as much as 80 percent.[237] This illuminates the importance of relatively immediate pre-exercise carbohydrate intake in common scenarios where competition begins in the morning.

However, there is a lack of consensus on amount and type of pre-exercise carbohydrate feeding within this time frame due to the wide variability of individual circumstances. Large carbohydrate doses (~200 to 300 grams) ingested two to four hours pre-exercise have been shown to enhance time trial performance and increase time to exhaustion.[237,238] Carbohydrate ingested within one hour pre-exercise has typically been dosed at ~1 g/kg, yielding a mix of results leaning toward the null.[237]

Concern has been raised over the potential for "rebound hypoglycemia" during exercise when carbohydrate is ingested during this time frame. However, the collective literature has not indicated this fluctuation in glycemia to threaten performance.

FLEXIBLE VOCAB

Glycemia

Glycemia is the concentration of sugar or glucose in the blood. As such, *hypoglycemia* and *hyperglycemia* refer to blood glucose levels that are too low or too high, respectively. Reactive hypoglycemia (also called postprandial glycemia) is the occurrence of low blood sugar levels two to five hours after a meal. This phenomenon is usually seen in diabetic and prediabetic states.

In the largest meta-analysis on this topic to date, Burdon and colleagues[239] found no clear benefit of low- versus high-GI pre-exercise meals for endurance performance. It should be noted that there is a lack of research directly comparing carbohydrate ingestion two to four hours versus one hour or less before exercise. In sum, ergogenic benefit is possible from a carbohydrate dose ranging from 1 to 4 g/kg within the four-hour window preceding higher-intensity ($\geq 70\%$ VO_2 max) events exceeding 90 minutes.[157] This represents a wide range of possibilities, so personal trial-and-error is important for individualizing protocols to optimize results.

During exercise

Position stands of the major scientific organizations converge on a during-exercise carbohydrate dosing range of 30 to 60 grams per hour for endurance events that last one hour or longer.[147,157] However, it should be noted that doses below and above this range have been effective for enhancing performance. As little as 15 grams per hour improved 20-km cycling time trial performance.[240] On the upper end of the spectrum, 90 grams per hour has been recommended for endurance events exceeding two and a half hours.[147,187]

A noteworthy trial by Smith and colleagues[241] examined the effect of 12 different carbohydrate doses in 10-gram increments (10 to 120 grams per hour) on cycling performance (two hours at 70.8% VO_2 max followed by a 20-km time trial). Performance increased alongside escalating doses until reaching a peak at 78 grams per hour. Beyond this dose, performance diminished.

Keep in mind that the research on during-exercise carbohydrate intake is confounded by the use of subjects in an overnight-fasted state, which is not representative of real-world competition conditions. Colombani and colleagues[242] recognized this lack of external validity in the existing body of research, so they aimed to examine real-world conditions. Their systematic review only included studies involving subjects in the postprandial/fed-state, in trials whose testing involved a fixed distance, fixed time, or fixed amount of work, or submaximal exercise followed by a time trial—rather than a time-to-exhaustion model. They concluded that carbohydrates ingested prior to or during exercise would not likely enhance performance for bouts shorter than 70 minutes and would result in a *"possible but not compelling ergogenic effect"* with durations longer than 70 minutes.

A meta-analysis by Pöchmüller and colleagues[243] used similar inclusion criteria (a meal consumed two to four hours prior to time trial–type testing) and found that in trained male cyclists, a 6 to 8 percent carbohydrate solution (also containing electrolytes) enhanced performance in bouts longer than 90 minutes. Taken together, these findings indicate that immediate pre- or during-exercise carbohydrate ingestion is not likely to enhance performance in postprandial conditions unless the bout exceeds 70 to 90 minutes.

Specific types of carbohydrate can impact performance through different mechanisms, depending on the nature of the bout. Glucose ingestion was recommended in earlier literature, but eventually, ingesting a combination of glucose and fructose was found to enhance performance. The co-ingestion of these two monosaccharides can increase their absorption rate by utilizing different intestinal transporters (GLUT5 and SGLT1, for the few of you interested). This has been called the *multiple transportable carbohydrate* model, where improved absorption leads to increased fuel delivery to working muscle.[244] The weight of the evidence supports the ingestion of a glucose-fructose ratio ranging from 1:1 to 2:1 during exercise, at a rate of 1.3 to 2.4 g/minute for maximizing endurance performance in bouts lasting two and a half to three hours, compared to ingesting a single type of sugar on its own.[245]

FLEXIBLE VOCAB

Carbohydrate transport

When you consume food containing carbohydrate, first your body digests it, then absorbs it, and then transports it. What this means is that as your body breaks down carbohydrate, it must transport those molecules to various tissues as usable energy. Skeletal muscle happens to be the major site of uptake and disposal of ingested glucose.

The advantage of the multiple transportable carbohydrate model might not apply to shorter exercise durations. A systematic review by Stellingwerff and Cox[185] concluded that in events lasting less than 60 minutes, it is possible that oral receptor exposure to carbohydrate, via either mouth rinse or consumption, stimulates the central nervous system reward centers, leading to enhanced performance.

In contrast, in events that are longer than 60 minutes (with conditions where glycogen availability can become a limiting factor), multiple transportable carbohydrate intake is warranted. The use of carbohydrate mouth rinse for enhancing endurance performance is an interesting but inconclusive area of study. A recent meta-analysis by Brietzke and colleagues[246] found that the use of carbohydrate mouth rinse increased mean power output in cycling trials but failed to improve time to complete the trials compared to placebo.

Proper hydration (fluid and electrolyte balance) is of crucial importance during endurance exercise. Carbohydrate concentrations ranging from 6 to 8 percent of the fluid solution (60 to 80 g/L, or 15 to 20 grams per 8-ounce cup) optimizes the rate of fluid and carbohydrate delivery to tissues.[83] Fluid intake should correspond with sweating rate, which varies across training intensities, environmental temperatures, and individual tolerances. Recommended rates of fluid intake are 0.4 to 0.8 L per hour, paced at 6 to 12 fluid ounces every 10 to 15 minutes throughout the exercise bout.

Sodium and chloride are the major electrolytes lost via sweat, with sodium being most critical to performance and functioning of organs and tissues. Exercise under an hour, especially if preceded by a meal containing sodium, is not likely to benefit from intraworkout sodium intake. However, endurance events lasting over an hour can benefit from a sodium intake of 20 to 40 mmol/L (460 to 920 mg/L).[247] For events that exceed two hours, a sodium concentration of 30 to 50 mmol/L (690 to 1,150 mg/L) can protect endurance athletes from a dangerous state of low blood sodium levels called hyponatremia.[248] A recent review by Vitale and Getzin[249] recommends an initial trial dose of sodium at 300 to 600 mg per hour of exercise, to be adjusted according to individual response. These authors reference the ISSN's position stand on exercise and sports nutrition,[83] which attributes the recommendation to the ACSM.

It should be emphasized that fluid and electrolyte balance must be tailored to the individual since sodium losses vary widely. The latter point is illustrated by Baker and colleagues,[250] who found that in athletes in various team sports, training-induced sodium losses per liter of sweat ranged from 418 to 1,628 mg. As an example of products mirroring research, Gatorade's original "Thirst Quencher" formula's sodium content is 457 mg/L, and its "Endurance" formula contains 832 mg/L. The latter is more appropriate for athletes in competitions that exceed two hours, while the original formula is suitable for shorter durations. Commercial formulas also contain one or more of the other electrolytes in sweat (potassium, calcium, and magnesium). However, there's a lack of evidence to support supplementing mid-training intake with anything beyond sodium and chloride; sweat losses of the other electrolytes are minuscule and inconsequential.

In light of mixed data and recommendations, it's reasonable to issue the following guidelines for achieving proper fluid and electrolyte balance during exercise: 6 to 8 percent carbohydrate solution ingested at a rate of 0.4 to 0.8 L per hour and sodium consumed at 300 to 600 mg/L (≥two-hour events 600 to 1,200 mg/L) at a pace of 6 to 12 ounces (~180 to 350 ml) every 10 to 15 minutes.

Post-exercise

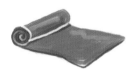

Immediate and strategic post-exercise carbohydrate ingestion in the context of endurance performance is critically important when there is time-urgency of restocking depleted glycogen stores. Classic work by Ivy[251] was perhaps the first to demonstrate the temporal impact of carbohydrate intake on post-exercise glycogen resynthesis after depletion. A 30-minute delay (as opposed to two hours) of ingesting carbohydrate (2 g/kg) resulted in ~50 percent faster glycogen repletion by the end of a four-hour period. Jentjens and Jeukendrup[252] recommended that tactics for refilling glycogen stores should be employed when there are eight hours or less between endurance events. Muscle glycogen synthesis rates are maximized when carbohydrate is consumed at 1 to 1.85 g/kg immediately post-exercise and at 15- to 60-minute intervals thereafter, for three to five hours. For the goal of maximizing rates of post-exercise glycogen resynthesis, the collective findings indicate immediate consumption of carbohydrate at 1.2 g/kg/hour for four to six hours post-exercise.

The type of carbohydrate consumed post-exercise can influence the speed of glycogen resynthesis. The GI of a given food indicates its ability to raise blood glucose levels and therefore its effectiveness at restocking glycogen. High-GI carbohydrate sources have thus been recommended in the post-exercise period under urgent time frames to recover between endurance exercise bouts.[252]

Glucose has a high GI while fructose has a low GI, so glucose and glucose polymers have traditionally been the prime choices for post-exercise endurance recovery. Indeed, direct comparison has shown superior glycogenic effects of post-exercise glucose versus fructose ingestion in isolation[253] and within mixed meals.[254] Interestingly, sucrose (a moderate-GI disaccharide composed of an even combination of glucose and fructose) has been shown to replenish glycogen at a similar rate to glucose when ≥1.2 g/kg/hour was consumed; this combo also minimized gastrointestinal distress.[255]

The king of the jungle for speed of glycogen replenishment is a high–molecular weight/low-osmolality carbohydrate by the brand Vitargo. It has outperformed glucose monomers and polymers in trials examining rate of gastric emptying,[256] rate of glycogen resynthesis,[257] work output during a 15-minute cycling time trial,[258] and power output during explosive resistance exercise preceded by glycogen depletion.[259]

FLEXIBLE VOCAB

Osmolality

Osmolality refers to the concentration of a substance in 1 liter of water divided by its molecular weight. For our purposes, this typically means concentrations of electrolytes and other chemicals in the blood.

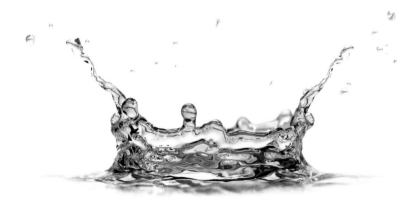

In light of these findings, it is worth reiterating that the speed of glycogen replenishment is of variable importance. Not all competitions involve the threat of glycogen depletion more than once in a day. Full glycogen repletion after depletion is possible within 24 hours simply by maintaining a high carbohydrate intake, without specific timing relative to the exercise bout.

Illustrating this, Starling and colleagues[260] reported that after 24 hours, an intake of carbohydrate dosed at 9.8 g/kg restored 93 percent of the muscle glycogen used during a prior two-hour cycling bout at 65 percent VO_2 max, while a low-carbohydrate intake (1.9 g/kg) restored only 13 percent. There was no specific carbohydrate timing protocol aside from evenly distributed energy intake at breakfast, lunch, and dinner.

Along these lines, Friedman et al.[261] reported that complete muscle glycogen resynthesis after prolonged moderate-intensity exercise is possible in 24 hours if ~500 to 700 grams of carbohydrate is consumed. Individuals who do not have immediate glycogen repletion requirements can relax their timing tactics, lift the emphasis from high-GI foods, and shift the focus to total daily intake.

On the note of flexibility, the physical form of the carbohydrate source (liquid versus solid) has shown a lack of influence on glycogen synthesis,[252] but this is when consumed in amounts ranging from 0.75 to 0.85 g/kg/hour. If consumed in amounts known to maximize rates of glycogen synthesis (~1.2 g/kg/hour), it's likely that the liquid form would be faster-acting in addition to providing hydration. Fluid loss through sweat (and urine) continues post-exercise, which necessitates a greater volume of fluid intake (125 to 150 percent) than the final fluid deficit.[147] So, for every 1 kg of bodyweight lost as a result of exercise, 1.25 to 1.5 L fluid should be consumed.

Emerging carbohydrate periodization strategies

Jeukendrup[262] recently defined periodized nutrition as *"the strategic combined use of exercise training and nutrition, or nutrition only, with the overall aim to obtain adaptations that support exercise performance."* There are a wide array of manipulations involving variations on the theme of training and/or recovering with low versus high exogenous and/or endogenous carbohydrate availability.[36]

The "Train High" model can be divided into three variants: 1) high glycogen levels, 2) high exogenous carbohydrate, and 3) high glycogen and exogenous carbohydrate. The latter variant has the strongest scientific support and thus reflects the recommendations of the authoritative consensus statements and position stands.[83,147,157]

The "Train Low" model can also be divided into three variants: 1) low glycogen levels, 2) fasted training, and 3) fasted with low exogenous carbohydrate. Training with low carbohydrate availability has the potential to increase the activation of key cell signaling kinases and transcription factors, which can result in mitochondrial biogenesis and the upregulation of lipid metabolism, thereby potentially improving exercise capacity. However, Train Low strategies (and carbohydrate restriction in general) should be used with caution due to risks including impaired exercise performance via decreased exercise economy[133] and impaired glycogen utilization,[263] which could be an unintended result of aiming to increase fat oxidation.[264] Other caveats of the Train Low variants include reduced training quality, increased risk of overreaching, and compromised immune response.

More recent models of carbohydrate periodization include the "Recover Low/Sleep Low" variant,[265] involving purposeful restriction of post-exercise carbohydrate intake to delay glycogen resynthesis. Post-exercise protein supplementation promoted MPS while preserving the effects of the low carbohydrate availability. A 10 km running performance and submaximal cycling efficiency were improved compared to the non-periodized condition.

Impey and colleagues[266] demonstrated a performance-enhancing model they call "fuel for the work required"—which combines elements of the Train Low variants but adds the twist of high carbohydrate availability for higher-intensity work and low carbohydrate availability (and high amino acid availability) for low-intensity/non-exhaustive work.

In contrast, Gejl and colleagues[267] tested a periodized protocol designed to provide ample glycogen availability for high-intensity bouts and periodic carbohydrate restriction for the lower-intensity bouts. Despite the strategic manipulation of carbohydrate, no endurance performance advantage was seen compared to a non-periodized carbohydrate intake.

Ultimately, carbohydrate periodization (as opposed to constant, linearly high or low intakes) makes sense from the standpoint of aligning carbohydrate needs with the demands of various types of training bouts (or phases). Varying energy/intensity demands require different carbohydrate levels, so fueling for the specific nature of the training bout is a sensible approach. However, extended periods of aggressive carbohydrate restriction in the hopes of forcing performance-enhancing adaptations lack research support. Box 5a summarizes carbohydrate dosing for athletic performance, including other fueling and fluid-balancing components.

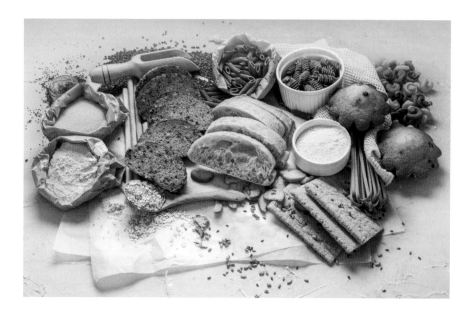

Daily Requirements

- Individuals without athletic performance goals have no minimum dosing requirement. Carbohydrate needs vary widely according to total energy requirements, personal preference, and tolerance.

- Individuals seeking to optimally support strength/power demands and/or hypertrophy goals: 3–8 g/kg of total bodyweight.

- Athletes seeking to optimize performance in sports with endurance demands: 6–12 g/kg of total bodyweight.

- Fiber: 14 g/1,000 kcal of dietary intake.

Acute/Time-Sensitive Fueling Requirements

PRE-EXERCISE:

Contemporary carbohydrate loading recommendations for endurance competition involve 7–12 g/kg of total bodyweight for 1–3 days prior to competition while training volume is tapered.

- Carbohydrate within the 4-hour window preceding events exceeding 90 minutes: 1–4 g/kg (this is a wide range requiring individual trial and error for both dose and timing).

- Protein is not directly ergogenic, but it's an opportunity to stimulate muscle protein synthesis (MPS) and inhibit muscle protein breakdown (MPB). It's also an opportunity for the trainee to partially fulfill the daily protein requirement (and help fulfill the protein feeding frequency target). Optimal protein dosing targets range from 0.4–0.6 g/kg.

DURING EXERCISE:

- Recommended rates of fluid intake are 0.4–0.8 L/hour, paced at 180–350 milliliters (6–12 ounces) every 10–15 minutes throughout the training bout or competition.

- Carbohydrate for endurance events that last 1 hour or longer: 30–60 g/hour within a 6–8 percent solution (60–80 g/L) containing sodium dosed at 300–600 mg/L of fluid.

- Carbohydrate for endurance events that last 2 hours or longer: 60–90 g/hour within a 6–8 percent solution (60–80 g/L), containing sodium dosed at 600–1200 mg/L of fluid and multiple transportable carbohydrates (glucose:fructose ratio ranging 1:1–2:1).

- Protein dosed at 0.15 g/kg/hour (~8–15 grams of protein or 5–10 grams of EAA) has been shown to suppress exercise-induced muscle damage. However, it should be noted that this finding was seen in the absence of pre-exercise protein intake, but it can nevertheless serve as an extra protective measure for prolonged endurance bouts (>2 hours).

POST-EXERCISE:

- Carbohydrate for maximizing the rate of post-exercise glycogen resynthesis, 1.2 g/kg/hour for 4–6 hours post-exercise, is warranted (especially when the recovery time between bouts is 8 hours or less).

- For every 1 kilogram of bodyweight lost as a result of exercise, 1.25–1.5 liters of fluid should be consumed. Sodium should not be restricted in the post-exercise period, especially after prolonged endurance events.

- Post-exercise protein feeding is not directly ergogenic, but it's an opportunity to stimulate MPS and inhibit MPB. It's also an opportunity for the trainee to partially fulfill the daily protein requirement (and to help fulfill the protein feeding frequency target). Optimal post-exercise protein dosing target ranges from 0.4–0.6 g/kg.

CHAPTER 5 IN A NUTSHELL

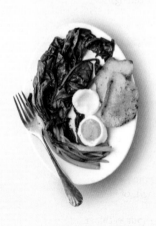

- Carbohydrate is one of the three macronutrients, providing 4 kcal per gram. It functions primarily as an energy source and is involved in glucose and insulin action, cholesterol and triglyceride metabolism, and fermentation.

- Dietary fiber is a plant-based compound that includes a wide range of nonstarch polysaccharides that are not fully digested in the human gut. The current evidence collectively supports a minimum fiber intake of 25 to 29 grams per day (about 14 grams per 1,000 kcal) for lowering the risk of all-cause and cardiovascular-related mortality and a wide range of chronic diseases.

- Fiber is technically not calorie-free; its metabolizable energy is ~2 kcal/g on average. Interestingly, higher fiber intakes have been found to promote greater weight loss and dietary adherence independently of macronutrient and caloric intake.

- Glycogen (the stored form of carbohydrate) can vary considerably depending on lean body mass (LBM), diet composition, and training demands. Adults store ~350 to 700 grams in skeletal muscle and 100 grams in the liver.

- Despite fat having nearly double the energy content of carbohydrate, the oxidation ("burning") of fat is an inefficient way to produce ATP (the body's energy currency). ATP production via glucose oxidation is two to five times faster than from fat oxidation. Carbohydrate availability becomes crucial for optimally performing exercise at greater than ~60 percent of maximal oxygen consumption (high-moderate intensity and beyond).

- Glycemic index (GI) is a ranking of a food's ability to raise blood glucose levels. Glycemic load (GL) takes into consideration both GI and amount of carbohydrate. Ultimately, GI and GL are irrelevant distractions when the big picture of optimizing macronutrition, minimizing highly refined/processed foods, and consuming adequate dietary fiber is accomplished.

- Added sugar recommendations by the major health organizations are inconsistent (ranging from 5 to 25 percent of total energy) and based on poor evidence. A practical solution hearkens back to Chapter 1, and that is to set a *discretionary* calorie allotment of 10 to 20 percent of total intake from essentially whatever you want; added sugar would fall within that allotment.

- Unlike protein and fat, carbohydrate is not necessary for survival. Thus, carbohydrate is not classified as an essential nutrient. The traditional, clinical definition of *essentiality* refers to survival, but essentiality can be goal-dependent. Within the context of maximizing athletic performance (especially at higher intensities) or muscle mass, it can be argued that carbohydrate is indeed essential.

- As in the case of protein, the collective evidence does not warrant different carbohydrate intake levels based on sex. The broad range of individual variation in carbohydrate needs reinforces the lack of utility in generalizing different requirements for men and women.

- Optimizing carbohydrate dose for muscle hypertrophy is a gray area filled mainly with observational inferences. However, a consistent finding is that restricting carbohydrate to ketogenic levels (less than 10 percent of total energy; roughly 50 grams or less) has resulted in either lean mass reduction or a compromised gain in lean mass. Thus, ketogenic levels of carbohydrate restriction are suboptimal for this purpose (not a deal breaker, but a compromise to maximal rates of growth).

- A wide range of carbohydrate–fat proportions are similarly effective for the goal of fat loss when protein and total calories are equated in diet comparisons. This leaves room for flexibly programming diets to suit the inevitable variability of individual needs. Thus, the amount of carbohydrate required for fat loss is whatever the individual can best adhere to.

- Traditional moderate-to-high carbohydrate dosing for enhancing athletic performance (both strength and endurance) has been challenged by recent research showing the potential for ketogenic diets to be similarly effective. However, in high-level competition, under-carbing carries performance risks that may not concern recreational trainees.

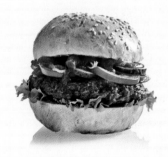

- Carbohydrate periodization (as opposed to constant, linearly high or low intakes) makes sense from the standpoint of aligning carbohydrate needs with the demands of various types of training bouts/phases.

- Carbohydrate dosing requirements on a daily basis as well as time-sensitive nutrient needs relative to training and competition are laid out in Box 5a.

FAT

6

The structure of this chapter differs from the structure of
the protein and carbohydrate chapters because fat has fewer
performance- and muscle-oriented applications; it simply lacks
that capability. Fat intake is mainly a default of calorie and protein
requirements (and carbohydrate requirements, in the case of
performance athletes). So, unlike protein and carbohydrate, the
discussion of fat intake for specific goals such as muscle gain, fat loss,
and athletic performance is more consolidated and generalized here.
The focus is primarily on total intake amount and type. I also discuss
the perpetual controversies surrounding dietary fat, which show no
signs of going away any time soon.

The key property that separates fats (also called lipids) from the other
macronutrients is their insolubility in water and their solubility in organic
solvents such as acetone, chloroform, and ether.[268] Several compounds
are classified as lipids, and only a minority of them are relevant to dietary
macronutrition. Simple lipids include fatty acids, triacylglycerols (more
commonly called triglycerides), and waxes. Compound lipids include
phospholipids, glycolipids, and lipoproteins. Derived lipids include sterols,
steroids, and the hydrolysis products of simple lipids and compound lipids.

Leading the macronutrients in energy density, fat yields ~9 kcal per gram,
while protein and carbohydrate have roughly 4 kcal per gram. Dietary fat
plays several physiological roles, including the metabolism of fat-soluble

vitamins, cell membrane function, the maintenance of structural integrity of the brain and nervous system, and hormone synthesis.

While carbohydrate is considered nonessential for survival (essentiality for optimizing high exercise performance is another story, as shown in chapter 5), fat—like protein—is considered an essential nutrient. This is because the body cannot manufacture sufficient amounts of fat for survival, so it needs to be dietarily derived.

The long-standing scientific consensus is that the two essential fatty acids (EFAs) are linoleic acid and alpha-linolenic acid (ALA), which the body cannot produce and thus must obtain from food. Linoleic acid is an omega-6 polyunsaturated fatty acid (PUFA), and ALA is an omega-3 PUFA. There is compelling evidence of the essentiality of arachidonic acid (AA) and docosahexaenoic acid (DHA) as well.[269,270]

TOTAL DAILY FAT REQUIREMENTS

So, what's the minimum amount of EFA needed to prevent deficiency? The Food and Nutrition Board of the Institute of Medicine (IOM) has set the adequate intake of linoleic acid for men at 17 grams per day, and ALA at 1.6 grams per day. These minimum standard intakes are based on the US population's median intake where deficiency is nonexistent in healthy individuals.

Although linoleic acid and ALA are considered essential nutrients, they are widely available in Western diets (especially linoleic acid), and EFA deficiency is rare outside of prolonged malnutrition or malabsorption syndromes. However, it's possible that EFA deficiency can occur when fat intakes are chronically below 10 percent of total calories.[271] With this said, the minimum amount of fat required to avoid deficiency should not be confused with the minimum amount of fat required to make a diet sustainable and optimal for promoting health and preventing disease. The IOM's AMDR for dietary fat is 20 to 35 percent of total daily calories.[49]

I don't have any major disagreement with the 20 percent lower-end cutoff, but it's noteworthy that studies on low-fat diets show that this is difficult to attain. Despite a target of 20 percent of total kcals from fat, subjects' actual intakes ranged from 26 to 28 percent.[59] The apparent difficulty to sustain this low fat target isn't necessarily a bad thing from the standpoint of preserving testosterone levels.

Cross-sectional studies have shown a consistent association of lower fat intakes with lower testosterone levels. Cross-sectional studies can provide useful food for thought, but observational findings are largely hypothesis-generating and subject to further testing in controlled interventions to determine causal relationships.

A recent systematic review by Whittaker and Wu[272] concluded that lower-fat diets (averaging 18 percent of total kcal, ranging from 6.8 to 25 percent) decreased testosterone levels compared to their higher-fat counterparts (averaging 39.3 percent of total kcal, ranging from 36.4 to 40.7 percent). This decrease was reported to be due to a reduction in testicular production of testosterone. The clinical or practical significance of this androgen-suppressive effect of low-fat diets is subject to individual goals and objectives.

FLEXIBLE VOCAB

Androgen

Androgen is a natural or synthetic steroid hormone that regulates male characteristic development and maintenance. It does so by binding androgenic hormones (like testosterone) to androgen receptors. Such hormones exist in men and women (though at lower levels in the latter) and can act as precursors to estrogens.

I do take issue with the AMDR's 35 percent upper-end cutoff. It's too restrictive in that it excludes proportions of dietary fat that are common in low-carbohydrate (and certainly ketogenic) diets. Excluding these options is not evidence-based, and certain factions of the general population indeed can benefit from diets with a fat intake above 35 percent (which is ultimately an arbitrary limit).

Let's imagine that someone is dieting on 2,000 kcal, 125 grams (500 kcal) of which is protein. Let's also imagine that this person is restricting carbohydrates to 125 grams (500 kcal). This leaves them with 1,000 kcal from fat (111 grams), which is 50 percent of their calories, significantly breaching the AMDR. What is inherently wrong with that? The answer is nothing.

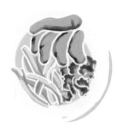

We can take it a step further and apply this example to someone restricting their carbohydrate intake to ketogenic levels (50 grams or less), which would put their fat proportion at 65 percent—nearly double the AMDR's upper limit. There's nothing inherently wrong with ketogenic diets; they are a tool in the toolbox. Just like any diet, the food sources can determine their relative healthfulness.

To reiterate, the 35 percent upper limit set by the IOM is arbitrary. When I headed the ISSN's position stand on diets and body composition, I included ketogenic diets as viable options based on the weight of the evidence on what has consistently shown efficacy. (Long-term sustainability is another matter.) The AMDRs exclude not only ketogenic diets, but non-ketogenic low-carbohydrate diets as well, and this simply is not reflective of the literature on what works for a range of clinical and nonclinical goals.

Dietary fat requirements in the literature are typically expressed as a percentage of total calories. Requirements are rarely expressed as grams per unit of bodyweight, let alone per unit of LBM. This is unlike protein and carbohydrate, which have numerous examples in the literature (including position stands of the major scientific organizations) where requirements are expressed in grams per kilogram of bodyweight. The scant publications that do list fat requirements in the aforementioned terms boil down to observational studies and narrative reviews on bodybuilders (which are also observational in nature). A recent review by Iraki and colleagues[273] on the nutritional requirements of physique competitors in the off-season (gaining/recovery phase) recommends a fat intake range of 0.5 to 1.5 g/kg. A late-breaking review by Ruiz-Castellano and colleagues[274] on dieting resistance-trained athletes recommends 0.5 to 1 g/kg.

While I don't take major issue with these recommendations (in fact, I was one of the authors of the latter paper[274]), I personally would recommend higher lower- and upper-end intakes. As the lead author—well, the only author—of this book, this is exactly what I'm doing. Given the collective evidence, an appropriate range of fat intake across the spectrum of populations and goals is 0.7 to 2.2 g/kg, or 0.32 to 1 g/lb.

My reasoning is similar to that of the previous example with the AMDR for fat intake; these ranges don't accommodate perfectly viable low-carbohydrate diets. Plus, dietary fat set at 0.5 g/kg could be too low to be sustainable for those who are already lean or within normal weight ranges; this figure is potentially applicable to extreme sport situations where the limits of leanness are sought for temporary periods. For example, Chappelle and colleagues[124] reported that high-level natural bodybuilding competitors who placed in the top five had fat intakes ranging from 0.4 to 0.8 g/kg during contest prep. In most cases, a minimum of 0.7 g/kg keeps fat intake from dropping below 20 percent of total calories, helping protect against the potential for excessive drops in testosterone.

Let's discuss the upper end of fat intake using some common numbers. Imagine that an 80 kg individual (or someone whose TBW is 80 kg) is consuming 2,400 kcal and has a preference for a non-ketogenic, low-carbohydrate, high-protein diet. With protein at 2 g/kg (160 grams; 640 kcal) and a carbohydrate intake of 130 grams (520 kcal), this leaves us with 1,160 kcal from fat, which amounts to 128.88 grams, which, divided by 80 kg, amounts to 1.61 g/kg. This breeches the 1.5 g/kg upper end recommended by Iraki and colleagues,[273] and it's a typical non-ketogenic, carbohydrate-restricted intake of 130 grams. Using this same example but with a ketogenic level of carbohydrate restriction (50 grams of carbs instead of 130 grams) would amount to a fat intake of 2.16 g/kg. There is nothing inherently wrong with this figure, but it breeches the proposed limit even further.

Therefore, to accommodate low- and very-low-carbohydrate regimens, I would broaden the dietary fat range and increase the upper end to 2.2 g/kg. Bear in mind that fat (and carbohydrate) intakes are ultimately at the mercy of total caloric intake. Proportions of fat and carbohydrate are flexible, depending on individual goals and preferences. This means that the upper end of fat intake I listed (2.2 g/kg) is subject to being exceeded in cases where higher total energy intakes dictate it. It's a soft limit, not a hard one. It just happens to be right in the ballpark of the upper end of most carb-restricted programs, which typically aim for weight loss and thus do not involve high total daily calories.

Furthermore, 2.2 g/kg is advantageous from a mnemonic standpoint, since the effective upper end of protein for maximizing muscle growth—in most cases—is also 2.2 g/kg.[66] Once again, if we want to be really thorough with our contingencies, then remember that dose recommendations based on grams per unit of bodyweight assume that we're discussing a "normal" bodyweight, or what I like to call TBW (goal or ideal bodyweight). If you're at the bodyweight you aim to maintain, then that's what the dose should be based on; otherwise, base the dose on TBW. Table 6a provides "official" fat intake recommendations from the major health agencies along with my personal recommendations.

Table 6a: Dietary Fat Requirements

RECOMMENDATIONS FROM MAJOR HEALTH AGENCIES					
Publication	Total	Saturated	Omega-3	Omega-6	Trans
Food and Nutrition Board, Institute of Medicine: Dietary reference intakes for energy, carbohydrate, fiber, fat, fatty acids, cholesterol, protein, and amino acids. *J Am Diet Assoc.* 2002 Nov;102(11):1621-30.	20–35% of total energy	Limit intake (amount not specified)	0.6–1.2% of total energy	5–10% of total energy	Limit intake (amount not specified)
Food and Agriculture Organization of the United Nations: Fats and fatty acids in human nutrition: report of an expert consultation. *FAO Food Nutr Pap.* 2010;91:1-166.	20–35% of total energy	<10% of total energy	0.5–2% of total energy	2.5–9% of total energy	<1%
Dietary fats and cardiovascular disease: a presidential advisory from the American Heart Association. *Circulation.* 2017 Jul 18;136(3):e1-e23.	*"Reduction in total dietary fat or a goal for total fat intake is not recommended."*	5–6%, in reference to the joint position stand of the AHA and ACC	Amount not specified	Amount not specified	Limit intake of industrial trans fats (amount not specified)

MY RECOMMENDATIONS BASED ON THE COLLECTIVE EVIDENCE (AND REAL-WORLD PRACTICALITY)					
Publication	Total	Saturated	Omega-3	Omega-6	Trans
These recommendations include influence from the *International Society of Sports Nutrition Position Stand: Diets and Body Composition* as well as the sum total of the research discussed in this chapter.	Instead of percentage of total energy, I prefer to recommend 0.7–2.2 g/kg (0.32–1 g/lb) of target bodyweight (TBW). This upper end is not set in stone (total energy intakes vary).	Stick to mostly lean meats and whole and minimally refined/processed food sources, taking note that "healthy" processed SFA sources include fermented milk products and dark chocolate, while extra-virgin coconut oil is mostly neutral.	Most populations can derive cardio-protective benefits from ~1–2 g EPA/DHA per day (3–6 g of fish oil) or 3–6 oz (85–170 g) of fatty fish.	There is no need to stress over a specific minimum of omega-6 fats as long as your total fat intake isn't chronically very low (<20%).	If your intake of processed baked goods, shortenings, and solid margarines is low, you don't have to worry about industrial trans fats.

Sex-based differences in fat metabolism

The current position stands of the major scientific organizations do not specify separate fat intake targets for men and women. This makes sense considering the wide-ranging goals and preferences across individuals, which essentially nullify the validity of generalized sex-specific targets. Nevertheless, differences in substrate utilization are worth discussing.

As mentioned in the carbohydrate chapter, a higher rate of fat oxidation during submaximal exercise occurs in women than in men.[188] While this might lead some folks to jump to the conclusion that female athletes require more dietary fat than men, this greater reliance on fat as fuel is the result of a greater amount of intramuscular triglyceride storage in women. Also, this greater rate of fat oxidation during exercise is counterbalanced by a lower rate of basal (resting) fat oxidation in women, which partially explains their higher net fat storage (and higher overall percentage of body fat).

Nevertheless, due to the greater exercise-mediated reliance on fat as fuel, literature reviews on this topic have asserted the importance of women avoiding extremes in low fat intake. Hausswirth and Le Meur[189] cautioned that a very low fat intake (10 to 15 percent of total daily calories) combined with a high volume of endurance training might impair performance by lowered intramuscular triglyceride storage. Similarly, Wohlgemuth and colleagues[275] recommended that female athletes consume at least 20 percent of total calories from fat in order to support substrate utilization during exercise, and also to support sex hormone regulation and fat-soluble vitamin bioavailability.

A final wrinkle I'll add is that women have shown a greater conversion of ALA[276] (a plant-derived omega-3 fatty acid) to eicosapentaenoic acid (EPA) and DHA, which are biologically important omega-3 fatty acids found most commonly in fatty fish. This detail is potentially relevant to vegans and individuals who do not eat any animal foods. However, this difference is somewhat immaterial in the face of a low conversion of ALA to EPA and DHA overall, regardless of sex. I'll discuss this further in the forthcoming section on omega-3 and omega-6 fatty acids.

Timing of fat relative to the exercise bout

Before and during exercise

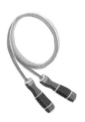

The practice of fat-loading was born from the idea that preferential fat utilization as fuel for exercise would improve endurance due to the vast stores of fat within the body, which could ostensibly "spare" glycogen and provide nearly limitless energy. Thus, in the days leading to an athletic event (typically an endurance competition), carbohydrate restriction combined with high fat intake has been done with the aim of becoming fat-adapted (also called keto-adapted).

However, this scheme has failed to produce performance enhancements in controlled experiments—and in fact has shown performance impairments. Havemann and colleagues[228] found that seven days of a high-fat diet followed by one day of high carbohydrate increased fat oxidation but decreased sprinting power output in well-trained cyclists.

A mechanistic explanation for this ergolytic effect was provided by Stellingwerff and colleagues,[263] who found that within a week, a high-fat diet increased fat oxidation but also lowered the activity of an enzyme called pyruvate dehydrogenase (PDH). Decreased PDH resulted in decreased glycogen breakdown and thus lower carbohydrate availability, which in turn compromised high-intensity work output.

Burke and colleagues[232] saw similar results, reporting that in elite endurance athletes, marked increases in fat oxidation occur within as little as five to six days on a ketogenic diet. However, the study also revealed a concurrent reduction in exercise economy (characterized by an increased oxygen "cost" per unit of time) at intensities relevant to real-life endurance events. This performance decrement persisted even in the face of resuming high carbohydrate availability to fuel the event. These short-term findings are corroborated in chronic studies on high fat intakes combined with carbohydrate restriction on endurance performance in carefully controlled studies (refer to chapter 5 for a detailed discussion).[133,230,231,264]

As for the more immediate pre-exercise period, only one study to date directly compared fat with the two other macronutrients on endurance performance. In 2002, Rowlands and Hopkins[151] compared the effects of mixed-macronutrient meals (~1,100 kcal each) that were either high-fat (mix of dairy cream, canola oil, coconut cream, and egg yolk), high-carbohydrate (sago starch and sucrose), or high-protein (soy protein isolate). Meals were ingested 90 minutes prior to a test involving sprinting and 50 km performance in competitive cyclists. No significant performance differences between the treatments were seen.

The topic of pre- and during-exercise fat ingestion warrants a discussion of medium-chain triglycerides (MCTs). MCTs are metabolized differently from longer-chain fats because they bypass lymphatic circulation and directly enter the portal system. As such, they are more readily used/oxidized rather than stored in adipose tissue.

Portal system

In anatomy, the portal system comprises the vessels that collect nutrient-rich blood from the digestive tract (except the lower rectum) and various other organs so it can be transported to the liver, where nutrients are metabolized and then sent to the parts of the body that need them.

The interest in MCTs has been fueled by their potential as a weight loss aid, where their effectiveness has accurately been described as "modest," with weight loss averaging 0.51 kg in a meta-analysis of 13 RCTs.[277] Anyway, as the hope and hype surrounding MCTs snowballed, interest in their ergogenic potential entered the fray. However, the momentum of this idea eventually dissipated alongside the accumulation of studies showing consistent failure of MCTs to enhance performance when consumed pre- and/or during exercise.[278] Furthermore, several studies have shown MCT ingestion to decrease exercise performance due to gastrointestinal upset.

This poor track record kicks MCTs out of the running as an ergogenic aid.[278] In general, it makes no sense to purposely add substantial amounts of fat to pre- and/or during-exercise meals if the goal is to enhance exercise performance (especially in endurance-oriented sports). Carbohydrate outperforms fat in the majority of trials, and fat also carries the risk of inducing gastrointestinal upset that can hinder performance.

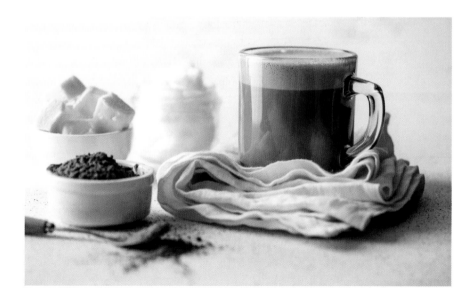

Post-exercise

A couple of decades back, when the post-exercise "anabolic window of opportunity" was all the rage, a popular recommendation was to avoid fat in the post-exercise meal. The reasons were based on concerns about slowing gastric emptying, which was supposed to interfere with glycogen resynthesis and hinder the anabolic response—collectively impairing recovery and growth. All of that is pretty much nonsense, unless you're a competitive endurance athlete with a very short time frame (<eight hours) between exhaustive, glycogen-depleting bouts.[252] In the latter case, it would benefit the athlete to employ all tactics necessary to expedite glycogen replenishment (this is discussed in the carbohydrate chapter).

Exemplifying the inconsequentiality of post-exercise fat on 24-hour glycogenesis, Burke and colleagues[279] compared a control diet consisting of high-glycemic carbohydrate (7g/kg) with two experimental treatments: 1) the control diet plus a substantial amount of added fat (1.6 g/kg) and protein (1.2 g/kg), and 2) a matched-energy diet, which was the control diet with added carbs to equal the calories of the other experimental treatment.

Subjects trained for two hours at 75 percent of VO_2 max, ending the session with four 30-second sprints. Despite a high fat intake in one of the experimental groups, the researchers discovered no differences in muscle glycogen content 24 hours after training compared to the two low-fat groups. Similarly, Fox and colleagues[280] found no difference in glycogen replenishment 24 hours after glycogen-depleting exercise in a high-fat post-exercise feeding scheme (165 grams of fat distributed across three meals) compared to a low-fat scheme (18 grams of fat across three meals).

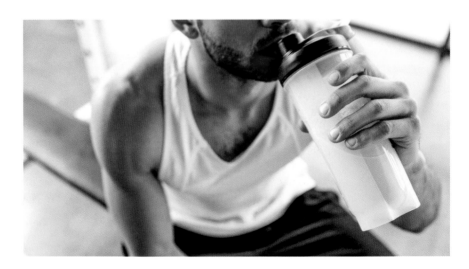

The concern about post-exercise fat is rooted in hypothetical foolishness about fat slowing absorption, blunting the insulin response and thus MPS. This idea has been refuted by studies comparing the anabolic response of protein-rich meals with differing fat contents.

Elliot and colleagues[281] compared the effect of fat-free milk, whole milk, and a higher dose of fat-free milk (to match the calories of the whole milk) taken 60 minutes post–resistance exercise. Whole milk was superior for increasing net protein balance. Interestingly, the calorie-matched dose of fat-free milk contained 14.5 grams of protein versus 8 grams in the whole milk (an 81 percent advantage), but whole milk still resulted in greater MPS. The investigators speculated about the possible mechanisms behind the outcome (insulin response, blood flow, subject response differences, fat content improving nitrogen retention) but ended up dismissing each one in favor of concluding that further research is necessary.

A similar story played out in van Vliet and colleagues'[282] comparison of post-exercise consumption of an isonitrogenous (protein-matched) dose of egg whites versus whole eggs—the latter was superior for stimulating MPS. These results are noteworthy because they occurred in resistance-trained subjects.

Subsequently, a 12-week trial by Bagheri and colleagues[87] compared the effects of three whole eggs versus six egg whites consumed post-exercise in resistance-trained men. Lean mass gain was greater in the whole egg group (3.7 kg versus 2.9 kg), but not to a degree of statistical significance. Fat mass decreased in both groups (2 kg and 1.1 kg in the whole egg and egg white groups, respectively), but this difference did not reach statistical significance.

However, body fat *percentage* decrease was significantly greater in the whole egg group. Whole eggs also resulted in significantly greater gains in knee extension and hand grip strength. Another potential factor working in the favor of whole eggs was their greater impact on testosterone, which increased by 240 ng/dL and 70 ng/dL in the whole egg and egg white groups, respectively. The clinical significance of this testosterone hike is open for debate, but it's plausible that it could have contributed to the anabolic process beyond the extra calories from the fat content of the yolks.

Does this mean there's actual "magic" in post-exercise fat consumption? I doubt it, but what's clear is that for muscle recovery and growth, it's not the inherently bad thing, as traditionally thought.

CONTROVERSIES

Saturated fat: villain or vindicated?

During the 1980s, dietary fat was uniformly vilified. "Chronologically advanced" readers can recall the ubiquity of fat-free products lining supermarket shelves. A lack of fat was their main selling point. The 1990s began to give fat a break but also ended up nurturing the dichotomous and reductionistic belief that unsaturated fatty acid consumption was good, and saturated fat consumption was bad for cardiovascular health.

Major health organizations have unanimously issued the public health message to minimize saturated fat intake. The current position paper by the American Heart Association (AHA)[283] calls for a saturated fat intake of 5 to 6 percent of total caloric intake for individuals seeking to lower low-density lipoprotein (LDL) cholesterol levels. The 2020–2025 Dietary Guidelines for Americans[284] continues its traditional recommendation of less than 10 percent of total caloric intake from saturated fat. This guideline is echoed internationally.[285] The latest systematic review and meta-analysis on this topic in the Cochrane database[286] included 15 RCTs and found that reducing saturated fat intake lowered the risk of combined cardiovascular events by 17 percent.

FLEXIBLE VOCAB

LDL and HDL cholesterol

Cholesterol is a substance found in your cells. It's waxy and fat-like and alongside fat has developed something of a bad reputation—low-density lipoprotein (LDL) cholesterol in particular, as too much can lead to buildup in arteries, whereas high-density lipoproteins (HDLs) carry cholesterol back to your liver, where it can be removed.

However, the long-standing vilification of saturated fat (and cholesterol) was based on incomplete/weak evidence that lacked context.[287,288] While there are still plenty of knowledge gaps in this area, it has become increasingly evident that we may have been punishing the wrong suspects—or at least taking a view that's too reductionistic and not holistic enough.[289,290]

In a recent review challenging the conventional perspective, Heileson[290] examined the literature on saturated fat intake and heart disease dating back to 2009. He reported that nine meta-analyses of observational studies were done, and none of them found that saturated fat intake was independently associated with heart disease. Furthermore, of the 10 meta-analyses of RCTs on this topic, none reported a significant increase in the "hard" end points such as heart disease mortality or total mortality.

There are important nuances and challenges to the blanket presumption that saturated fat is "bad." It's necessary to consider the vehicle of the fat, the food source, and the overall dietary context rather than fixating on the type of fatty acid. For example, Shih and colleagues[291] did a secondary analysis of the 12-month DIETFITS weight loss trial[292] to evaluate the associations between saturated fat intake and blood lipid profile in subjects assigned a healthy low-carbohydrate diet. Subjects in both the healthy low-carb group and its comparator (a healthy low-fat diet) were specifically instructed to maximize vegetable intake; focus on nutrient-dense, whole/minimally processed foods; prepare food at home whenever possible; and minimize added sugars, refined flours, and trans fats. Despite the low-carb group's diet consisting of 12 to 18 percent saturated fat, overall lipid profile improved, including a reduction in triglycerides, while HDL and LDL cholesterol levels remained unchanged. Current saturated fat intakes among US adults average 11 percent of total calories,[283] so it's not as if the push toward decreasing intakes below 10 percent is in the midst of alarming degrees of saturated fatty acid (SFA) overconsumption.

We need to start looking at individual foods rather than oversimplistically lumping saturated fat itself and saturated fat–containing foods together in a homologous heap. The main singular food sources of saturated fat are cheese, butter, fatty cuts of meat, cream, lard, and plant sources such as palm oil and coconut oil.[285,293] The hierarchy of the US population's intake of saturated fat–containing foods within (and independently of) the context of mixed dishes/entrees are as follows, beginning with the greatest contributor: regular cheese, pizza, grain-based desserts, dairy-based desserts, chicken and chicken-based mixed dishes, sausage/franks/bacon/ribs, burgers, and Mexican mixed dishes.[293] Notice the diversity and range of foods as well as the recurrence of fatty meats and dairy as part of mixed foods (both dessert and non-dessert foods).

Dairy

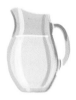

In a recent systematic review of RCTs, Duarte and colleagues[294] reported that although dairy foods can be rich in SFA, they are a diverse group with varying effects on health parameters, depending on the specific food. An excerpt from a recent review by Poppitt describes the concept eloquently:[295]

> *"Notably, it is no longer adequate to consider nutrients in isolation, with evidence that the complex matrix of a food may be equally or more important than the fatty acid content and composition alone when predicting cardiometabolic risk. It has been proposed that in a complex dairy food such as cheese, for example, the effect of SFAs on blood lipids and disease risk may be counterbalanced by the content of protein, calcium, or other dietary components."*

I'm going to lean into the dairy topic since it's a prominent aspect of the saturated fat controversy—which exists largely due to our tendency to oversimplify things in order to understand them. The dairy question illustrates our human tendency to compartmentalize in a binary (good/bad) fashion (remember dichotomous thinking?). It also illustrates the contextual role of the food matrix. For example, plain yogurt and ice cream are both dairy foods with nearly opposite cardiometabolic consequences when consumed liberally. This is due not just to differences in macronutrition but to micronutrition as well. A 26-study meta-analysis by O'Sullivan and colleagues[296] found that high intakes of milk, cheese, yogurt, and butter were not associated with increased risk of mortality compared with low intakes. Importantly, the authors used the data for full-fat versions of the products in the analysis.

Speaking of full-fat dairy, Hirahatake and colleagues[297] recently reported that overall, the data from meta-analyses of observational and interventional studies do not indicate harmful effects of full-fat dairy consumption on cardiometabolic disease outcomes and risk factors. In fact, the totality of evidence from meta-analyses and prospective observational studies show a protective effect of fermented dairy foods (full-fat yogurt and cheese) against cardiovascular diseases and T2D.[298-300] Yogurt and cheese consistently have not caused adverse effects on blood lipids and blood pressure despite their saturated fat (and sodium) content.[297]

Again, the whole is more than the sum of its parts, and the concept of the food matrix—rather than nutrients in isolation—comes into play. Ultimately, the public health push toward consuming low-fat and fat-free dairy and avoiding full-fat dairy foods to support cardiometabolic health lacks compelling support.[297]

Butter

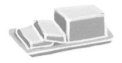

Unlike other full-fat milk products, the collective evidence doesn't give butter the stamp of approval. Doesn't making everything taste better count for something? It should. Anyway, the reason for this circles us back to the food matrix concept. Butter tends to have adverse effects on blood lipids (increased LDL cholesterol) compared to other dairy foods like cheese and cream, which have neutral (and in some cases beneficial) effects on blood lipids.

Rosqvist and colleagues[301] investigated this discrepancy by directly comparing the effects of butter and cream. Cream had a neutral effect on blood lipids. However, butter adversely affected blood lipids by increasing LDL cholesterol as well as the ratio of apolipoprotein B to apolipoprotein A1, which raises concerns for cardiovascular health since the apo-B/apo-A1 ratio may be a more accurate index of heart disease risk than conventional lipid ratios.[302-304]

FLEXIBLE VOCAB

Apolipoproteins

These proteins bind with lipids to create lipoproteins and transport lipids through the body. They do so by surrounding the lipid, which is insoluble in water, to make it water-soluble and transportable in the blood.

A possible explanation is that cream contains a higher milk fat globule membrane (MFGM) content. MFGM has been shown to have protective and beneficial health effects.[305,306] In butter, much of the MFGM is removed in the churning process. This doesn't mean butter needs to be avoided. It just means that it should be moderated judiciously given its adverse potential when consumed in abundance. It also means that the hype behind butter as some sort of superfood (or health-promoting addition to coffee) is unsubstantiated.

Chocolate

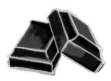

Chocolate is an intriguing food steeped in legend, history, and—yes—science. Of relevance here, chocolate is rich in saturated fat. Despite this, chocolate (especially dark chocolate) has an interesting body of evidence consistently showing positive effects on indexes of cardiovascular health, including the lowering of LDL cholesterol[307] and blood pressure.[308] Prospective observational studies have found chocolate consumption to lower risk for diabetes, stroke, and coronary heart disease.[309]

The main types of fatty acids chocolate contains are stearic and palmitic fatty acid;[310] both are SFAs. Among the types, dark chocolate has the highest levels of oleic acid (a monounsaturated fatty acid famous for being predominant in olive oil) and linoleic acid (an omega-6 fatty acid that's notoriously vilified by keyboard warriors).[310] Dark chocolate also has the lowest levels of myristic acid (an SFA) among the chocolate variants.

As we delve further, we can again invoke the concept of the food matrix, where health benefits result from the interaction of multiple components rather than isolated components such as fatty acids. Due to a higher cocoa content, dark chocolate is rich in polyphenols called catechins, anthocyanins, and proanthocyanidins (these are powerful antioxidants and are sometimes referred to as flavonols).[311] These compounds within chocolate are associated with improved endothelial function, which is integral to vascular function and health. In addition, chocolate is a source of magnesium, potassium, copper, and iron.[311]

FLEXIBLE VOCAB

Endothelial

Endothelial cells make up the barrier between tissues and vessels, regulating the flow of substances into and out of tissue. As such, impaired endothelial function can lead to serious health issues in the human body.

A meta-analysis by Ebaditabar and colleagues[312] involving 17 RCTs found that dark chocolate consumption increased flow-mediated dilatation (a measure of endothelial function). The collective evidence indicates that dark chocolate's saturated fat content is a non-issue, thanks to the overall-positive health effects of the food matrix.

Coconut oil

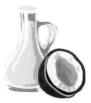

Coconut oil shares a similar story with chocolate in terms of the role of the food matrix in measures of health. The most recent position paper by the AHA[283] advised against the consumption of coconut oil, citing its ability to raise LDL cholesterol. A recent meta-analysis of RCTs also concluded that coconut oil raises LDL more than other non-tropical vegetable oils.[313]

However, neither of the aforementioned publications separately examined the studies on extra-virgin coconut oil (EVCO). Most of the studies comprising the unfavorable conclusions included a majority that did not specify the type of coconut oil used. This is a major confounder since the possibility of using refined/bleached/deodorized coconut oil and/or hydrogenated coconut oil remains.

EVCO is purposely produced to avoid these aspects of processing and refinement. It's made by pressing/squeezing out the coconut milk and oil from the wet coconut kernel. EVCO is distinctly different from refined, bleached, deodorized coconut oil (RBD-CO), which is processed with high temperatures of free fatty acid distillation and deodorization and can destroy or reduce nutritive value and antioxidant polyphenol content, which is retained by EVCO.[314]

With scant exception,[315] the current literature consistently shows the neutral-to-positive effects of EVCO on blood lipids[316-320]—specifically, neutral effects on LDL accompanied by either no change or an increase in HDL cholesterol. Despite its saturated fat content, a potential mechanism underlying EVCO's favorable effects is its antioxidant capacity due to the phenolic compounds it contains.[321]

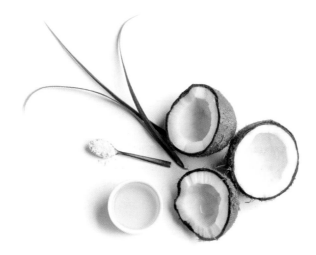

Steak and eggs

I'd be remiss not to include steak and eggs in this discussion. Let's first cover red meat, which is yet another magnet for controversy, providing a never-ending cycle of lurid headlines and debate among both academics and laypeople. Despite it being a good source of high-quality protein, iron, zinc, selenium, niacin, and B12, the prevailing public health narrative about red meat is that it should be consumed with caution.

Quoting the latest Dietary Guidelines for Americans:[284]

> *"...dietary patterns characterized by higher intake of red and processed meats, sugar-sweetened foods and beverages, and refined grains are, in and of themselves, associated with detrimental health outcomes."*

A joint recommendation by the World Cancer Research Fund and the American Institute for Cancer Research is to limit consumption to a maximum of roughly three servings per week, specified as a total of 350 to 500 grams (~12 to 18 ounces) cooked weight.[322] Similarly, the National Health Service of the UK recommends a maximum red meat intake of 70 grams per day (350 grams or 12 ounces per week).[323]

While these recommendations don't call for flat-out avoidance, there is considerable controversy over the strength of their scientific basis, especially in the case of lean, unprocessed red meat. A relatively recent meta-analysis by O'Connor and colleagues[324] included 24 RCTs and found that half a serving (35 grams or 1.25 ounces) or more per day does not influence blood lipids or blood pressure compared to less than half a serving. Importantly, no differences between the control and intervention groups were seen when consuming 1 to 1.9, 2 to 2.9, or ≥3 servings (210 grams or 7.5 ounces) of red meat per day, with the exception of HDL cholesterol being higher with ≥3 servings per day.

Other concerns about red meat have centered on colorectal cancer, but this is not without debate. Kruger and Zhou[325] reviewed the evidence behind the claims that N-nitroso compounds, heterocyclic aromatic amines, and heme iron comprise the mechanistic link between red meat and cancer. The authors concluded that there's a lack of evidence to support these claims. Overall, the mechanistic studies' underlying claims of risk failed to assess conditions remotely representative of realistic human consumption of red meat.

The dietary context of red meat consumption is important to consider. Maximova and colleagues[326] recently reported that a high intake of nonstarchy vegetables and fruits mitigated cancer risk despite the presence of red meat in the diet. But there's a consistency of research showing cardiometabolic benefits of healthy dietary patterns that contain lean, unprocessed red meat.[327-331]

Eggs—yolks, specifically—are another perpetually debated topic. While eggs do contain saturated fat, their dominant fat is oleic acid, which is the same monounsaturated fatty acid dominant in olive oil. However, it's the cholesterol content of egg yolks that garners all of the caution. A single whole egg can contain 200 to 300 mg of cholesterol, which practically zaps the daily limit of 300 mg traditionally recommended by major health agencies. However, the purported threat level of dietary cholesterol has diminished in recent years. This is reflected in the removal of dietary cholesterol from the USDA's list of "nutrients of concern for overconsumption" in the Dietary Guidelines for Americans as of the past two editions. (New editions are issued every five years.)

Recently, Mah and colleagues[332] conducted an umbrella review encompassing seven systematic reviews and 15 meta-analyses examining the relationship of egg consumption and cardiometabolic outcomes. To the certain disappointment of egg haters, they concluded that increased egg consumption is not associated with cardiovascular disease risk in the general population, but this relationship was inconclusive in individuals with T2D.

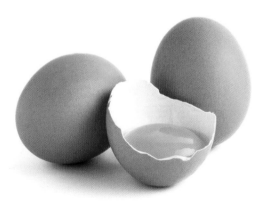

Another recent meta-analysis by Drouin-Chartier and colleagues[333] involving three large prospective cohort studies concluded that up to one egg per day is not associated with cardiovascular disease risk and is actually associated with lower cardiovascular disease risk in Asian populations. Yet another recent meta-analysis by Krittanawong and colleagues[334] included 23 observational studies and concluded that higher egg consumption (more than one egg per day) was associated with a significant *reduction* in risk of coronary artery disease. The authors conceded to the main limitation of their findings, which is that observational studies—unlike controlled intervention studies—cannot demonstrate causality.

Speaking of controlled interventions, a substantial blow to the widespread fear of eggs is the relatively recent DIABEGG study by Fuller and colleagues,[335] a well-controlled intervention trial that compared a high-egg diet (at least 12 eggs per week) with a low-egg diet (less than two eggs per week) in subjects with prediabetes and T2D. The trial had an initial three-month weight loss phase, with six- and 12-month follow-up checkpoints at weight maintenance. Macronutrition was equated between diets, as was an emphasis on keeping to a "healthy" dietary pattern. No between-group differences were seen by the end of the trial. The high-egg diet had no detrimental effects on cardiovascular risk factors, including lipids and lipoproteins, inflammatory markers, and glycemic control. An average of 12.2 and 10.5 eggs per week were consumed at six and 12 months, respectively. These findings are particularly noteworthy since they were seen in people with prediabetes and T2D, who are more vulnerable to the supposed adverse effects of eggs—yet none were seen.

There are still cautions to consider for those on the optimistic side of the egg debate. While the generations-long egg scare has indeed been challenged by accumulating research evidence, all of the published data in the world must bow to individual response. Study results are reported as group means (averages), and there inevitably are individuals who fall below and above the mean. Of special relevance here are a minority of "hyper-responders" to egg consumption. Hyper-responders experience increased total cholesterol, but this is typically due to a rise in both HDL and LDL cholesterol.[336]

If you love eggs and are concerned about exceeding the commonly reported safe limit of up to one per day,[337,338] a pragmatic approach would be to get your blood tested regularly and take note of any concerning trends in your blood lipids. In any case, several studies have shown neutral-to-beneficial effects on blood lipids with three eggs per day in a variety of populations.[339-348]

Trans fats

The malice toward saturated fat and cholesterol spawned a plethora of butter substitutes designed to save the population from cardiovascular health issues. That didn't happen. Engineering vegetable oils to have better spreadability and a longer shelf life involves a process called *hydrogenation.* To hydrogenate means to combine an unsaturated oil with highly pressurized hydrogen, producing a solid fat. This is done to thicken oils (and is specifically how vegetable oil is turned into margarine), thereby increasing heat tolerance and shelf life.

An unfavorable result of hydrogenation is the formation of trans fatty acids (TFAs). These TFAs are also referred to as industrially derived TFAs. Industrial TFAs have been implicated in adverse outcomes such as systemic inflammation, endothelial dysfunction, arrhythmia, and insulin resistance.[349] TFAs have been a favorite target for trashing by the public health media. The World Health Organization has called for a TFA intake of less than 1 percent of total kcal.

A systematic review and meta-regression by Gayet-Boyer and colleagues[350] found that naturally occurring TFAs in meat and dairy ("ruminant TFAs") have neutral health effects in moderate amounts (up to 4.19 percent of total daily calories). In a subsequent meta-regression by Allen and colleagues,[351] industrially derived TFAs intake levels that do not adversely affect blood lipid profile are significantly lower (2.2 to 2.9 percent).

There is an abundance of negative press surrounding TFAs, but it's important to put this topic into the proper perspective. The major sources of industrial TFAs are processed baked goods, shortenings, and stick margarines. The threat of TFAs is relatively immaterial within the context of a diet that's predominated by whole and minimally refined/processed foods and low in the aforementioned vehicles of industrially derived TFAs. The general public's intake of ruminant and industrial TFAs is estimated to be 0.5 to 1 percent[350] and 0.5 percent,[351] respectively. These intakes are well below the ranges expected to adversely affect blood lipids. So, it looks like constant alarm bells about TFAs don't apply to the majority of you reading this book (the health/fitness community with far better habits than the general public).

OMEGA-3 AND OMEGA-6 FATTY ACIDS: RANTS, RAVES, AND RATIOS

Polyunsaturated fatty acids (PUFAs) have been a darling of public health recommendations for several decades. The scientific support for the push for replacing saturated fat with PUFA has been consistent.[285]

Of the PUFAs, omega-3 fatty acids (abbreviated in the literature as n-3 PUFA) have become a household name, synonymous with good health. The omega-3 fatty acids of interest are EPA and DHA, which are most efficiently derivable from marine-based oils. EPA and DHA are involved in a multitude of biological processes essential to cardiovascular health but are perhaps best known for their anti-inflammatory effects. Topping off the favorability of fishy burps, Hu and colleagues[352] updated previous meta-analyses by adding three large, recently published RCTs[353-355] missing from previous meta-analyses and concluded that marine-based omega-3 supplementation significantly lowered most measures of cardiovascular risk in a dose-dependent manner.

The American Heart Association recommends at least two servings of fish per week for the general population. Back in 2002, the AHA recommended 0.5 to 1.8 grams per day of combined EPA and DHA.[356] This recommendation hasn't changed much. In a recent update, Kris-Etherton and colleagues[357] recommend at least one to two servings of fish per week, with additional primary prevention benefits from adding 1 gram of EPA/DHA on top of the fish intake. This is not tough to attain for regular fish consumers or for folks willing to commit to about three to six 1-gram capsules of fish oil per day (a typical 1-gram capsule contains 300 mg of EPA/DHA). For those with high triacylglycerol levels, a supplemental 2 to 4 grams of combined EPA/DHA is the AHA's suggested therapeutic dose (attainable through six to twelve 1-gram capsules of fish oil).[356] Based on results from the REDUCE-IT trial,[355] the upper end of that range (4 grams per day of EPA/DHA) is recommended for statin-treated patients who have cardiovascular disease or diabetes and elevated triglycerides.[357]

An important consideration for individuals planning to rely exclusively on plant foods for omega-3s is the body's inefficient conversion of ALA (the plant-derived omega-3) to the biologically active omega-3 fatty acids, EPA and DHA. Baker and colleagues[358] reported that overall, the conversion of ALA to EPA is estimated at 8 to 12 percent, and ALA to DHA is estimated to be 1 percent. Childs and colleagues[276] reported significant sex-based differences, where stable isotope studies have shown that conversion rates of ALA to EPA in men and women are 8 percent and 21 percent and ALA to DHA is 0 percent and 9 percent, respectively. So, this conversion from ALA to EPA and DHA is poor in general, but the conversion to DHA is particularly dismal, especially in men.

FLEXIBLE VOCAB

Stable isotopes

Isotopes refers to the two or more forms most elements possess, having the same number of protons but different numbers of neutrons and thus different masses. Stable isotopes do not decay into other elements. As such, studying stable isotopes in food allows scientists to track the impact of that food on the animal that consumes it.

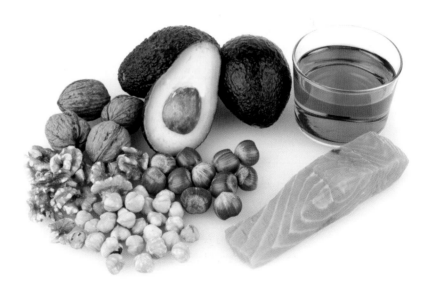

A review by Lane and colleagues[359] reported that over the course of seven key intervention studies during the past decade, *"ALA from nut and seed oils was not converted to DHA at all."* A solution for those who refuse to eat fish, supplement with fish oil, or consume any animal foods is oil from marine algae, which can be bought as a supplement. However, caution is warranted since algal supplementation has mainly been effective in providing DHA while lacking in EPA,[360] so check labels carefully.

If omega-3 PUFAs are the yin, omega-6 PUFAs are the yang. Whereas omega-3s are anti-inflammatory, omega-6 FAs (linoleic acid specifically) are a precursor to AA, which has inflammatory properties. Because of this—along with their potential to produce harmful oxidation products—omega-6–rich vegetable oils have been vilified, perhaps most vociferously by folks on the fringes of the Paleo and low-carb communities.

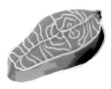

If you've done enough browsing of diet debates online, you've undoubtedly seen people blaming vegetable/seed oils (and, by extension, linoleic acid) for all of humanity's ills. So, what's the evidence of concern? It has been speculated that the largely opposite functions of omega-3 and omega-6 fatty acids warrant a greater degree of balance in the diet. The optimal omega-6:3 ratio has been speculated to be somewhere between 1:1 and 4:1.[361] The Western diet's typical ratio of omega-6:3 is roughly 15:1 to 20:1.[362]

The predominance of omega-6 in the Western diet has been blamed for the conglomerate of diseases of civilization. Despite this hypothesis being fairly reasonable, it's based on uncontrolled observation, which is insufficient grounds for deifying omega-3 intake while demonizing omega-6 intake. Along with oxidative stress, inflammation is thought to be a key component in the etiology of cardiovascular disease. In a systematic review of RCTs, Johnson and Fritsche[363] reported that there is "virtually no evidence" that linoleic acid consumption increases inflammatory markers (including levels of AA and pro-inflammatory eicosanoids) in healthy, non-infant humans.

FLEXIBLE VOCAB

Eicosanoids

Eicosanoids are a bit like hormones in that they act as chemical signaling molecules, but, unlike hormones, they stay local wherever they were created via the oxidation of arachidonic acid (AA) or other PUFAs. As a result, they play a role in (and serve in the research of) inflammation.

Ramsden and colleagues[364-366] have built a case against linoleic acid over a series of publications. However, their position relies heavily on the retrospective analysis of data from the Sydney Diet Heart Study and the Minnesota Coronary Experiment. Both of these studies were initiated in the mid-1960s and had several important limitations.

Those in the Sydney Diet Heart Study included a lack of delineation between hydrogenated versus non-hydrogenated linoleic acid sources, artificially high linoleic acid intake (double that of the general population), and a patient population with preexistent heart disease that was 70 percent smokers and more than a third moderate-to-heavy drinkers. The Minnesota Coronary Experiment involved nursing home and psychiatric patients and was confounded by a non-continuous patient stay (subjects were followed only while in the hospital), a high dropout rate, a lack of assessment of LDL cholesterol, and a lack of specification of trans fat intake.

The most rigorous and extensive publication on this topic thus far is a Cochrane systematic review and meta-analysis by Hooper and colleagues[367] involving 19 RCTs (totaling 6,461 subjects), with trial durations ranging from one to eight years. Unlike the adverse findings in Ramsden's work, increasing omega-6 intake had little or no influence on all-cause mortality or cardiovascular disease events.

Recent meta-analyses of observational studies further challenge the idea of linoleic acid's proposed danger. Farvid and colleagues[368] meta-analyzed 13 prospective cohort studies and concluded that linoleic acid intake is inversely associated with coronary heart disease risk in a dose-response manner. Subsequently, Li and colleagues[369] meta-analyzed 38 prospective cohort studies and found that higher linoleic acid intakes were associated with lower risk of all-cause mortality, cardiovascular disease, and cancer. Collectively, the evidence does not support the red flags raised against non-hydrogenated omega-6 intake—and, yes, this applies to seed oils.

FLEXIBLE VOCAB

Dose-response

As a central concept in toxicology, the dose-response framework allows for hazard assessment testing, dose-response model extrapolations, and environmental regulations. In short, it describes the relationship between the intensity of a treatment and its effect on a living organism. In the context of nutrition, dose-response is the relationship between amounts of ingested foods or supplements and their effects on metabolic processes.

In addition to the linoleic acid caution campaign lacking scientific support,[367-371] the traditional call to achieve a more balanced ratio of omega-3 to omega-6 intake struggles against the evidence. Importantly, this line of reasoning fails to acknowledge that some omega-6-rich foods also have well-established health benefits.

An immediate standout in this area is nuts. For example, almonds—which have consistently shown positive health effects[372]—are a significant source of omega-6 (about 12 percent of total kcal), and their omega-3 content is almost nonexistent, making their omega-6:3 ratio 2,011:1.

This is a common story with nuts; they are significant dietary sources of omega-6, and their omega-6 content almost always is many times greater than their omega-3 content. Nevertheless, nut consumption is associated with numerous favorable health outcomes, including antioxidant, anti-diabetic, hypolipidemic, anti-atherogenic, anti-inflammatory, anti-carcinogenic, and anti-obesogenic effects.[373-376] It's therefore unfounded to minimize or avoid nuts due to their high omega-6:3 ratio.

Supporting the idea of ditching the omega-3:6 ratio is a relatively recent review by Harris,[377] who made the valid points that this ratio is imprecise/nonspecific and is based on the invalid assumption that omega-6 fatty acids are pro-inflammatory and detrimental to cardiovascular health. An alternative to the omega-3:6 ratio is an objective, physiological measure of omega-3 status, the *omega-3 index*,[377] which is the EPA+DHA content of red blood cells (expressed as a percentage of the total mass of membrane fatty acids).

And that's a wrap for this chapter on fat. Figure 6a, inspired by the work of Forouhi and colleagues,[378] should help tie together the health-related concepts surrounding dietary fat.

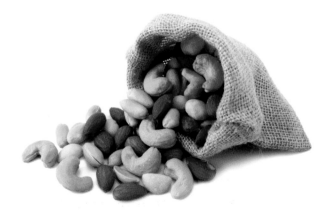

Figure 6a: Evolving Understanding of Dietary Fats and Cardiovascular Disease

EVOLVING UNDERSTANDING

EARLIER HYPOTHESES

RECENT & CURRENT HYPOTHESES

Dietary fat

Unsaturated & saturated fats

Omega-3 & -6 PUFA, MUFA, SFA, TFA, isolated nutrients

Food/food matrix in addition to isolated nutrients, dietary patterns, synergy of diet & exercise

Total cholesterol

LDL & HDL cholesterol

LDL is a single lipid parameter; others, such as non-HDL, total:HDL ratio, TG:HDL ratio, apolipoproteins, LDL size & particle number, should also be considered (more research is needed)

Lipid & non-lipid parameters, including endothelial function, inflammation, oxidative stress, glycemic control/insulin sensitivity, body composition, etc. (more research is needed)

CARDIOVASCULAR DISEASE

CHAPTER 6 IN A NUTSHELL

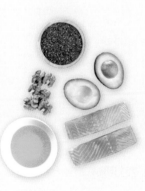

- Fat is one of the three macronutrients, providing 9 kcal per gram. Dietary fat has several physiological roles, including the metabolism of fat-soluble vitamins, cell membrane function, structural integrity of the brain and nervous system, and hormone synthesis. Fat is considered an essential nutrient because the body cannot manufacture sufficient amounts of it for survival, so fat needs to be dietarily derived.

- A fat intake of 10 percent of total kcal has been proposed as a practical minimum for avoiding clinical symptoms of EFA deficiency. However, the minimum amount of fat required to avoid deficiency should not be confused with the minimum amount of fat required to make a diet sustainable and optimal for promoting health and preventing disease. My recommended range of total daily fat intake is 0.7 to 2.2 g/kg (0.32 to 2.2 g/lb). Refer to Table 6a for the major health organizations' recommendations for the intakes of fats and fatty acids.

- The major scientific organizations do not specify separate fat intake requirements for men and women. Wide-ranging goals and preferences across individuals nullify the validity of generalized sex-specific targets. While there are differences in substrate utilization during exercise (due to greater intramuscular fat stores in women), this doesn't change the targeted intake ranges and objectives for fueling athletic performance or optimizing health.

- Pre-exercise "fat-loading" in the days (and/or hours) leading up to endurance competition has a passably plausible theoretical basis but has failed when objectively tested. In fact, a high-fat/low-carb diet can impair glycogen breakdown (and thus glucose availability), which compromises high-intensity work output. Post-exercise fat intake does not hinder 24-hour glycogen resynthesis, nor does it inhibit MPS.

- Major health organizations have unanimously issued the public health message to minimize saturated fat intake. The most prevalent recommendation is to keep saturated fat intake below 10 percent of total caloric intake. However, there are important nuances and challenges to the traditional view that saturated fat is "bad."

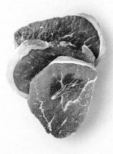

- The effects of red meat on cardiovascular disease and cancer risk remain controversial, with evidence for and against limiting intake to various degrees. It's questionable whether mechanistic studies' underlying claims of cancer risk reflect conditions representative of realistic human consumption of red meat. Controlled human intervention trials have consistently shown that lean, unprocessed red meat can be included in healthy dietary patterns that impart favorable effects on various cardiovascular risk markers.

- Eggs have a rocky history with public health agencies and their messages based on the cholesterol content of yolks. However, this concern has fallen into question in recent years. The bulk of the current evidence from meta-analyses shows a lack of cardiovascular risk for one egg per day, with several studies showing no adverse effects with three eggs per day. If you love eggs and insist on eating large amounts, a pragmatic approach would be to get your blood tested regularly to keep an eye on any adverse trends.

- There's a fair amount of hysteria surrounding trans fatty acids (TFAs), but it's important to keep them in the right perspective. Ruminant TFAs (naturally occurring TFAs in dairy and meat) have largely benign effects, while industrially derived TFAs (from hydrogenated vegetable oils) have more adverse potential on blood lipids. The general public's intake of ruminant and industrial TFAs are well below the ranges thought to adversely affect blood lipids.

- The omega-3 fatty acids of greatest relevance are EPA and DHA, which are most efficiently derivable from marine-based oils. EPA and DHA are essential to cardiovascular health. Most populations can derive cardio-protective benefits from ~1–2 grams of EPA/DHA (3–6 grams of fish oil) or 3–6 ounces (85–170 grams) of fatty fish per day.

- The Western diet's high proportion of omega-6 to omega-3 fatty acid intake (seed oil consumption in particular) has been blamed for the full range of cardiometabolic diseases in the industrialized world. Linoleic acid is the prime omega-6 fat in question. However, this hypothesis has not stood up to the collective scientific evidence. Once again, food source and context matter in the omega-6 discussion.

- Figure 6a depicts our evolving understanding of the role of dietary fats in cardiovascular health. As the cliché goes, more research is needed to fill in the wide (but steadily narrowing) gaps in our knowledge.

EXERCISE PERFORMANCE– ENHANCING SUPPLEMENTS

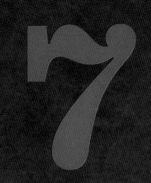

Ah, the wonderful world of pills, powders, and potions.

Regulation of dietary supplements at the federal level dates back to 1906 with the passage of the Federal Food and Drugs Act. Under this law, the Bureau of Chemistry (the predecessor to the FDA) was assigned the responsibility of prohibiting interstate and foreign commerce in adulterated and misbranded food and drugs.[379]

The next major ripple in the regulation universe didn't occur until nearly a century later. The Dietary Supplement Health and Education Act (DSHEA), signed by President Clinton on October 25, 1994, was perhaps the most significant legal victory for the supplement industry in modern history. The primary goals of the DSHEA were to ensure continued consumer access to a wide variety of dietary supplements and to provide consumers with valid information about their intended use.[380] Well, those were the DSHEA's main selling points, anyway.

The most significant effect of the DSHEA was that it limited the FDA to regulate dietary supplements as foods, not drugs. So, the burden of proof of a lack of safety of a given supplement was placed on the FDA, which was relegated to functioning as a policing entity, rather than approval for entry. With enough evidence, however, the FDA can yank a product off the market if it's proven harmful. Ultimately, the supplement industry landscape is analogous to the Wild West. There's a combination of effective, ineffective, and dangerous products on the market. Thanks to the DSHEA, all supplements are innocent until proven guilty. This is a double-edged sword for consumers, who have been granted maximal access to a growing array of products—both good and bad.

The DSHEA inevitably played a major role in facilitating the enormous financial growth of the dietary supplement industry in the US, which is estimated to be worth nearly $353 billion as of 2019.[381] The ascending trajectory continues. Since the start of the COVID-19 pandemic, worldwide supplement sales have spiked, reflecting consumers' concerns for bolstering immune protection from the disease. This chapter covers supplements for the primary purpose of enhancing athletic performance, although these agents have inevitable effects on body composition and health.

A WORD ABOUT WEIGHT LOSS SUPPLEMENTS ("FAT-BURNERS")

Given the interlocking crises of obesity, diabetes, and heart disease, a ton of research has been done on the impact of dietary sugars. Keep in mind we're talking about *added* sugars (also called extrinsic sugars), not sugars intrinsic to foods such as milk/milk products and fruit.

The underlying motivation of this book is to provide practical knowledge. In practice, I don't recommend "fat-burner" or weight loss supplements. The greatest fat loss supplement ever created is a sustained net caloric deficit. I say that facetiously, but also seriously. The "magic pill" for fat loss—aside from the recomp that newbies and intermediate-level trainees can experience—is expending more energy than you consume over the course of the week and stringing many weeks together within an adherence-friendly program.

I'm not claiming that no fat loss supplement has shown effectiveness. It's the degree of effectiveness weighed against the cost and risk that I find to be a deal breaker. And this is not to say that the muscle-building supplement world is free of worthless compounds. BCAAs, and leucine in particular, are a prime example. BCAAs are touted for enhancing muscle-related outcomes. However, high-quality protein is already abundant in BCAA, making supplementation redundant. BCAA has repeatedly failed to benefit muscle size or strength in resistance trainees consuming sufficient total daily protein (1.6 g/kg).[382,383] A recent systematic review by Marcon and Zanella[384] concluded that *"Performance, strength, and muscle mass seems not affected by BCAA supplementation."*

Back to fat loss supplements, a thorough review by Manore[385] aptly titled "Dietary supplements for improving body composition and reducing bodyweight: where is the evidence?" makes a strong case for the title's implications. There's a lack of strong research evidence (and replication of findings) of supplements causing significant weight loss (>2 kg) in the long term. However, certain foods or supplements (e.g., green tea, fiber, and dairy products) may contribute to good health and modestly facilitate weight loss and prevention of weight gain. Manore cautions that supplements containing central nervous system stimulants (e.g., caffeine, ephedra, and synephrine) are most likely to produce adverse side effects—due to a number of variables, including lack of consistent quality control or unexpected interactions with preexisting conditions. Her strongly worded conclusion is worth quoting:[385]

> *"With no effective weight-loss supplements on the market, it is the responsibility of the health profession to educate the public on diet, exercise, and lifestyle changes for weight loss or maintenance. Athletes and active individuals also need to be educated on how best to reach their performance and weight goals without resorting to stimulants. Finally, many of the weight-loss supplements can have serious health effects, for little or no benefit, and many are banned substances."*

On the flip side of Manore's paper is a review by Stohs and Badmaev.[386] Among other substances (including stimulants), the authors advocate for non-stimulant thermogenic substances, including p-synephrine (bitter orange extracts), forskolin, chlorogenic acid (green coffee bean extracts), and capsaicin. Despite being non-stimulant substances, they still qualify for Manore's criticisms of small weight loss effects lacking clinical significance despite having statistical significance, at best only a few supporting RCTs, and a lack of long-term RCTs.

A recent, rather massive review by Watanabe and colleagues[387] examined 21 weight loss supplements whose mechanisms of action included appetite suppression, thermogenesis, inhibition of fat absorption, and inhibition of carbohydrate absorption. The following excerpt from their conclusion is significant:

"Given the present literature revision, it is possible to conclude that many of the presented food supplements are likely to exert an anti-obesogenic effect in the absence of significant adverse events. However, none of this is capable of inducing a clinically relevant weight loss, with the most effective ones leading to a mere 2-kg reduction."

This zinger from Watanabe's review reinforces one of the core criticisms expressed in Manore's review, which was published in 2012. Some things don't change, and the relative failure of weight loss supplements to produce clinically meaningful weight loss appears to be one of them. I'm going to ignore the fact that Watanabe's paper closes with an unintentionally humorous proposal to try combining all of the fat loss supplements from each of the four aforementioned mechanisms to see if they'll work in concert (despite falling flat independently). A more recent systematic review and meta-analysis by Clark and Welch[388] adds another nail in the coffin by reporting that weight loss supplements were less effective than exercise, or diet and exercise, without weight loss supplementation.

An *incidental* fat loss supplement whose performance effects are discussed in the next section is caffeine. A recent systematic review and meta-analysis by Tabrizi and colleagues[389] found that caffeine consumption reduced weight, BMI, and body fat in a dose-dependent manner. Doubling the daily dose of caffeine resulted in 22 percent, 17 percent, and 28 percent greater reductions in weight, BMI, and fat, respectively.

These findings are not too surprising since caffeine has been demonstrated to increase energy expenditure and fat oxidation and decrease appetite. However, I wouldn't recommend using caffeine specifically for the goal of weight loss; other program variables offer more bang for their buck and don't tread lines of risk. As in the case of all central nervous system stimulants, caffeine dosing has a point of diminishing returns that quickly crosses into the danger zone (discussion forthcoming in the caffeine section).

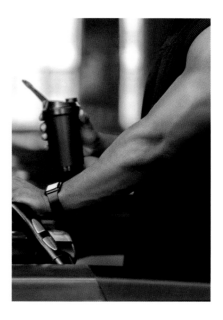

Lift heavy and take a multi

"Just lift heavy and take a multi" is an intentionally funny (and obviously oversimplistic) bit of advice from the dark days of bodybuilding message boards 10 to 15 years ago. It originated as sincere advice in response to people overcomplicating things and ended up becoming a meme because of its subtle and absurd humor. Ironically, it's not bad advice, assuming it's not delivered in the context of neglecting diet quality.

Before we go into the next section, I'll impose my opinion about the silliness of taking performance supplements but neglecting to consider covering the bases of essential micronutrition. This is yet another topic of controversy with support on both sides. However, an honest examination of the full range of evidence does not draw those flippantly dismissive conclusions about multivitamin-mineral (MVM) supplements, especially when we consider populations that clearly and consistently run low on several essential nutrients.

There's a common presumption that taking an MVM is a waste of money. Indeed, this is yet another topic of controversy, since there is research literature supporting the position of dismissing MVMs due to a failure to prevent chronic disease and bring about lower mortality in the general population.[390,391] For example, a recent meta-analysis by Kim and colleagues[391] concluded that MVM supplementation does not improve cardiovascular outcomes in the general population. While this publication often gets wielded as a weapon against taking MVMs, it certainly isn't unassailable gospel. To qualify as an MVM, a supplement had to contain at least four vitamin and/or mineral ingredients. This low barrier of entry raises many questions, especially since only five of the 18 trials specified the ingredients of the supplement used. Of the 18 trials, 16 were prospective cohort studies and two were RCTs that had conflicting outcomes (one RCT showed null effects[392] and the other showed favorable effects[393]). These are not minor limitations to sweep under the rug while we jump to the conclusion that MVMs are useless. As with all controversial topics, there's evidence on the other side of the debate in support of MVM use.

Here's the crux of the problem. The majority of the general public—and I'd suspect a large portion of health and fitness enthusiasts—either a) could not describe, in terms of food, what constitutes a micronutritionally complete diet, b) do not consume a micronutritionally complete diet themselves, or c) both a) and b), which is likely the case.

Let's be real; most of the general public's dietary habits are crappy, and most of the fitness community's diets—especially those who are dieting—are limited in food variety and total amount. Both of these populations commonly subsist on diets with multiple micronutritional shortcomings. Speaking of which, micronutrients "of concern" (due to nationwide underconsumption), as specified by the Dietary Guidelines Committee, are numerous: vitamin A, vitamin C, vitamin D, vitamin E, calcium, choline, iron, magnesium, and potassium.[394] The committee also lists fiber as an underconsumed nutrient at the population level. I would add omega-3 fatty acids to that list as well.

With this said, the solution is not to go out and buy these nutrients individually in supplement form. An optimal approach is to maximize the sufficiency of micronutrition from foods and then, if/where necessary, supplement the diet. An MVM can at least partially alleviate the common and persistent problem of multiple nutrient shortcomings. But don't just take my word for it; let's review some research.

It's not at all far-fetched to think that MVM supplement use can prevent chronic disease in individuals with poor or suboptimal nutritional status.[395] The heterogeneity (diversity of conditions and habits) in the study populations prevents bold, sweeping generalizations that universally apply to all individuals. In any case, multiple concurrent micronutrient inadequacies are widespread. Bird and colleagues[396] reported that 40 percent of dietary supplement non-users had the highest risk of nutrient deficiency, compared to 14 percent of users of full-spectrum MVM supplements.

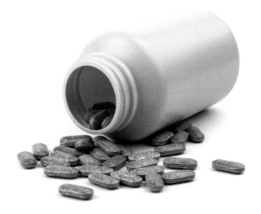

It's mere reality that suboptimal nutritional status is rampant among dieters, athletes (both recreational and competitive), and certainly dieting athletes—not to mention older adults and diseased populations. A study by Calton[397] compared sufficiency of the 27 essential micronutrients in four popular diets with what's recommended by Reference Daily Intake (RDI) standards. On average, the diets fell 56.48 percent short of RDI sufficiency and lacked 15 of the 27 essential micronutrients analyzed. Similarly, Engel and colleagues[398] found several micronutrient inadequacies in three popular diet programs, even after adjusting the plans to 2,000 kcal per day.

FLEXIBLE VOCAB

Dietary Reference Intake

Reference Daily Intake (RDI) and Recommended Dietary Allowance (RDA) are both part of the Dietary Reference Intake system, which is used on nutrition labels in the US and in some other countries to indicate a nutrient's daily healthy intake level—specifically, how much of that nutrient is needed to meet the nutritional requirements of the majority of healthy individuals.

Athletic populations—as obsessed with health and nutrition as they might be—still tend to create their own sets of problems with nutrient deficiencies. Bodybuilders are a good example since they are known for their food particularities, both in extremes of food exclusion and food abundance.

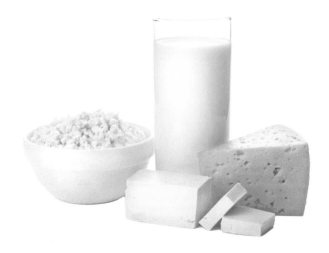

Kleiner and colleagues[399] examined the pre-contest dietary habits of junior national and national-level competitors. Despite consuming adequate total calories, women were described as "remarkably deficient" in calcium intake. This isn't surprising since dairy is commonly absent in pre-contest meal plans.

Subsequent work by Kleiner and colleagues[400] on national-level bodybuilders found that men consumed only 46 percent of the RDA for vitamin D, while women consumed 0 percent of the RDA for vitamin D and only 52 percent of the RDA for calcium, in addition to inadequate intakes of zinc, copper, and chromium. Serum magnesium levels in women were low despite dietary magnesium intakes above the RDA.

An eye-opening study by Misner[401] investigated the adequacy of food alone for providing 100 percent of the RDA/RDI of the daily micronutrient requirements in the diets of a mix of professional endurance athletes, amateur endurance athletes, and sedentary subjects. Men had deficiencies in 40 percent of the vitamins and 54.2 percent of the minerals. Women had deficiencies in 29 percent of the vitamins and 44.2 percent of the minerals. Athletes had higher nutrient deficiency rates than sedentary subjects. None of the subjects met all of the RDA-based micronutrient requirements for preventing deficiency diseases. It's evident that the risk of nutrient deficiency is compounded when high energy expenditure is combined with a poor or incomplete selection of foods.

It's important to note that a poor diet supplemented with an MVM is still a poor diet. However, a poor diet with an MVM is a step up, despite falling far short of optimal. Even well-planned diets can fail to meet multiple essential nutrient needs, and the potential of MVMs as a simple, preventive countermeasure should not be ignored.[274] I'll wrap things up by relaying the concluding excerpt from a review by Ward[402] that presents a particularly lucid perspective of the utility of MVMs. I also quoted Ward in a review paper I did with Ruiz-Castellano and colleagues[274] because I feel it boldly states the obvious in the face of controversy:

> *"When deciding whether to recommend the use of dietary supplements, it is important to consider the benefit:risk ratio. Current data suggest minimal, if any, risk associated with MVM preparations containing 10 or more vitamins and minerals at recommended daily intake levels in healthy people and a possibility of modest benefits that include a reduced risk of cancer and nuclear cataract, for a relatively low financial cost."*

There is a vast sea of sports supplements out there, but I'll focus on the effective agents instead of the quacky and iffy ones. Supplements have varying degrees of evidential strength, and this chapter will concentrate on the ones with the greatest consistency of RCTs in their favor. Research is ongoing, and supplements currently showing glimmers of promise (from a small number of RCTs) might be more heavily weighted for consideration in the future as evidence accumulates. What follows this overview are the heavyweights of the evidence-based performance-enhancing supplement arena, summed up in Table 7a at the end of the chapter.

ROLE IN ATHLETIC PERFORMANCE

Creatine

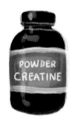

Let's begin with the king of (legal) ergogenic aids for the goal of gains in muscle size, strength, and power. Creatine stems from the Greek word *kréas,* which means meat.[403] Michel Eugène Chevreul, a French chemist who was the first to isolate creatine in the 1830s, gave it this name. Creatine is by far the most prolifically studied sports performance supplement, and its effectiveness has been replicated across a multitude of independent labs and various athletic populations.[23] A review by Kreider[404] relayed an astonishing estimate of at least 500 studies on creatine supplementation. Well, Kreider's review was published in 2003, and here we are nearly two decades later.

Creatine is a naturally occurring compound derived from glycine and arginine via the formation of guanidinoacetate and ornithine.[405] Skeletal muscle stores the vast majority (95 percent) of the endogenous creatine pool. Dietary provision and endogenous production contribute equally to the body's creatine stores.[403] Specifically, the body biosynthesizes roughly 1 gram of creatine per day and derives roughly another 1 gram per day from the diet.[406] Most of the body's creatine is synthesized in the liver, but it's possible that the brain synthesizes its own creatine.[407]

An emerging body of research shows creatine's potential for clinical applications, including the treatment and prevention of neurological disorders, sarcopenia, and inflammatory diseases such as arthritis.[408]

There's even the potential for creatine supplementation to improve cognitive processing in the context of brain creatine deficits due to acute conditions (e.g., sleep deprivation and exercise) as well as chronic conditions (e.g., traumatic brain injury, Alzheimer's disease, and aging).[409]

Supplemental creatine enhances exercise performance by saturating muscle phosphocreatine stores.[404] This allows greater short-term/anaerobic work capacity by prolonging ATP availability and buffering pH changes occurring from the accumulation of lactate and hydrogen ions.[408]

The collective data shows the efficacy of creatine supplementation for enhancing maximal muscular efforts ranging from 30 to 150 seconds.[406] Lifting, sprinting, and any type of intermittent high-intensity work derives particular benefit. Muscle hypertrophy is the inevitable result of progressive increases in lifting capacity, but there are other mechanisms potentially at work that contribute to creatine's effectiveness.

Creatine increases cellular volume via increased hydration, which can provide extra leverage for anabolic processes. Due to the creatine molecule's hydrophilic nature, cellular hyperhydration is not conducive to weight loss. Weight gain (in the form of lean mass) is a nearly inevitable side effect, particularly if hypocaloric conditions are not purposely targeted while creatine loading. It's possible for roughly 2 percent of total starting bodyweight to be gained during the loading phase alone.[410] Other potential mechanisms underpinning creatine's effects include increases in satellite cells, myonuclei, myogenic gene transcription, and MPS, along with decreased MPB.

Dosing

When a loading phase is implemented (20 to 25 grams per day for five to seven days), lean mass gains of 1 to 2 kg can occur within four to 28 days.[405] Maintenance dosing is ~3 to 5 grams per day (0.04 to 0.07 g/kg/day); larger individuals may require more. A loading phase is not necessary if there is no urgency to reach muscle saturation, which happens in approximately four weeks at maintenance dosing.

There are no hard and fast rules for creatine loading. The classic weeklong loading phase can be prolonged by a week with the dose decreased to 10 grams per day, and saturation is reached in two weeks instead of one, while potentially avoiding the gastrointestinal upset that some individuals might experience.

Only a few studies have directly compared different creatine timing strategies relative to the exercise bout. Two studies showed that immediate post-exercise dosing is superior to immediate pre-exercise dosing for size and/or strength gain,[411,412] and one study showed no difference.[413] A recent review by Ribeiro and colleagues[414] concludes that existing data are scarce and contradictory, so specific creatine timing relative to exercise *"...is not currently supported by solid evidence and should not be considered a real concern for now."* In my view, creatine's effectiveness depends upon saturation of muscle creatine levels, so timing relative to training matters only for the goal of expediting saturation during the loading phase (in which case, post-exercise dosing could be the ticket). Once you're creatine-loaded, timing relative to training is unlikely to have any meaningful impact.

Occasionally, I get the question of how much time off of creatine supplementation results in a significant decrease in muscle levels (and presumably effectiveness). Keep in mind that once muscle creatine stores are saturated after loading, a return to baseline levels after discontinuing supplementation (washout) is a slow process. Full washout has been reported to take four to six weeks.[415]

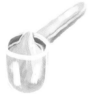

Rawson and colleagues[416] observed a 45 percent increase in muscle creatine stores after a loading phase consisting of 20 grams per day for five days, and this decreased only 22 percent during a 30-day washout period. So, if you don't keep to a daily creatine dosing schedule, instead choosing a less regular one (e.g., a total of 14 to 35 grams per week distributed evenly across three to five days), you'll still reap ergogenic benefits. Even if you take periodic "breaks" from creatine supplementation that are significantly shorter than a month, your muscle creatine levels are not likely to decrease to pre-supplementation levels.

Creatine is found in small amounts in animal foods (muscle meats of beef, pork, poultry, fish, etc.) and, to a lesser extent, dairy products.[407] Vegan diets are devoid of creatine without supplementation. Vegetarians have lower plasma and muscle creatine levels but similar brain creatine levels to omnivores.[407] Omnivorous diets typically contain only about 1 gram. Therefore, it's highly inefficient to attempt to attain supplemental levels of creatine (3 to 5 grams per day) through diet unless you eat about a kilogram of meat per day.

Several types of creatine are available commercially, but the *monohydrate* form is the most stable and most widely studied and confirmed for efficacy.[23] Creatine monohydrate is not only the most reliable form in terms of safety, efficacy, and regulatory status,[417] but it's also the most economical.

Safety and caveats

Creatine has a consistent track record for safety, including effects on kidney function in healthy individuals without preexisting renal disease.[418] Dosing as high as 30 grams per day for five years has shown no ill effects.[23]

Concern has been raised over a potential conflict of action between caffeine and creatine when taken concurrently, where the effects of creatine are diminished. However, creatine has been shown to be effective when taken with coffee or tea, and several studies have shown the effectiveness of multi-ingredient supplements containing creatine and caffeine for increasing strength, power, and LBM.[419] Furthermore, a recent 10-study systematic review by Marinho and colleagues[420] reported that the combination of caffeine and creatine improves exercise performance when caffeine is ingested after creatine loading is complete, but not when consumed during the loading period.

Concerns have also been raised about the potential for creatine supplementation to exacerbate hair loss. This stems from a study by van der Merwe and colleagues,[421] who reported a significant increase in dihydrotestosterone (DHT) in college-aged male rugby players who supplemented with creatine (25 grams per day for seven days followed by 5 grams per day for an additional 14 days). DHT is a key androgen involved with the development of male-pattern baldness,[422] so readers of van der Merwe's study leaped to the speculation that creatine supplementation causes hair loss.

Of course, this became a rumor that spread quickly and struck fear in the hearts (and heads) of individuals guarding their precious locks. However, these results are thus far unreplicated. Importantly, DHT levels were still within the normal range. Furthermore, the existing research on creatine's effects on testosterone (at least 12 studies to date) fails to show increases in free testosterone, a precursor to DHT.[418] So far, the idea that creatine drives hair loss is far-fetched and remains to be demonstrated in a controlled study.

Beta-alanine

Beta-alanine is a nonessential amino acid produced endogenously as well as derived in small amounts from animal flesh foods. Beta-alanine availability is the rate-limiting factor for the synthesis of intramuscular carnosine.[423] The significance of this is that carnosine plays a key role in regulating intramuscular pH and acts as a buffer against intramuscular acidosis—thereby increasing work capacity. Vegetarians have been reported to store 26 percent less muscle carnosine than omnivores.[424]

Beta-alanine can be viewed as an agent that enhances high-intensity endurance, more toward the middle of the strength-endurance continuum, with increased aerobic demands. A 15-study meta-analysis by Hobson and colleagues[425] found that supplemental beta-alanine improves exercise performance further toward the middle range of the strength-endurance continuum (high-intensity exercise lasting 60 to 240 seconds). In a more recent 40-study meta-analysis, Saunders and colleagues[426] reported that beta-alanine benefits exercise bouts of an even broader range (0.5 to 10 minutes).

An even more recent review by Brisola and Zagatto[427] examined the discrepancies between these two publications and concluded that the greatest effectiveness of beta-alanine supplementation occurs in exercises lasting between 60 and 240 seconds. And this makes sense considering beta-alanine's primary mechanism of action of buffering acidity generated by high-intensity work. The authors inferred that there is strong evidence for beta-alanine supplementation benefiting cycling (4 km), swimming (100 and 200 m), rowing (2,000 m), combat modalities, and water polo.

Dosing

Increased exercise performance has occurred at doses ranging from 3.2 to 6.4 grams per day for four to 12 weeks.[426] It should be noted that the commonly recommended four-week duration of beta-alanine dosing at ~3 to 6 grams per day can't be viewed as a period where maximal "loading" of intramuscular carnosine occurs.

To illustrate my point, a four-week trial by Harris and colleagues[428] reported intramuscular carnosine increases of 42.1 and 64.2 percent via beta-alanine dosed at 3.2 and 6.4 grams per day, respectively. Saunders and colleagues[429] found that the average duration to reach peak intramuscular carnosine levels (119.2 percent) was 18 weeks, at 6.4 grams per day. Interestingly, five of the 25 subjects did not plateau in carnosine content by the end of the 24-week trial, suggesting that longer durations and/or higher doses are necessary for some individuals to saturate carnosine stores.

Investigating a maintenance dose, Stegen and colleagues[430] found that 49 days of dosing beta-alanine at 3.2 grams per day caused a moderate increase (30 to 50 percent) in intramuscular carnosine, and 1.2 grams per day was able to maintain this increased carnosine level for the remainder of the trial, which lasted another six weeks. Washout is a slow process,[410,426,427] with the low end ranging from six to nine weeks and the high end ranging from 16 to 20 weeks, depending largely on the degree of carnosine increase from baseline.

FLEXIBLE VOCAB

Washout

When using supplements, reaching optimal concentrations within the body typically takes a certain amount of time. *Washout* refers to the opposite effect— when concentrations decrease to pre-supplementation levels—and it often takes even longer.

Safety and caveats

Beta-alanine thus far has a good safety track record. Dolan and colleagues[431] performed a systematic risk assessment and meta-analysis of beta-alanine supplementation. They assessed five main outcomes: 1) side effects in longitudinal trials, 2) side effects in acute trials, 3) effect on circulating biomarkers, 4) effect of muscle taurine and histidine levels, and 5) outcomes from animal trials. The analysis included over a hundred human studies, and the only side effect reported was paresthesia (an itchy, prickling/tingling sensation that's been described as "pins and needles"). No other adverse effects were found within the doses used in the studies.

Paresthesia can be minimized or avoided by taking divided doses of beta-alanine every few hours throughout the day at a maximum of 800 milligrams.[432] The slow-release form of beta-alanine has shown tolerability in doses as high as 1.6 grams,[433] which makes dosing less of a chore.

A recent crossover study by de Salazar and colleagues[434] compared 8 grams of commonly used slow-release beta-alanine tablets with a novel controlled-release formulation (8 grams of beta-alanine, 300 milligrams of L-histidine, and 100 milligrams of carnosine). The rationale of including histidine in this formula is theoretically sound, since carnosine is a dipeptide composed of carnosine and histidine, and histidine availability can decline with chronic beta-alanine supplementation.[435] The novel formulation was 2.1 times more bioavailable than the conventional treatment. However, paresthesia was also higher with the novel formula. Perhaps future developments in this area will alleviate the paresthesia problem, which is the limiting factor in beta-alanine dosing. This will allow greater progress with more efficient/less arduous dosing protocols.

FLEXIBLE VOCAB

Bioavailable

Bioavailability describes the rate at which or degree to which a substance (such as a supplement) is absorbed by the body and becomes available for use—that is, when and how much of the substance reaches systemic circulation.

Sodium bicarbonate

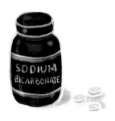

Sodium bicarbonate is better known as baking soda. Yes, that box of white powder in the back of your fridge. Sodium bicarbonate increases performance capacity by raising blood levels of bicarbonate. This increases blood pH and mitigates fatigue by buffering exercise-mediated acidosis.

Sodium bicarbonate has been extensively studied and has accumulated enough interest to spawn several meta-analyses[436-440] and a recent ISSN position stand.[441] Similar to beta-alanine, sodium bicarbonate's applicability is toward the middle of the strength-endurance continuum, with a lean toward the high-intensity side.

Despite sodium bicarbonate and beta-alanine sharing a similar ergogenic mechanism, combining the two has shown greater benefit for sprinting performance than sodium bicarbonate alone.[442] Combining sodium bicarbonate with creatine or beta-alanine may have additive effects, but it's not clear whether additive effects occur in combination with caffeine or nitrates.[441] The benefits of sodium bicarbonate are seen in muscular endurance activities ranging from 30 seconds to 12 minutes. These include combat sports and high-intensity cycling, rowing, running, and swimming.

Dosing

The most recent meta-analysis by Calvo and colleagues[437] involved 17 studies and focused specifically on energy metabolism. The authors concluded that sodium bicarbonate mainly affects/benefits the anaerobic energy system, dosed at 0.3 g/kg via gelatin capsule, taken 90 minutes before exercise. The ISSN position stand recommends a dosing range of 0.2 to 0.5 g/kg, with the caveat that doses beyond 0.4 g/kg significantly raise the risk for gastrointestinal upset and accompanying decreases in performance.[441]

Sodium bicarbonate can be dosed singularly or chronically, with the latter being preferred for reducing the risk of gastrointestinal distress. Single-dose protocols (~0.3 g/kg) are best timed 60 to 180 minutes before the bout. Chronic protocols involve a daily dose of 0.4 to 0.5 g/kg (in divided doses of 0.1 to 0.2 gram with each meal) for three to seven days leading to the event.

Safety and caveats

The Achilles' heel of sodium bicarbonate is its potential for gastrointestinal upset, including nausea, vomiting, stomach pain, and diarrhea.[443] However, these risks are mainly a function of dose. In my observations, competitors who've had bad experiences with sodium bicarbonate supplementation were most resentful about the fear of pooping their pants.

Tactics for minimizing the risk of side effects include ingesting sodium bicarbonate in smaller doses, with meals, in enteric coated capsules, and with sufficient time allotted between ingestion and competition. It's prudent to engage in trial runs (no pun intended) of different dosing and timing schemes that suit individual response.

Nitrate

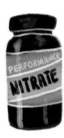

Dietary nitrate is available from green leafy vegetables and root vegetables, with beetroot being a common source in performance research. Ingested nitrate results in the production of nitric oxide, which imparts performance-enhancing effects through increased vasodilation (widening of blood vessels), blood flow, mitochondrial biogenesis, and muscular contractility.[444-446]

Nitrate supplementation benefits the performance of exercise in the mid-range of the strength-endurance continuum, in activities ranging from ~12 to 40 minutes.[444] Ergogenic effects above and below this range are equivocal.

Nitrate supplementation has been studied extensively. A 76-study meta-analysis by McMahon and colleagues[445] found that nitrate benefited endurance capacity (time to exhaustion), but not time trial performance. In the most recent meta-analysis on dietary nitrate involving 73 studies, Gao and colleagues[446] reported similar results. Nitrate supplementation improved power output, time to exhaustion, and distance traveled but had no significant effects on perceived exertion, time trial performance, or work done.

Dosing

The consensus statement of the International Olympic Committee (IOC)[444] recommends 5 to 9 mmol (310 to 560 mg) ingested two to three hours prior to exercise. This is the equivalent of roughly 500 to 750 milliliters (2 to 3 cups) of beetroot juice.[447] Chronic nitrate intake (>three days) at this dose leading to an event may also benefit performance. Similarly, a review by Clements and colleagues[448] reported a dosing range of 300 to 600 milligrams either in a single bolus or up to 15 days of consistent consumption prior to competition.

For those who prefer to take the food route rather than the supplement or juice route, celery, chervil, cress, lettuce, red beetroot, spinach, and arugula (also called rocket or rucola) all contain more than 250 milligrams per 100 grams of fresh weight.[449] A cup of raw spinach contains 926 milligrams of nitrate (Popeye was ahead of his time).

Safety and caveats

Nitrate ingestion/supplementation overall has been demonstrated as effective for endurance applications. However, it has a somewhat dichotomous set of findings, where it appears to consistently benefit endurance capacity but not time trial performance. Furthermore, nitrate supplementation has shown a lack of effect in several studies using highly trained endurance athletes. Some concern was raised after a crossover trial by Larsen and colleagues[450] found that nitrate dosed at 0.1 mmol/kg (6.2 mg/kg) for three days lowered resting metabolic rate (RMR) by 4.2 percent compared to placebo. However, a subsequent meta-analysis by Pawlak-Chaouch and colleagues[451] involving 29 RCTs found that the collective evidence shows that nitrate does not affect RMR.

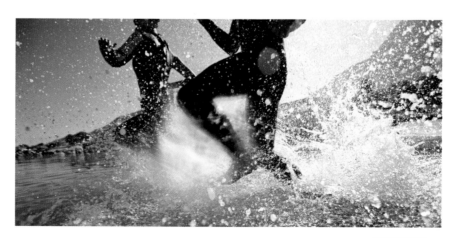

Caffeine

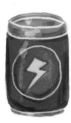

Caffeine is somewhat out of place in discussions about dietary supplements because technically, it's a psychoactive drug as well as a central nervous system stimulant.[452] Perhaps unsurprisingly, caffeine is also the most widely used drug in the world.[453]

Caffeine is a methylxanthine that naturally occurs in the leaves, seeds, and fruits of a multitude of commonly consumed plants. Caffeine is an adenosine receptor antagonist. So, it works by mitigating the fatigue and drowsiness associated with adenosine activity. Other potential mechanisms for performance enhancement include calcium release from the sarcoplasmic reticulum,[454] a glycogen-sparing shift in substrate utilization toward the oxidation of fatty acids, and stimulation of beta-endorphins, which lower the perception of pain or fatigue.[455]

FLEXIBLE VOCAB

Adenosine

You might recall this word as part of adenosine triphosphate, the body's energy currency. That's one of the three forms adenosine takes. It is present in every human cell and has a multitude of uses both diagnostic and therapeutic. In the brain, it is a central nervous system depressant associated with healthy sleep patterns.

Caffeine traditionally has been recognized as an endurance enhancer,[455] but a 10-study meta-analysis by Grgic and colleagues[456] reported that caffeine imparts significant improvements in maximal muscle strength of upper body and muscle power. Grgic and colleagues[457] recently conducted an umbrella review encompassing 21 meta-analyses on the effects of caffeine supplementation on exercise performance. They concluded that caffeine improves performance for a broad range of demands, including strength, endurance, anaerobic power, and aerobic endurance. The magnitude of effect tended to be greater for aerobic compared to anaerobic exercise.

Similar conclusions have been drawn by the most recent ISSN position stand on caffeine and athletic performance,[458] which states that caffeine use benefits a wide range of aerobic and anaerobic sport-specific applications, but aerobic endurance reaps the largest/most consistent benefits.

Dosing

For enhancing exercise performance, the latest ISSN position stand on caffeine[458] and the IOC consensus statement on supplements for athletes[444] converge on a dosing recommendation of 3 to 6 mg/kg of bodyweight ingested 60 minutes pre-exercise. Very high dosing (e.g., 9 mg/kg) carries a high risk of side effects. Minimum effective dosing where ergogenic effects are still detectable are not definitively known, but 2 mg/kg has been suggested.[458]

Safety and caveats

Potential side effects of caffeine include insomnia, nervousness, anxiety, nausea, gastrointestinal upset, tremors, and tachycardia—which have been reported at doses as low as 250 to 300 milligrams.[459] The growing energy drink industry relies on caffeine as its active ingredient, with doses ranging from 47 to 80 milligrams per 8 ounces to 207 milligrams per 2 ounces.[460] It is therefore unsurprising that energy drink consumption is associated with several adverse cardiovascular, metabolic, skeletal, and mental health outcomes.[461] Most of these effects can be largely attributed to excessive caffeine intake.

Calling caffeine an addictive drug is controversial and has been disputed in the literature.[462] The counterpoint is that caffeine causes behavioral and physiological effects similar to those caused by other drugs of dependence—including a persistent desire, unsuccessful efforts to cut down or control use, continued use despite harm, and physiological withdrawal.[453,463]

In contrast to caffeinated energy drinks (which have highly adverse potential—especially since they're heavily marketed toward adolescents[464]), foods and beverages with naturally occurring caffeine tend to be less risky from a health standpoint. For example, coffee has net positive health effects when consumed in moderation (2 to 4 cups a day).[465] Upper safe limits of caffeine intake are 400 milligrams per day for healthy adults, 300 milligrams per day for pregnant women, and 2.5 mg/kg of bodyweight per day for adolescents and children.[466] The acute lethal dose is estimated to be 10 grams. Commonly consumed "natural" caffeine sources are coffee (~100 mg/cup), espresso (~64 mg/shot), tea (~27 mg/cup), and chocolate (~12 mg/ounce).

The anhydrous (crystalline) form of caffeine has been used in the majority of the research since the use of coffee presents variations in caffeine content and a lack of standardization. However, coffee is still a viable delivery vehicle for caffeine's ergogenic effects. A review by Higgins and colleagues[467] reported that there is moderate evidence supporting the use of coffee (providing a caffeine dose of 3 to 8.1 mg/kg) to improve performance in endurance cycling and running. In agreement, the aforementioned umbrella review by Grgic and colleagues[457] reported that the average cup of coffee contains 100 milligrams of caffeine, so 2 cups would cross into the ergogenic dosing zone by delivering 200 milligrams, or ~3 mg/kg for a 70-kilogram individual.

The IOC and World Anti-Doping Agency removed caffeine from the "controlled substance" list in 2004. However, caffeine is still monitored by the World Anti-Doping Agency, and athletes are encouraged to keep urinary caffeine levels below the 12 µg/ml limit.[458] The latter would require ingesting 10 mg/kg, which is substantially beyond the dosing range known to be ergogenic (3 to 6 mg/kg).

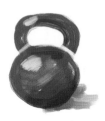

A common presumption is that habituating (becoming physiologically accustomed) to regular caffeine use will diminish its ergogenic effect. This is not necessarily true; it's a gray area in the literature. I'll quote the current ISSN position stand on caffeine and athletic performance:[458]

> *"There does not appear to be a consistent difference in the performance effects of acute caffeine ingestion between habitual and non-habitual caffeine users, and study findings remain equivocal."*

Another unresolved topic surrounding caffeine and exercise performance is the role of genetic predisposition, which might explain some of the different responses across individuals. The gene CYP1A2 encodes cytochrome P450 1A2 (an enzyme responsible for roughly 95 percent of caffeine metabolism), so it's been the target of ongoing study. However, a recent meta-analysis by Grgic and colleagues[468] on the CYP1A2 genotype concluded that small and inconsistent differences challenge the utility of genotyping to guide caffeine use in athletes.

And that's a wrap for this chapter. Refer to Table 7a for a summary of the exercise performance–enhancing supplements. Figure 7a is a graphic representation of the role of these supplements on the strength-endurance continuum. Note that I placed question marks on sodium bicarbonate (lots of anecdotes of stomach upset/urgent poops) and nitrate (questionable benefit in highly trained endurance athletes). Nevertheless, I included sodium bicarbonate and nitrate because they are consistently placed in the top tier in published articles and position stands of evidence-based sports supplements.

Table 7a: Exercise Performance–Enhancing Supplements

SUPPLEMENT	ERGOGENIC EFFECTS	DOSING	CAVEATS
Creatine monohydrate	Increases muscle size, strength, power (including sprint-type activities) in maximal efforts lasting 30–150 seconds.	Loading phase optional (20–25 g/day for 5–7 days), followed by a maintenance dose (3–5 g/day or ~0.04–0.07 g/kg of bodyweight).	Weight gain (as lean mass) is difficult to avoid during loading; caution is warranted when used for weight-sensitive endurance sports.
Beta-alanine	Increases high-intensity endurance capacity (bouts lasting 1–4 minutes, possibly up to 10 minutes).	3.2–6.4 g/day for 4–12 weeks, possibly 24+ weeks to fully load. Divided doses of 0.8 g (reg form) or 1.6 g (timed release form) can minimize paresthesia.	Paresthesia (unpleasant sensation of "pins and needles") is the limiting factor in simple/efficient dosing schemes.
Sodium bicarbonate	Increases high-intensity endurance capacity (bouts lasting 30 seconds to 12 minutes).	Single-dose protocols (~0.3 g/kg) timed 60–180 minutes pre-bout. Or a daily dose of 0.4–0.5 g/kg (0.1–0.2 g with each meal) for 3–7 days leading up to the bout.	Potential for gastrointestinal upset, including nausea, vomiting, stomach pain, and diarrhea.
Dietary nitrate	Increases mid-range endurance capacity (bouts ranging from 12–40 minutes).	300–600 mg, either in a single bolus or up to 15 days of consistent consumption of this dose prior to competition.	Inconsistent effectiveness for time trial performance in highly trained endurance athletes.
Caffeine	Increases exercise performance across the entirety of the strength-endurance continuum, although improvements in aerobic exercise are greater than anaerobic exercise.	3–6 mg/kg ingested 60 minutes before the bout.	A potent and potentially risky/addictive drug. Non-pregnant adults should not exceed 400 mg/day. Refer to the full section on caffeine for the details on its risks.

Figure 7a: Supplementation Along the Strength-Endurance Continuum

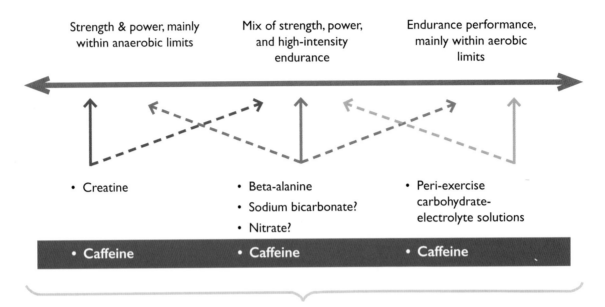

CHAPTER 7 IN A NUTSHELL

- The wild world of dietary supplements is both a blessing and a curse. Thanks to the DSHEA of 1994, consumers have virtually unlimited access to various helpful (and harmful) products.

- Weight/fat loss supplements range from slightly useful to just plain dangerous. Collectively, they have a poor risk-to-benefit balance. The best weight loss supplement is a caloric deficit (and, yes, I realize this statement may upset some readers).

- Multivitamin-mineral (MVM) supplements are a topic of controversy, with literature both for and against them. From a pragmatic standpoint as well as weighing risk versus benefit, MVMs are warranted despite doubts cast by null-result research. MVMs can be particularly useful for a wide range of populations, the most relevant for the readers of this book being physically active folks who go through hypocaloric phases and/or consume a limited spectrum of foods within and across the food groups.

- Based on the current weight of the evidence, which includes the position stands of the major athletic organizations, I've boiled down the "heavyweights" of evidence-based performance supplementation to creatine, beta-alanine, sodium bicarbonate, nitrate, and caffeine.

- Refer to Table 7a for a summary of effects, dosing, and caveats, and refer to Figure 7a for a graphic representation of the role of these supplements on the strength-endurance continuum.

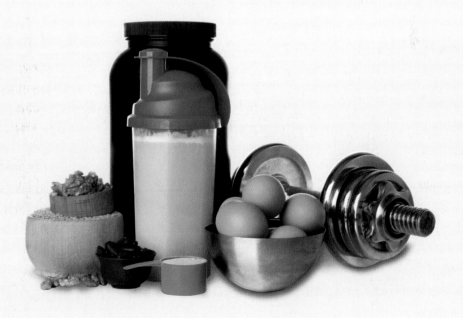

PART 4

PROGRAMMING THE COMPONENTS

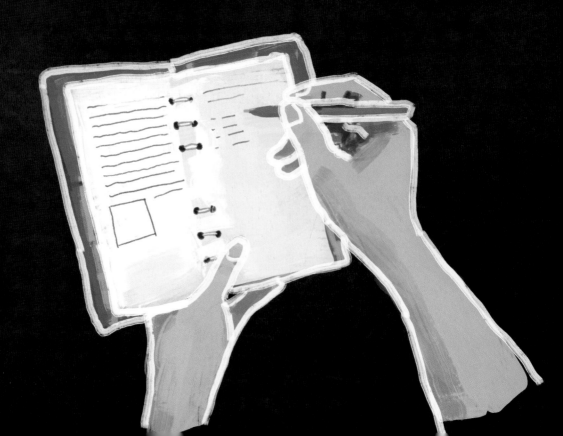

DIETARY PROGRAMMING

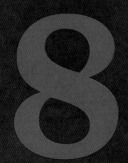

The dietary programming frameworks I've used throughout the course of my career are not particularly exciting; they just make the most sense. Also, keep in mind that in some of the figures and formulas, I use pounds instead of kilograms (divide pounds by 2.2 to get kilograms).

I'll cover qualitative approaches of programming in the final chapter of this book, but as far as quantitative approaches go, there are two main frameworks, both of which depend on the goals of the individual. The first framework is appropriate for programs where athletic performance goals are not of primary importance. We can creatively call it *Athletic Performance: Secondary* (APS). This process is applicable to the majority of the general population and the majority of the clients that health/fitness/nutrition professionals work with (Box 8a).

BOX 8A: ATHLETIC PERFORMANCE: SECONDARY

1. Set the goal and time frame.

2. Set calories.

3. Set protein.

4. Set fat.

5. Fill in the remainder with carbohydrate.

Now, here's the programming framework we can creatively call *Athletic Performance: Primary* (APP). This framework is applicable to competitive athletes whose primary goal is performance. Note the subtle but important difference in the order of the programming steps in Box 8b.

BOX 8B: ATHLETIC PERFORMANCE: PRIMARY

1. Set the goal and time frame.

2. Set calories.

3. Set protein.

4. Set carbohydrate.

5. Fill in the remainder with fat.

As you can see, the difference between APS and APP is the order of steps 4 and 5. If you're stumped about the rationale for this difference, let me direct you to the carbohydrate chapter (Chapter 5) and specifically Box 5a. Briefly, carbohydrate dosing for individuals seeking to optimally support strength/power demands and/or hypertrophy goals is 3 to 8 g/kg of bodyweight. Athletes seeking to optimize performance in sports primarily involving high volumes of endurance work require 6 to 12 g/kg of total bodyweight. Individuals whose athletic performance goals are secondary to nonexistent can effectively choose any carb-fat proportion they personally prefer (and can best adhere to). With that, we can move on to the steps of the programming frameworks.

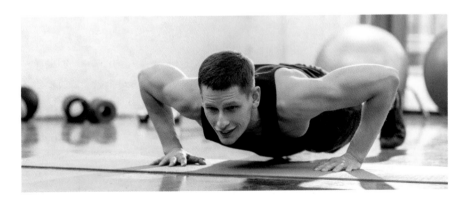

STEP 1: SETTING THE GOAL AND TIME FRAME

Putting "recomp" into perspective

I'll be discussing two main goals in this chapter: muscle gain and fat loss. In the following chapter, I'll discuss maintenance. I'd like to talk about recomposition (or recomp) first since it's a common goal—yet one that we have minimal control over compared to the other two goals.

Recomp is simultaneous muscle gain and fat loss. The topic of recomp was first touched upon in the fat loss section of the protein chapter, where I also discussed the proposed mechanisms. It's important to know the hierarchy of recomp capacity—in other words, the pecking order of the populations that can experience recomp, from greatest to least (Box 8c).

BOX 8C: HIERARCHY OF RECOMPOSITION CAPACITY

1. Formerly fit/trained folks with excess body fat

2. Overweight novices

3. Intermediates

4. Advanced trainees who are relatively lean

Notes on training status

A frustratingly difficult question to answer definitively is what determines training status, since the question can apply either to physique or to sports performance goals. The latter is easier to stratify than the former.

The problem of classifying trainees involved with physique endeavors is compounded by a lack of objective performance requirements. In conceptual terms, the closer you are to your potential for muscular size (and/or leanness), the more advanced you are. It's fair to say that professional bodybuilders (those who earn prize money within major organizations such as the International Federation of Bodybuilding and Fitness) are advanced trainees, as are national- and state-level competitors. As we proceed down the ranks, things get progressively muddier, the subjectivity increases, and the lines between intermediate and advanced begin to blur—even in formal competition.

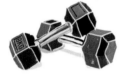

The imprecision of these constructs makes thresholds of categorization extremely difficult to establish. As we move away from the competitive realm, what if you are one of the ten most jacked people at your gym, and we're talking about a gym in southern California at peak capacity? What if you are undisputedly the most jacked person at the public pool? It's complicated.

A common benchmark for the limit of natural muscular development (thus "advanced" status) is a fat-free mass index (FFMI) of 25. FFMI is the ratio of FFM (in kilograms) to height (in meters squared). The cutoff point of 25 stems from an observational study by Kouri and colleagues,[469] who examined a sample of 157 male athletes: 83 users of anabolic-androgenic steroids (AAS) and 74 non-users. This sample included Mr. America winners from the pre-AAS era (1939 to 1959), whose FFMI averaged 25.4. Ultimately, the authors concluded that the FFMI cutoff of 25 represents a useful screening tool for AAS use. Despite the study's limitations, which include self-reported details and indirect estimates, an FFMI of 25 is a satisfactory benchmark for gauging proximity to the limits of muscular development for natural trainees wondering about their training status.

In line with Kouri's findings, Chappell and colleagues[124] reported that male elite-level, top-five-placing natural bodybuilders in contest condition had an average FFMI of 22.7. Only two of the ten competitors exceeded an FFMI of 25. Female elite natural competitors' FFMI averaged 18.1. The authors mentioned that an FFMI screening benchmark for the natural limit of female athletes has not been established but suggest that it's likely to be 19 to 20. By comparison, in the general/untrained, normal-weight population, FFMI ranges from 16.7 to 19.8 in men and 14.6 to 16.8 in women.

A more recent study by Trexler and colleagues[470] reported that in a sample of 235 NCAA Division I and II football players, 62 individuals (26.4 percent) had FFMI values above 25. Six linemen had FFMIs of 28.1, and the highest FFMI was 31.7. While these findings have been waved around in an attempt to debunk the FFMI-25 "natty cutoff," there's no certainty that all of the athletes were natural. But, more importantly, the FFMI-25 benchmark applies to athletes in their leanest state. The subjects in Trexler's study averaged 12 percent body fat, while elite natural bodybuilding competitors average about 4 to 5 percent body fat on contest day. Therefore, Trexler's data is not a fair comparison or a viable refutation of the FFMI-25 benchmark. Another example of athletes exceeding FFMI-25 is professional sumo wrestlers, who have an FFMI averaging 26.6.[471]

With that said, let's just be clear that outliers do exist in the animal kingdom. An FFMI above 25 isn't automatic grounds to presume certainty of AAS use in very lean individuals. Though not peer-reviewed, one of the most rigorous analytical explorations of FFMI and the limits of naturally attainable muscle growth is an ebook called *Your Muscular Potential* by Casey Butt. I highly recommend this book for anyone who wants to take a deeper dive into the fine details of the limits of natural muscular potential and its related anthropometrics.

It's tempting to automatically link training status to how long you've been training, but to quote my friend and colleague Brad Schoenfeld, "I know people who after several months of training are more 'advanced' than those with years of training." This underscores the importance of considering how consistent someone has been with making progress without significant time off, injuries, or setbacks.

I would also add that we can't completely separate time from training status. Although it's inevitably subjective (and observational), the transition from beginner to intermediate status typically occurs within the first year of consistent training. The road from intermediate to advanced never happens with the vast majority of recreational/non-competitive trainees. However, in my observations, those who dedicate themselves to the goal of muscular development with minimal layoffs and setbacks can spend as little as two to three years as intermediate trainees before graduating to advanced. Others may take at least twice as long to approach advanced status.

There are many influencing variables, not the least of which are life stability in general, genetic predisposition, optimization of nutrition and training, and supplement/drug use. An example of a rapid ascent through the ranks is seven-time Mr. Olympia Phil Heath. Although unlikely to be natural, he stands out for reportedly engaging in bodybuilding-specific training for only three years before winning the National Physique Committee (NPC) Nationals. He won his first pro show the next year. The rest is history.

Notes on recomp

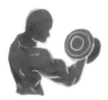

The potential for recomp exists on a sliding scale of magnitude depending on body composition and training status. While the literature indeed has several reports of recomp in male subjects classified as lean and trained, their starting body comp averaged in the mid-teens. The implementation of a novel, better designed diet and training program can indeed cause recomp in this population. However, the more advanced your training status, the more you need to focus on one goal at a time.

An exception is the case of advanced trainees engaging in novel supplementation or pharmaceutical help. While recomp in advanced trainees is not impossible, it's just not a practical pursuit, especially for those who have been training consistently and progressively for several consecutive years.

From a programming perspective, recomp is more of a bonus than a targeted pursuit. The prime candidates for recomp (beginning trainees and formerly fit folks with excess body fat) are obviously free to choose recomp as a primary goal. However, I would keep in mind that always hoping for recomp can progressively set the stage for inefficiency of action and ultimately lead to frustration. The goals involving maintenance are different from recomping and are not subject to the same competing objectives.

With that all said, there are things you can do to maximize your chances of recomp. Box 8d lists the relevant elements, relayed from a recent paper by Barakat and colleagues on the topic.[125] (Keep in mind that these are observational rather than causal elements, but they are valuable nonetheless.)

Now that I've talked you out of actively pursuing recomp (and instead accepting it as a bonus that's dependent on initial training status and body composition), let's talk about the goal of muscle gain.

Muscle gain

Potential gains over the long term

Muscle gain is a relatively straightforward goal, especially compared to recomp. Nevertheless, it's important to maintain realistic progress expectations. It's common for people to have expectations of amount and rate of muscle gain that far exceed what's possible for most.

You might think a good place to start would be knowing how much muscle an untrained adult can build naturally, but this is impossible to answer definitively or with a high degree of precision. Trying to unearth a universally applicable maximal rate of muscle gain in resistance trainees in the peer-reviewed literature is a futile endeavor. On the high end, there are publications showing spectacular gains in lean mass within short time frames, such as Wilson and colleagues' reporting a lean mass gain of 7.4 kilograms (16.28 pounds) in 12 weeks.[472] On the other end, a recent meta-analysis by Benito and colleagues[382] reports a disappointing average gain of 1.5 kilograms (3.3 pounds) in resistance-training men. Studies in the meta-analysis ranged from two weeks to one year. A caveat to this finding is that having muscle hypertrophy as a targeted outcome wasn't part of the inclusion criteria for the studies.

Given the lack of published data on this question, it's reasonable to draw inferences from FFMI differences between high-level natural bodybuilders and the general population. In the general population of men aged 18 to 39, the average FFMI is 19.[473] In elite-level drug-free male bodybuilders, FFMI is 22.7 to 25, with few exceptions.[124] This is 17.4 to 24 percent greater than untrained men in the general population. In the general population of women aged 18 to 39, average FFMI is 15.6.[473] In elite-level drug-free female bodybuilders, FFMI is 18.1 to 19.5.[124,474] This is 16 to 25 percent greater than untrained women in the general population. Box 8e puts these numbers toward concrete examples.

BOX 8E: EXAMPLES OF MAXIMAL DRUG-FREE MUSCLE GAIN POTENTIAL IN ADULTS

- A completely untrained man at 85 kg (187 lbs) with 20% body fat has 68 kg (149.6 lbs) of FFM. Increasing FFM by 17.4–24% would add 11.8–16.3 kg (26–35.9 lbs).

- A completely untrained woman at 65 kg (143 lbs) with 30% body fat has 45.5 kg (100.1 lbs) of FFM. Increasing FFM by 16–25% would add 7.3–11.4 kg (16.1–25.1 lbs).

In summary, men have the (natural) potential to gain ~17 to 24 percent more muscle when starting from an untrained state. The example I gave shows ~26 to 36 pounds. Women have the (natural) potential to gain ~16 to 25 percent more muscle when starting from an untrained state. The example I gave shows ~16 to 25 pounds. These are realistic ranges based on comparing general population stats with the stats of elite-level natural bodybuilders. In line with findings in the published research, men and women have similar proportional gains, although the net amounts differ.[475]

People rarely find these numbers to be way off-base, but those who do tend to sneer at them and claim they can do way better. If you think you can, then good—have at it. Just keep in mind that realistic expectations set people up for success and further motivation. Failure and frustration due to unrealistic goals are unfortunately the norm. Also keep in mind that the data on "enhanced" individuals (on AAS and/or other anabolic or performance-enhancing drugs) are scarce. In my observations, you can safely add another 20 to 25 percent (or more) to these figures when estimating the totals for "enhanced" trainees.

Rate of muscle gain determines the time frame

A realistic perspective of progress rate is crucial to maintaining motivation and mitigating frustration. A simple guideline for intermediate trainees is 1 to 2 pounds per month. Where you fall within that range depends on your initial training status. The 1 to 2 pounds per month figure is a simplification that can be applied to beginners and intermediate-level trainees, who comprise the vast majority.

Keep in mind that this is in reference to lean mass, not total mass. For intermediate trainees, it's difficult, but not impossible, to make strictly lean gains. For novices, it's more common to experience strictly lean gains without concurrent fat gains (and in some cases, fat loss as well). Per our discussion about recomp, it's possible in intermediates, but to a lesser degree, as it's typically not a practical pursuit.

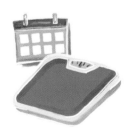

A realistic lean:fat mass gain ratio in intermediates is 1:0.5 to 1. In other words, for every pound of muscle you gain, it's likely and acceptable to gain a half to a whole pound of fat. Ideally, it would be kept to a maximum of 1:0.5 (a half pound of fat mass for every pound of lean mass gained), but this gets progressively less realistic as you mature in muscle mass and/or leanness.

Once again, this goes back to the principle that the more advanced you are, the more exclusive the focus needs to be on either muscle gain or fat loss. Box 8f presents a good-case scenario of muscle gain for the first year of consistent progressive training, starting from a completely untrained (or detrained) state.

BOX 8F: REALISTIC RATES OF MUSCLE GAIN IN MEN

1–2 pounds/month in beginners and intermediates, 0.5–1 pound/month in late-intermediates and advanced trainees

One-year really good-case scenario, starting untrained:

Months 1–3: 2 pounds/month (6 pounds total)

Months 4–6: 1.5 pounds/month (4.5 pounds total)

Months 7–12: 1 pound/month (6 pounds total)

———————————

Grand total: 16.5 pounds

Overall average monthly gain: 1.37 pounds

This is a really good-case scenario, where all the programming variables are geared toward growth. It includes net caloric surplus conditions. While muscle growth is possible without maintaining a purposeful caloric surplus, the process is not maximized. Muscle growth is indeed possible in hypocaloric conditions, although this phenomenon is limited mostly to untrained subjects. Therefore, hypercaloric (caloric surplus) conditions should be maintained if the goal is to maximize rates of muscle gain. The further you progress from novice status, the less aggressive the caloric surplus can be without fat gain.

A good rule of thumb is a 10 to 20 percent caloric surplus (roughly 250 to 500 kcal above maintenance needs) for intermediates and more advanced trainees, and a 20 to 40 percent caloric surplus (500 to 1,000 kcal) for novices seeking to maximize muscle gains.[57] If, as a novice trainee, the 1,000 kcal surplus figure scares you, then try the 500 kcal surplus to see if it's enough to facilitate the rate of gains outlined in Box 8f.

The high end of these surplus recommendations is mainly suitable for those who have difficulty maintaining hypercaloric conditions due to subconscious ramp-ups in non-exercise activity thermogenesis (NEAT) in response to overfeeding. The latter is what underlies the phenomenon of "hard-gainers," or those who work out hard but have difficulty putting on muscle. Their NEAT levels tend to increase alongside attempts to remain hypercaloric.

FLEXIBLE VOCAB

Non-exercise activity thermogenesis (NEAT)

NEAT is used to describe the calories we burn and the energy we use via movements necessary for going about our daily lives, including physical movement like occupational tasks, fidgeting, maintaining body posture, spontaneous movement—anything that isn't planned exercise.

Illustrating the NEAT ramp-up of hard-gainers, Levine and colleagues[476] fed normal-weight adults 1,000 kcal above their maintenance needs for eight weeks. On average, 432 kcal were stored and 531 kcal were burned. Nearly two-thirds of this (336 kcal) was attributable to NEAT. One of the subjects had a NEAT ramp-up of 692 kcal per day in response to the 1,000 kcal per day surplus. This finding explains why some individuals can increase their daily caloric intake—in some cases substantially—and not gain weight. A subconscious increase in NEAT can nullify the attempted caloric surplus.

As trainees progress toward advanced levels, the rate of gain is half of the 1 to 2 pounds/month attainable by intermediates and beginners—at best. Illustrating this point are elite-level competitive bodybuilders. It's rare to see them step onstage more than 5 to 10 pounds heavier with each year of competition as a national-level or professional competitor. This is the triumphant tragedy of being so close to one's ultimate potential.

Notes on muscle gain in women

Women have similar capability for muscle gain compared to men, on a proportional basis.[475] The same is true with strength gains.[477] However, in terms of absolute (net) amounts, men tend to carry substantially more muscle mass than women.

Janssen and colleagues[478] reported that in the general population, men ranging in age from 18 to 88 years carry ~57 percent more muscle mass than women, on average. In contrast, Abe and colleagues[479] examined the differences between male and female athletes with a high degree of muscle mass and reported an average of 30 percent more muscle mass in men.

For our purposes (which involve resistance training), it's more appropriate to go with Abe and colleagues' findings when estimating sex-based differences. This means that the 1 to 2 pounds/month benchmark in novice and intermediate men would need to be modified to 0.7 to 1.4 pounds/month in order to more accurately apply to women (Box 8g).

BOX 8G: REALISTIC RATES OF MUSCLE GAIN IN WOMEN

0.7–1.4 pounds/month in beginners and intermediates, 0.35–0.7 pound/month in late intermediates and advanced trainees

One-year really good-case scenario, starting untrained:

Months 1–3: 1.4 pounds/month (4.2 pounds total)

Months 4–6: 1 pound/month (3 pounds total)

Months 7–12: 0.9 pound/month (5.4 pounds total)

_____

Grand total: 12.6 pounds

Overall average monthly gain: 1.05 pounds

Fat loss

Notes about calories versus hormones

Let's first get it straight that, despite the abundance of fairy tales floating around the diet and nutrition media, calories matter for the goal of fat loss. There is a common and misleading idea that calories don't matter, hormones do. This either-or proposition is false. Bear with me as I explain why.

The body's relative state of energy balance—whether it's a caloric surplus or deficit—can puppeteer hormone levels in lockstep with shifts in said energy balance. This keeps caloric balance and the hormonal environment inextricably entwined. A prime example of their interconnectedness is how under- and overeating to various degrees affects levels of hunger and satiety hormones. Appetite affects eating behavior (including under- and overeating), which circles right back to relative energy balance. The macronutrients differ in their ability to affect hunger and satiety and in their inherent caloric costs of processing within the body (protein being the most metabolically expensive and the most satiating).

Hormones play intimate roles in energy homeostasis. Pitting hormones and calories against each other by claiming that weight/fat loss is all about hormones and not calories is a false dichotomy. With that said, sustaining a net caloric deficit is necessary for achieving and maintaining significant weight (fat) loss in the long term.[59] It's true that fat loss can occur in the absence of a caloric deficit, as in the case of recomp seen in beginners and early intermediate trainees. However, failing to program a caloric deficit when the main goal is fat loss will ultimately sabotage the mission.

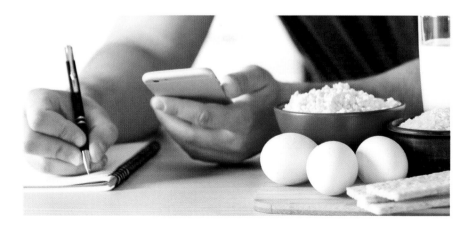

Realistic body fat percentage (BF%) targets

Once again, unrealistic targets are a common source of frustration and cessation of endeavors to reach fat loss goals. Minimal levels of body fat for optimally supporting women's fertility and reproductive capability (17 to 22 percent)[480] are substantially higher than minimal levels for mere survival. The limits of leanness in women without approaching imminent death (though not by much) are represented in physique competitors (see Box 8h), which can be as low as ~11 to 12 percent BF. This is by no means a healthy level of leanness to sustain for more than brief periods. It's unsettling that a similar level of leanness is seen in women with the restrictive variant of anorexia nervosa, ranging from ~10 to 13 percent BF, at a bodyweight of ~40 to 44 kilograms (88 to 97 pounds).[481,482] Normal/healthy body fat levels for women in the general population range from ~20 to 30 percent. Male physique competitors get down to ~4 to 5 percent on contest day, while normal/healthy body fat levels of men in the general population range from 10 to 20 percent. Box 8h outlines the BF% targets documented in the peer-reviewed literature for various populations.[473,480,483-486]

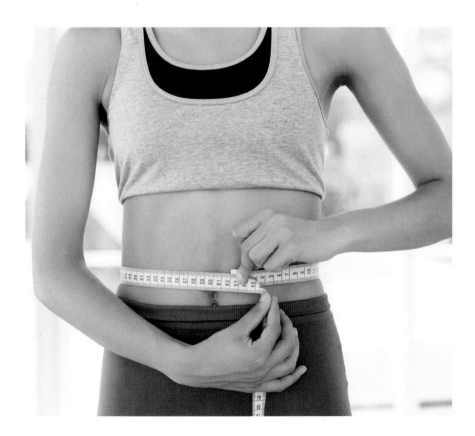

Normal/Healthy BF% Standards for the General Population

BMI-based values (Abernathy & Black, 1996):

- Women: 20–30%

- Men: 12–20%

FFM and body fat mass index-based (Kyle et al., 2003):

- Women: 21.7–33.2%

- Men: 10.8–21.7%

BF% of Elite Olympic Athletes (Fleck, 1983)

- Men in the 100- and 200-meter sprints: 6.5%

- Male boxers and wrestlers: 6.9–7.9%

- Women in the 100-, 200-, and 400-meter sprints: 13.7%

- Canoe and kayak: men 13%; women 22.2%

- Swimmers: men 12.4%; women 19.5%

BF% of Elite-Level Female Physique Competitors (Hulmi et al., 2016)

Amateur female physique competitors in the IFBB, competitors per division: 17 bikini, 9 body fitness, 1 fitness

- Body fat reduction results of a 20-week prep period, from baseline to contest day, according to three different methods:

  - DXA: 23.1 to 12.7%

  - BIA: 19.7 to 11.6%

  - Skinfold: 25.2 to 18.3%

12-Month Body Composition Changes of a Professional Natural Bodybuilder (Rossow et al., 2013)

- At the start of the six-month prep, DXA-measured body comp: 14.8% body fat

- Contest day: 4.5% body fat

- Six months post-contest: 14.6% body fat

Rate of fat loss determines the time frame

In obese populations, rapid initial weight loss has been associated with greater long-term success in weight loss maintenance.[487] The more body fat there is to lose at the outset, the faster weight loss can occur without unfavorable repercussions. However, as dieters get leaner and advance in their training status, rapid rates of weight loss can threaten the preservation of lean mass.[488]

A simple guideline for fat loss aimed at maximally preserving lean mass is 1 to 2 pounds per week (or a decrease of roughly 0.5 to 1 percent of total bodyweight per week).[489] Where you fall within that range depends on your initial body fat level (the more you have, the faster the loss). The 1 to 2 pounds per week figure can be applied to states of overweight and obesity. And keep in mind that while the "per-week" view doesn't seem like much, it's actually on the rapid side when the big picture is considered (26 to 52 pounds a year). Remember that the 1 to 2 pounds per week standard needs to be cut in half (0.5 to 1 pound per week) for estimating rates of fat loss in lean and normal-weight individuals. Box 8i presents a good-case scenario of weight loss for the first six months, starting from a state of obesity.

BOX 8I: REALISTIC RATE OF FAT LOSS

**1–2 pounds/week in those with overweight or obesity;
0.25–0.5 pound/week in lean and normal-weight trainees**

Six-month really good-case scenario, starting with obesity:

Month 1: 3 pounds/week (12 pounds total)

Month 2: 2 pounds/week (8 pounds total)

Months 3–6: 1 pound/week (16 pounds total)

_____

Grand total: 36 pounds

Average monthly loss: 6 pounds

Average weekly loss: 1.5 pounds

It's important to note that this is merely an example of a really good-case scenario. It's impossible for a six-month weight loss curve to be the same for everyone. Some will lose more linearly, and some will experience less linearity. For some, the progress curve will be more dramatic, and for others it will be flatter.

In any case, averaging a 1- to 2-pound loss per week is an excellent rate of progress. Imagine losing 25 to 50 pounds in six to 12 months. That is a tremendous drop by any standard. Consider that it means reversing in six to 12 months what typically took many years (or even decades) to accumulate. So, when setting realistic goals, refer to Boxes 8f and 8g. For realistic time frames, refer to Boxes 8f and 8h. Now let's move on to the next step: setting total daily calories.

STEP 2: SETTING CALORIES

Before we dive in...

I need to cover some background before we start crunching numbers. I'll first relay the conventional approach and then go over my personally developed method, so hopefully you can appreciate the hows and whys underpinning my methods.

The conventional approach to dietary programming is to estimate current calorie needs and then either add or subtract from there. One way to estimate total daily intake is the old-fashioned way, which is to record everything you eat and drink for a number of days (a week is preferable over two to three days, especially if your intake varies from day to day). Take an average of your daily records, and there you have it—an estimation of your maintenance needs. The problem with this method is that merely knowing you're recording everything you eat and drink has the potential to change your behavior, where you subconsciously eat "better" during the journaling process.

The other conventional method of determining total daily caloric needs is typically a three-step process:

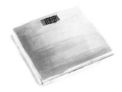

1. Estimate RMR, or run it through one of the standard equations such as the Harris-Benedict or Mifflin St. Jeor (online calculators abound for these). Alternatively, you could multiply your current bodyweight (in pounds) by 10 and arrive at a very similar RMR estimate. One caveat here is that multiplying current bodyweight by 10 is valid for RMR estimations only if your bodyweight is within normal range. Individuals with obesity would need to multiply "ideal" or goal bodyweight by 10 so as not to spuriously skew the estimate upward.

2. Multiply RMR by a physical activity level ranging from 1.2 to 2.2 (sometimes as high as 2.4).[490] Common sedentary physical activity level range is 1.2 to 1.3; moderate activity levels range from 1.4 to 1.7; and high activity levels range from 1.8 to 2.2. After completing this step, you've arrived at an educated guess of your total daily caloric requirement to maintain your current weight.

3. Adjust your maintenance requirement by adding or subtracting calories (typically plus or minus 10 to 20 percent, or about 250 to 500 kcal), depending on your goal. Individuals with obesity can choose to target a 20 to 30 percent deficit since they have more leeway for fat loss without undue lean mass loss. Leave the number as is if you're fine with knowing what theoretically maintains your weight.

There's nothing inherently wrong with this conventional method. To its credit, it has withstood the test of time. However, its shortcomings lie in its subjectivity and lack of precision. Ballparking is OK, but I've found that the conventional method is often skipped over and replaced by quick-and-dirty estimations. If you're going to go through some calculations, they might as well account for a more complete set of variables. Importantly, I prefer basing needs on TBW. Using TBW allows us to set macronutrient and energy intakes based on the maintenance requirements of the status we're aiming to achieve rather than simply imposing an arbitrary surplus or deficit of calories on the present status.

As far as I know, I was the first to develop systematic formulas for determining calorie needs based on TBW and hours of physical activity. These formulas were first made public in my collab with Lou Schuler, *The Lean Muscle Diet*, but a similar version was first available in the February

2011 issue of AARR (my monthly research review). I refined the formulas in the April 2018 issue of AARR, where I was also the first to develop calorie formulas that accounted for training hours, TBW, and NEAT. In this book is the latest refinement of my calorie formulas. They were pretty darn good in 2018, but I found a way to streamline the factoring of NEAT levels.

Target bodyweight (TBW)

A foundational component of my method of estimating calorie needs is determining your TBW. In order to set that goal, it's crucial to get a grip on the stuff you just learned: realistic goals (fat loss or muscle gain) with realistic time frames.

Targeting net amounts of muscle gain or fat loss by settling on a TBW is a little trickier. For muscle gain, I suggest looking ahead a minimum of six to 12 months at a time. For fat loss, I recommend looking ahead at least three to six months. There are two basic methods for determining TBW. The simple way is to recall what you weighed the last time you had the body composition that you liked (Box 8j).

BOX 8J: THE SIMPLE WAY OF DETERMINING TARGET BODYWEIGHT

- Pick an adult bodyweight at which you've been happy with your physique in the past. Remember that changes in LBM can also influence the viability of that target, not just body fat. To keep the target as realistic as possible, keep in mind how your body may have changed over the period between now and when you were at this weight. Don't pick a weight from your teens, because it's possible that you may have gained some skeletal weight (bone density) since then. If you pick a TBW from the peak of your competitive/athletic prime, hey—that's on you. ☺

- This method is straightforward if there actually was a previous point in your adult life when you were satisfied with your weight or body comp. If there was no such point in your past, then you can simply project how much weight change you want to target, referring to Boxes 8f and 8h for realistic time frames in which this can be accomplished.

- If your current weight happens to be your target, that's fine—just stick with that for the calculations.

If the simple method described in Box 8j isn't feasible, then you can take a methodical, stepwise approach to figuring out TBW, which I'll explain next. Please note that this exercise is fun for some but an eye-roller for others who don't enjoy number-crunching. For this reason, I'll reiterate that the simpler way of setting TBW is just fine.

Now, for the more quantitative/analytical types, here are the steps in order—briefly at first (Box 8k), and then I'll cover case examples that go into more detail. I encourage you to plug some different numbers and scenarios into this exercise; it's kind of fun to see where the chips fall total bodyweight–wise for different body composition variations.

BOX 8K: THE METHODICAL WAY OF DETERMINING TARGET BODYWEIGHT (TBW)

1. Calculate your lean body mass (LBM).

2. Select a target LBM, then multiply this number by 100.

3. Select a target BF%, then subtract this number from 100.

4. Divide the result of Step 2 by the result of Step 3 to get your TBW.

We're now going to go through the paces of establishing TBW, then calories and macronutrients, and finally put it into a diet/menu-type format. I can't really call it a diet or menu because it doesn't dictate specific foods. This is a good thing, since it won't anger dietitians too much when trainers/coaches read this book and use my format. Also, note that there is an online calculator to simplify this process (alanaragon.com/calculator), but I'd like you to go through it manually so you can solidify this skill. Without further ado, let's get to know our client/subject/friend, Brody.

Case Subject: Brody

- Healthy adult

- 190 pounds at 20% BF

- Former college athlete

- Training status: intermediate, has kept decent mass, accumulated excess fat

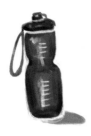

- Total training hours per week: 4

- NEAT level (non-exercise activity): low

- Goal: fat loss

Brody is a middle-aged adult, but I purposely did not bake any presumptions about his age into the programming. Disparities between chronological age and biological age are common. (If I may use myself as an example, I'm 50, but stronger and much more fit than I was at 25—never mind that in terms of emotional maturity, I'm about 18.) My point is that you can easily misprogram or include unnecessary caveats with age-based presumptions. For a child or an elderly person (especially one who's frail or sarcopenic), then a case could be built for special dietary considerations/tactics, but that falls outside the scope of this book.

Brody (like just about everyone) would love to recomp, but I explained to him that at this stage in the game, it would be better for him to focus on one goal at a time since he's an intermediate-level trainee with some lifting experience under his belt. Of the two goals, he leaned more in favor of fat loss. We established the understanding that muscle gains in the midst of accomplishing his goal would be a bonus rather than a purposeful pursuit, but keeping LBM while reducing body fat would be a major win on its own.

Here's an important point I'd really like to drive home when someone is not a complete beginner or completely untrained but has the dual goal of recomp. If the person's desire for fat loss outweighs the desire for muscle gain, it's best to be as cautious as possible when baking LBM gains into the determination of TBW. The safest route is to shoot for maintenance of LBM in order to ensure that a caloric deficit is established. On the other hand, if someone is a complete beginner (or is completely detrained/deconditioned), then you can justify a targeted lean mass that's greater than their current lean mass (refer to Boxes 8f and 8g). For Brody, we are playing it safe.

Step 1: Calculate your LBM. Calculating LBM requires estimating BF%. And yes, it's an estimation, since measuring it directly would involve dissection, which is obviously a deal breaker.

There are several ways to estimate BF%, and all of them—no matter how sophisticated—are ultimately educated guesses. There is no single best method; they all have their strengths and limitations. What matters is choosing the method that's most practical for your circumstances.

In my private practice, I used the three-site digital skinfold calipers by Skyndex and a digital scale. What I liked about calipers was the ability to choose the sites on the body that made most sense to track the progress of. When I moved my practice online, I had my remote clients use girth measurements and a scale and relied more heavily on photos for progress checks.

For now, I'll treat you to something I created in the midst of writing this book. The "android" distribution of body fat is characterized by the greatest concentration of fat storage occurring in the abdominal area. In other words, men tend to wear most of their body fat on their beltline. So, I present to you the proprietary Measurement-Free Body Fat Calculator for Men (Box 8l). Please note that it's not 100 percent serious, but it's surprisingly accurate for the limited range that it covers. I almost didn't include it, but I figure that my audience can handle this level of slapstick.

BOX 8L: MEASUREMENT-FREE BODY FAT CALCULATOR FOR MEN*

- 4–5% – Sharp, crisp six-pack, contest ready, dangerously near death.

- 6–8% – Solid six-pack, all abdominal rows clearly visible, life clearly miserable, camera-ready.

- 9–12% – Softer six-pack, bottom row not as sharp but still visible, no one cares but you.

- 13–16% – Bottom row not visible, "blurry four-pack" of the gods, no one's really impressed, but no one's really offended either.

- 17–20% – Only top row visible, still has plenty of mojo.

- >20% – No visible abs, still has a great personality.

*This is a combination of satire and reality.

Back to Brody. His estimated body fat level is 20 percent. Given his weight of 190 pounds, the calculation to determine LBM looks like this:

190 lbs × 0.20 = 38 lbs fat

190 – 38 = 152 lbs LBM

Step 2: Select a target LBM, then multiply this number by 100. This involves selecting a "target" or goal LBM. Going the conservative route since his primary goal is fat loss, we established that Brody's goal is to keep his LBM, so we simply do the following calculation: 152 × 100 = 15,200.

Step 3: Select a target BF%, then subtract this number from 100.
Brody determined that his goal body fat is 12 percent. So, 100 – 12 = 88.

Step 4: Divide the result of Step 2 by the result of Step 3 to get your TBW.

Here we go, the final step to determining TBW: 15,200 ÷ 88 = 172.7 lbs

Looking at the road in front of Brody, his TBW is about 17 pounds less than his current weight of 190 pounds. Remember that a realistic rate of fat loss is 1 to 2 pounds per week when starting from a state of overweight or obesity. This means that a realistic time frame for Brody to reach his goal is 8.5 to 17 weeks.

In practice, I encourage clients to accept the longer time frame and slower progress rate (1 pound per week) and view it as a bonus if they happen to reach their goal sooner. This keeps expectations realistic and sets people up to succeed without sacrificing undue amounts of muscle mass and quality of life.

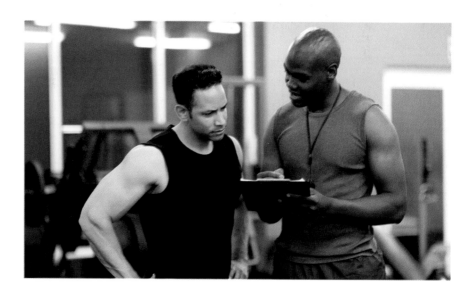

Estimating total calorie requirement based on training volume, TBW, and NEAT

Important notes about formulas: Formulas exist mainly to help people who have a historically haphazard intake or do not have an inkling of the calories that maintain their current or targeted (goal) circumstances. As proud as I am about the formulas I have developed, I have to admit that folks with a keen familiarity of their habitual or historical intake don't need to run them. Formulas are merely ballpark starting points from which to adjust according to individual response. They are not Gospel; in fact, the numbers derived from formulas are hypothetical at best. If the numbers derived from any formula do not sit well with your sensibilities or historically effective intake, then you're free to scrap them or try another approach.

Most formulas are designed to estimate maintenance needs. In order to adjust for weight loss or weight gain, an arbitrary surplus or deficit must be assigned, and it's usually about 250 to 500 kcal up or down. In contrast, my formula (Box 8m) accounts for training volume, NEAT level, and TBW, which can also be thought of as ideal bodyweight. The previous subsection was designed to give you a realistic idea of the total bodyweight you are aiming at based on your targeted body composition. Again, there is an online calculator for my formula for those who need it (alanaragon.com/calculator).

BOX 8M: THE ARAGON FORMULA FOR DETERMINING TOTAL DAILY CALORIES

Step 1:

Do the calculation in parentheses first: TBW x (10 + total weekly training hours)

Step 2:

Multiply the result of Step 1 by the appropriate NEAT factor.

TBW: target bodyweight in pounds

NEAT factor: 1.0, 1.1, 1.2, or 1.4 depending on low, moderate, high, or very high level of non-exercise activity

Step 3:

This is what I call the "fudge factor." If you tend to overestimate your intake while dieting, subtract 10 percent from the total daily caloric target calculated in Step 2. If you tend to underestimate while aiming for gains, add 10 percent to the target calculated in step 2. Otherwise, skip the 10 percent fudge factor.

Step 1: Plug the numbers into the Aragon formula. We'll use Brody's TBW of 172.7 pounds, which I'll round to 173 pounds. Remember to do the calculation in parentheses first and then multiply it by TBW.

Note: When adding up your hours of formal exercise, make sure to include any formal, sweat-inducing cardio or sports as well as resistance training. Well, Brody is a classic "desk jockey" and is very sedentary aside from his gym time, where he averages four training hours per week.

TBW × (10 + total weekly training hours)

173 × (10 + 4)

173 × 14 = 2,422 kcal

Step 2: Multiply the answer arrived at in Step 1 by the NEAT factor that corresponds with your non-exercise activity level, described in Box 8n. Brody has a low NEAT level, so he doesn't have to alter his target of 2,422 kcal. Next comes the process of calculating his macros.

BOX 8N: NEAT LEVELS SPECIFIC TO THE ARAGON FORMULA

Low NEAT: 1.0

Occupation: low movement, mostly sitting, desk work. Life outside of work: low physical activity, mostly sitting or lying around with occasional bouts on your feet for low-intensity tasks. *Note:* The majority of people with fat loss goals fit into this category.

Moderate NEAT: 1.1

Either your job or your home life (but not both) involves moderate physical activity or work on your feet. Or both your job and your time away from work involve a consistent stream of moderate physical activity.

High NEAT: 1.2

Either your job or your home life involves substantial/continuous physical activity (on your feet and moving) aside from formal exercise.

Very High NEAT: 1.4 (or more)

Both your job and your home life involve substantial/continuous, strenuous/exhaustive physical activity aside from formal exercise. If your full-time job involves continuous and strenuous physical labor, you're in this category.

STEPS 3 TO 5: SETTING THE MACROS

The previous chapters covering protein, carbohydrate, and fat had separate summary boxes covering the needs for various populations and goals. Box 80 is a quick-reference summary of the total daily requirement for each macronutrient.

BOX 80: MACRONUTRIENT REQUIREMENTS AND ORDER OF PROGRAMMING STEPS

Note that programming macronutrition involves basing needs on TBW (ideal or goal bodyweight), not current bodyweight, unless maintenance is the goal.

Protein (4 kcal per gram)

- Minimal requirement for the general population without specific athletic or body composition–oriented goals aside from general health: 1.2–1.6 g/kg (0.54–0.7 g/lb)
- General/most commonly applicable range for those engaged in regular exercise: 1.6–2.2 g/kg (0.7–1 g/lb)
- Pushing the envelope of muscle gain or retention under physiologically stressful circumstances (i.e., athletic competition combined with hypocaloric conditions): 2.2–3.3 g/kg (1–1.5 g/lb)

Carbohydrate (4 kcal per gram)

- Individuals without athletic performance goals have no minimum dosing requirement. Carbohydrate needs vary widely according to total energy requirements, personal preference, and tolerance.
- Individuals seeking to optimally support strength/power demands and/or hypertrophy goals: 3–8 g/kg (1.4–3.6 g/lb) of total bodyweight
- Athletes seeking to optimize performance in sports with endurance demands: 6–12 g/kg (2.7–5.4 g/lb) of total bodyweight

Fat (9 kcal per gram)

Catchall range based on personal preference, tolerance, and goal: 0.7–2.2 g/kg (0.32–1 g/lb)

Order of programming (from Boxes 8a and 8b)*

1. Set the goal and time frame.
2. Set calories.
3. Set protein.
4. Set fat.
5. Fill in the remainder with carbohydrate.

*If athletic performance is of primary importance, you'd swap steps 4 and 5, calculating carbohydrate needs first and then filling in the remaining calories with fat.

How to build a plan

Protein

In Brody's case, he wants fat loss first and foremost, but he also wants more muscle. We know that recomp is possible in intermediates, but it's not a pragmatic goal to actively pursue. Still, higher protein intakes increase the chances of recomp happening in resistance trainees. My executive decision is to assign him 2.2 g/kg (1 g/lb). A high protein intake will help control hunger and maximally preserve lean mass (and in this case, possibly facilitate muscle growth as a bonus). Remember the programming theme of using TBW in pounds. Brody's TBW is 173, so our calculation is 173 × 1 = 173 grams of protein. To calculate the number of calories in this amount of protein, we simply multiply that number by 4, as follows: 173 × 4 = 692 kcal.

Fat

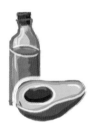

At this point, let me remind you that if we were creating a program for a competitive athlete with specific performance goals, we'd set the carb target before setting the fat target. This is not the case with Brody. Based on his preference for a moderate amount of fat, I'm shooting just under the midpoint of the 0.7 to 2.2 g/kg (0.32 to 1 g/lb) range and setting fat at 0.6 g/lb. Brody's TBW is 173, so our calculation is 173 × 0.6 = 103.8 grams of fat, which I'll round to 104 grams. To calculate fat calories, we multiply fat grams by 9, as follows: 104 × 9 = 936 kcal.

Carbohydrate

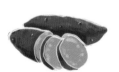

Programming carbohydrate in Brody's case is a matter of filling in the remaining calories with carbohydrate. We figure carbohydrate grams in the reverse order of the other macros, which are figured first in grams and then in calories. With carbs, we figure calories, and then we can calculate grams. In other words, we add up the protein and fat calories and subtract that number from the total caloric requirement (in Brody's case, it's 2,422 kcal), and then we convert that calorie number to carb grams by dividing by 4 (since carbs have 4 calories per gram). It sounds more complicated than it actually is. Here are the steps:

First we add up protein and fat kcals:

692 + 936 = 1,628 kcal

Then we subtract this number from total daily calories (2,422 kcal) to figure carbohydrate calories, which we then divide by 4 to arrive at carbohydrate grams:

2,422 – 1,628 = 794 kcal

794 ÷ 4 = 198.5 g, which I'll round to 198 g.

And we're done. Here are Brody's targets:

- Total daily calories: 2,422 kcal

- Protein: 173 g

- Carbs: 198 g

- Fat: 104 g

Note: If you math-out these macros (4 kcal/g of protein and carbohydrate, 9 kcal/g of fat), you'll find that they amount to 2,420 kcal rather than 2,422 kcal. This is due to rounding the macronutrient grams in the calculation process. Since the difference is too minuscule to matter, and it's virtually impossible to nail the caloric total exactly every day, I'll list the original target (2,422 kcal) in the following plan.

Establishing calories and macros is typically the final step for coaches, aside from delivering general guidance on how to hit those macros by the end of the day. While there's nothing inherently wrong with just having a set of macros to hit, it can help to get an idea of how to construct a more concrete plan, or a framework that involves foods.

The way I format my clients' diets is another unique development from my decades in practice. I have never been a fan of handing clients menus listing specific foods to eat. Instead, I prefer to allow them the freedom of choice across the food groups, within "floating" meals and snacks, while meeting certain serving targets per food group. What follows is how Brody's plan looks in the way I format diets for clients as well as research subjects.

Brody's plan

Targeted total: 2,422 kcal, 173 g P, 198 g C, 104 g F

FLOATING MEAL A: 401 kcal, 22 g P, 40 g C, 17 g F

- 3 whole eggs, any style (or) 6 egg whites + 1/2 medium avocado (or) 3 ounces meat, fish, or poultry of any fat level (or) 1 scoop protein powder (in water) + 2 tbsp nut butter, any type (or) 1 scoop protein powder + 2 tbsp nuts (a scant handful), any type

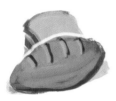

- 2 slices of bread, any type (or) 3/4 cup dry ready-to-eat cereal, any type (or) 3/4 cup cooked starch such as rice, pasta, peas, beans, corn, oatmeal, or grits (or) 1 medium or 2 small (egg-size) potato(es), ~6 ounces (or) ~160 kcal of your favorite cereal grain product (or) 160 "wildcard" kcal

- Nonstarchy veggies can be added if/as desired; shoot for at least 3 servings per day (a serving of fibrous veggies is ~1 cup raw or 1/2 cup cooked).

FLOATING MEAL B: 587 kcal, 46 g P, 40 g C, 27 g F

- 6 ounces lean meat or poultry (or) 6 ounces fish, any type (or) 2 cups tofu, firm (or) 3.5 veggie patties (or) 2 scoops protein powder + 2 tbsp nuts (a scant handful), any type (or) 2 scoops protein powder + 1 tbsp nut butter, any type

- 2 slices of bread, any type (or) 3/4 cup dry ready-to-eat cereal, any type (or) 3/4 cup cooked starch such as rice, pasta, peas, beans, corn, oatmeal, or grits (or) 1 medium or 2 small (egg-size) potato(es), ~6 ounces (or) ~160 kcal of your favorite cereal grain product (or) 160 "wildcard" kcal

- Nonstarchy veggies can be added if/as desired; shoot for at least 3 servings per day (a serving of fibrous veggies is ~1 cup raw or 1/2 cup cooked).

FLOATING SNACKS: 835 kcal, 60 g P, 70 g C, 35 g F *(Note that these can go anywhere in the day, or you may add them, either separately or in combination, to either lunch or dinner.)*

- 3 servings of milk, yogurt, and/or cheese, any fat level; 1 serving = 1 cup milk (or) 3/4 cup yogurt (or) 1 ounce cheese, any type (double up or mix/match any of these choices)

- 3 servings of fruit; 1 serving = 1 large fruit, any type, such as an apple, banana, or orange (or) 1.5 cups chopped fresh fruit (or) 1/4 cup dried fruit (or) 2 small fruits, any type, such as apricots, figs, kiwis, or tangerines

- 6 ounces lean meat or poultry (or) 6 ounces fish, any type (or) 2 scoops protein powder + 2 tbsp nuts (a scant handful), any type (or) 2 scoops protein powder + 1 tbsp nut butter, any type

- 1/4 cup nuts, any type (or) 2 tbsp nut butter, any type (or) 1/2 small avocado

FLOATING MEAL C: 597 kcal, 45 g P, 48 g C, 25 g F

- 6 ounces lean meat or poultry (or) 6 ounces fish, any type (or) 2 cups tofu, firm (or) 2 scoops protein powder + 2 tbsp nuts (a scant handful), any type (or) 3.5 veggie patties (or) 2 scoops protein powder + 1 tbsp nut butter, any type

- 2 slices of bread, any type (or) 3/4 cup dry ready-to-eat cereal, any type (or) 3/4 cup cooked starch such as rice, pasta, peas, beans, corn, oatmeal, or grits (or) 1 medium or 2 small (egg-size) potato(es), ~6 ounces (or) ~160 kcal of your favorite cereal grain product (or) 160 "wildcard" kcal

- Nonstarchy veggies can be added if/as desired; shoot for at least 3 servings per day (a serving of fibrous veggies is ~1 cup raw or 1/2 cup cooked).

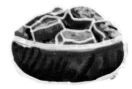

Simplifying the process

Let's run through another scenario. I'll streamline it this time with less commentary so you can see the uninterrupted flow of the process. Meet Brenda, who is a beginner; completely untrained. She too wants to lose fat and gain muscle, but she is in a better position to do so by virtue of her newbie training status. Notice in the following description that I put "projected" training hours per week since she is starting from zero.

Case Subject: Brenda

- Healthy adult

- 145 pounds at 35% BF

- Training status: untrained/complete beginner

- Total (projected) training hours per week: 4

- NEAT level (non-exercise activity): low

- Goals: fat loss (primary), muscle gain (secondary)

Step 1: Calculate your LBM. Calculating LBM requires estimating BF%. Since Brenda has 35 percent body fat and weighs 145, the calculation is:

145 lbs × 0.35 = 50.75 lbs fat

145 − 50.75 = 94.25 lbs LBM

Step 2: Select a target LBM, then multiply this number by 100. This involves selecting a "target" or goal LBM. Because Brenda is an untrained newbie with muscle gain as a secondary goal, we can refer to Box 8g and target a three-month estimation of 3 pounds. This is a relatively bold target as she won't be in a caloric surplus, but it's still realistic, and we're going to go for it. This brings her target LBM from 94.25 to 97.25. Multiplying this by 100, we get 9,725.

Step 3: Select a target BF%, then subtract this number from 100. Brenda determined that her goal body fat is 25 percent. So, 100 − 25 = 75.

Step 4: Divide the result of Step 2 by the result of Step 3 to get your TBW. Final step: 9,725 ÷ 75 = 129.6, which I'll round to 130 pounds.

Brenda's TBW is 15 pounds less than her current weight of 145. Since a realistic rate of fat loss is 1 to 2 pounds per week when starting from a state of overweight or obesity, a realistic time frame for Brenda is 7.5 to 15 weeks. Again, I prefer to set clients up to accept the longer time frame and slower progress rate (1 pound per week) and encourage them to view it as a bonus if they happen to reach the goal sooner. Now we can proceed by plugging the numbers into the Aragon Formula, doing the calculation within parentheses first:

TBW × (10 + total weekly training hours)

130 × (10 + 4)

130 × 14 = 1,820 kcal

The next step is to multiply this number by a NEAT factor, but because it's 1.0 for the Low NEAT level, we can leave it as is. The next step is to fill it in with macros.

Protein

The optimal range for protein intake is 1.6 to 2.2 g/kg (0.7 to 1 g/lb). I chose 0.9 g/lb as a realistic target for Brenda. She wants recomp, so we're going high, but she's accustomed to a low protein intake, so we're not going to do the upper end. The calculation is as follows: 130 × 0.9 = 117 g. Protein is 4 calories per gram, so figuring protein calories is as follows: 117 × 4 = 468 kcal.

Fat

Based on Brenda's preference for a moderately high fat intake (the range is 0.32 to 1 g/lb), we're setting fat at 0.7 g/lb. Her TBW is 130 pounds, so our calculation is 130 × 0.7 = 91 grams of fat. Since fat is 9 calories per gram, calculating fat calories is as follows: 91 × 9 = 819 kcal.

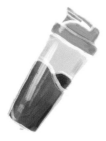

Carbohydrate

Now we simply fill the remaining calories with carbohydrate.

First, we add up the protein and fat kcals:

468 + 819 = 1,287 kcal

Then we subtract this number from total daily calories (1,820 kcal) to figure carbohydrate calories, which we divide by 4 to arrive at carbohydrate grams:

1,820 – 1,287 = 533 kcal

533 ÷ 4 = 133.25 g (I'll round this to 133 g)

And we're done. Here are Brenda's targets:

- Total daily calories: 1,820 kcal

- Protein: 117 g

- Carbs: 133 g

- Fat: 91 g

Note: If you math-out the macros above, you'll find that they amount to 1,819 kcal rather than 1,820 kcal; this is due to rounding the macronutrient grams in the calculation process. Since the difference is minuscule, and it's virtually impossible to nail the caloric total exactly every day anyway, I'll list it as the original target (1,820 kcal) in the following plan.

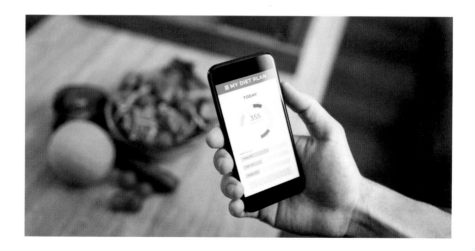

Brenda's plan

Targeted totals: 1,820 kcal, 117 g P, 133 g C, 91 g F

FLOATING MEAL A: 472 kcal, 23 g P, 41 g C, 24 g F

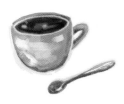

- Coffee + 1/4 cup half-and-half.

- 3 whole eggs, any style (or) 6 egg whites + 1/2 medium avocado (or) 3 ounces meat, fish, or poultry, any type (or) 1 scoop protein powder + 1 tbsp nut butter, any type (or) 1 scoop protein powder + 2 tbsp nuts (a scant handful), any type

- 2 slices of bread, any type (or) 3/4 cup dry ready-to-eat cereal, any type (or) 3/4 cup cooked starch such as rice, pasta, peas, beans, corn, oatmeal, or grits (or) 1 medium or 2 small (egg-size) potato(es), ~6 ounces (or) ~160 kcal of your favorite cereal grain product (or) 160 "wildcard" kcal

- Nonstarchy veggies can be added if/as desired; shoot for at least 3 servings per day (a serving of fibrous veggies is ~1 cup raw or 1/2 cup cooked).

FLOATING MEAL B: 450 kcal, 32 g P, 40 g C, 18 g F

- 4 ounces meat, fish, or poultry, any type (or) 1.5 cups tofu, firm (or) 2.5 veggie patties (or) 1.5 scoops protein powder + 2 tbsp nuts (a scant handful), any type (or) 1.5 scoops protein powder + 1 tbsp nut butter, any type

- 2 slices of bread, any type (or) 3/4 cup dry ready-to-eat cereal, any type (or) 3/4 cup cooked starch such as rice, pasta, peas, beans, corn, oatmeal, or grits (or) 1 medium or 2 small (egg-size) potato(es), ~6 ounces (or) ~160 kcal of your favorite cereal grain product (or) 160 "wildcard" kcal

- Nonstarchy veggies can be added if/as desired; shoot for at least 3 servings per day (a serving of fibrous veggies is ~1 cup raw or 1/2 cup cooked).

FLOATING SNACKS: 491 kcal, 20 g P, 42 g C, 27 g F *(Note that these can go anywhere in the day, or you may add them, either separately or in combination, to either lunch or dinner.)*

- 2 servings of milk, yogurt, and/or cheese, any fat level; 1 serving = 1 cup milk (or) 3/4 cup yogurt (or) 1 ounce cheese, any type (double up or mix/match any of these choices)

- 2 servings of fruit; 1 serving = 1 large fruit, such as an apple, banana, or orange (or) 1.5 cups chopped fresh fruit (or) 1/4 cup dried fruit (or) 2 small fruits, any type, such as apricots, figs, tangerines, or kiwis

- 1/4 cup nuts, any type (or) 2 tbsp nut butter, any type (or) 1/2 small avocado

FLOATING MEAL C: 406 kcal, 42 g P, 10 g C, 22 g F

- 6 ounces meat, fish, or poultry, any type (or) 2 cups tofu, firm (or) 2 scoops protein powder + 2 tbsp nuts (a scant handful), any type (or) 3.5 veggie patties (or) 2 scoops protein powder + 1 tbsp nut butter, any type

- Nonstarchy veggies can be added if/as desired; shoot for at least 3 servings per day (a serving of fibrous veggies is ~1 cup raw or 1/2 cup cooked).

Notes about Brody and Brenda's plans

Note that it says "(or)" in the bullet points

At first glance, the plan looks like a mountain of food. However, each meal is a set of bullet points with several serving equivalents to choose from. You get one choice per point. I attempted to offer choices that are macronutritionally similar, but that's not always possible—and that's fine. What matters is that you adopt an effective pattern that you can follow consistently.

Also, Brody's and Brenda's plans are just two examples of many possibilities, depending on individual goals and circumstances. Resist the natural tendency to think of them as archetypical or model programs. Individuals vary widely in their needs; some men might need fewer calories than Brody, and some women might need more calories than Brenda.

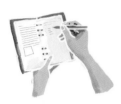

Grouping and separating the meals and their components

I can't emphasize enough how this diet plan is a flexible example of how to cover your dietary bases and hit the various targets of the program. I split it into three meals and a set of floating snacks as a baseline suggestion that happens to work well. You are free to move the meals (and bullet points) around as you wish. If you want to group together all of your assigned bullet points into a total of two meals per day, have at it. You probably wouldn't want to attempt to do it all in one meal, but in theory, you could, if that's what makes you consistently feel and perform best.

Optional indulgence leeway

If/when desired, you may substitute one or more of the starch bullet points with a 160-kcal "wildcard." This includes desserts and alcohol—basically whatever you intuitively perceive as junk food or a source of empty or "naughty" calories. Brody's plan contains optional wildcards in meals A, B, and C, amounting to a maximum of 480 kcal per day. Brenda's plan contains optional wildcards in meals A and B, amounting to a maximum of 320 kcal per day. Both of these optional "indulgence" allotments fall within the guideline of discretionary calories comprising 20 percent or less of the total.

Measuring

Weighing food is not necessary (unless you insist, in which case I won't stop you), but use measuring cups whenever possible for at least the first two weeks. This will give you an objective perspective of what the targeted portion size should be. Once you have a good idea of ounce estimates for meat, etc., you can use the area and thickness of your open palm to represent 5 to 7 ounces and your four fingers to represent 3 to 4 ounces. You might also notice that the fat amounts per meal are slightly higher than the foods let on. I do this on purpose because a nominal amount of fat will be used for cooking or dressing.

Ballparking

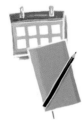

Not every meal you run into while you're out and about will fit nicely into the outlined format. Use your best judgment to stick as closely to the format of the scheduled meal as you can. If there's a significant deviation, make a note of it in your records.

Fluid intake

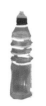

Drink a minimum of 4 cups of fluid (about 1 liter, or 32 ounces) per day. Unsweetened tea, coffee, and noncaloric beverages count toward this total. An easy way to individualize and autoregulate fluid intake is to consume at least three "water meals" throughout the course of the day, where you drink to comfortable fullness each time. Note that this is in addition to the fluid you consume during training.

Fibrous/nonstarchy vegetables

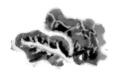

There is no limit to the amount of fibrous and nonstarchy vegetables you may consume, since they contain only minor amounts of metabolizable energy. Furthermore, attempting to eat a ton of them tends to displace other foods that are more calorically dense. I'm therefore not worried about excessive veggie intake. Note that fibrous vegetables may be added to any meal and consumed at any point in the day. The goal is to get a minimum of three servings per day.

Nonstarchy veggies

- All leafy greens
- All lettuces
- All peppers
- All sprouts
- Artichokes
- Arugula
- Asparagus
- Bok choi

- Broccoli
- Brussels sprouts
- Cabbage
- Carrots
- Cauliflower
- Celery
- Collards
- Cucumbers

- Dandelion greens
- Garlic
- Green beans
- Kale
- Leeks
- Mushrooms
- Mustard greens

- Onions
- Radishes
- Spinach
- String beans
- Tomatoes
- Zucchini

Additional notes

It's understood that inconsistencies in food availability may result in differences between what's on the plan and what you actually consume. It's also understood that it's nearly impossible to hit the precise gram targets of protein, carbohydrate, and fat each day. The goal is to stay in the ballpark. If you do, you will knock your goals out of the ballpark.

Notes on trial and adjustment

Putting a plan to trial involves a consistent and focused effort to hit the assigned targets. It's worth reiterating that the goal is to stay in the ballpark, not obsess over perfection. When putting a plan to trial, the "golden" time frame is one month. Weight/fat loss time frames are the same for men and women: 1–2 pounds per week from a starting point of overweight or obesity.

Despite this weekly outlook for weight loss, I recommend withholding judgment until the one-month mark. In people who menstruate, body water shifts due to the menstrual cycle can yield deceptive scale changes if a comparison is made between different points of a given month. Otherwise, a case can be made for making adjustments to a program that doesn't yield adequate progress in the first two weeks (especially if there is a particularly urgent deadline for the results).

Still, my preference leans toward putting programs to trial for a full month before coming to conclusions. If the rate of progress at four weeks is sufficient, the move is simple: keep the program the same. If fat loss shows signs of slowing, I recommend riding that progress into a bona fide plateau, which is four full weeks of stagnation, before making program adjustments to re-establish a caloric deficit. The specifics of handling progress plateaus are discussed in the next chapter.

CHAPTER 8 IN A NUTSHELL

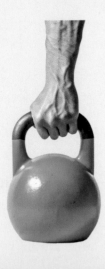

- My quantitative dietary programming approach involves first setting the goal and time frame, then calories, then protein, and then the other macronutrients. Athletic goals require prioritizing carbohydrate programming before fat programming (refer to Boxes 8a and 8b).

- Training status in physique development is difficult to determine due to an abundance of subjectivity. However, FFMI thresholds can serve as a rough screening tool for assessing how close you are to your potential for muscle growth. Of course, there are a lot of caveats that I encourage you to review.

- From a programming perspective, recomposition (simultaneous fat loss and muscle gain) is better considered a bonus rather than a targeted pursuit. Exceptions are beginning trainees and formerly fit folks with excess body fat. Boxes 8c and 8d summarize the hierarchy of recomp capacity and the steps to maximize the likelihood of recomp, respectively.

- Men have the (natural) potential to gain ~17 to 24 percent more muscle when starting from an untrained state. Women have the (natural) potential to gain ~16 to 25 percent more muscle when starting from an untrained state (see Box 8e). Men and women have similar proportional gains, although the net amounts differ.

- A realistic perspective of progress rate is crucial for maintaining motivation and mitigating frustration. A simple guideline for rate of muscle growth in intermediates and beginners is 1 to 2 pounds per month. Women have a similar proportional rate of muscle growth to men, but net amounts are about 30 percent less (see Boxes 8f and 8g).

- Normal/healthy body fat levels for women in the general population range from 20 to 30 percent. Normal/healthy body fat levels for men in the general population range from 10 to 20 percent. See Box 8h for the body fat ranges of an assortment of athlete populations.

- A simple guideline for fat loss aimed at maximally preserving lean mass is 1 to 2 pounds per week (or roughly 0.5 to 1 percent of total bodyweight decrease per week). The more starting body fat you have, the faster the loss (see Box 8i).

- Setting calories can be done in a number of ways. I go over the traditional way and then a method I originated that factors in TBW, weekly training hours, and non-exercise activity thermogenesis (NEAT).

- The case studies of Brody and Brenda illustrate the finer points of my method of programming. Also note that there is an online calculator for my formula (alanaragon.com/calculator).

ADHERENCE, MAINTENANCE & WEANING OFF OF TRACKING

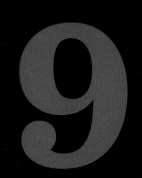

I'm going to shift gears and return to speaking in general terms. It's tough, but we have to let go of Brody and Brenda for the time being. This is the final leg of the journey where we discuss the work involved with living happily ever after. That begins with dietary adherence to the program. A step beyond that is adherence to the successful habits that the program is designed to nurture.

When we think of "The Program," it's usually a script printed out on a piece of paper that you attempt to follow to the letter. That's fine for the short term, but the long term is a whole different animal.

We'll first cover adherence to the scripted program. Then we'll cover how to sustain successful habits that facilitate the "weaning off" of micromanagement (quantifying and tracking everything). Let's be clear: the latter is beneficial—at least initially. However, for most people, a life that involves constant daily monitoring of calories and macros is somewhere between unideal and a miserable existence.

Some people love attempting to quantify everything and actually enjoy the micromanagement. (I know and love some of you.) Some use several apps and devices to track every bodily process. I'm not against these apps and devices. In fact, much of the literature is in favor of monitoring in some shape or form. What I am against is the monitoring instruments owning and controlling a person instead of vice versa. Now that I've rustled some jimmies, let's talk about adherence.

DIETARY ADHERENCE

Adherence is everything. A program or plan is only as good as its ability to be followed for the length of time intended. We've all heard some version of the disappointing failure rate among dieters driving the general belief that diets don't work. I think that's a needlessly pessimistic oversimplification. I would modify it to say that cookie-cutter, one-approach-fits-all diets lack sustainability, and these are what comprise the majority of dieting attempts by the confused general public.

So, yes, it's true; the success rate is dismal. A review by Wing and Phelan[491] reported that the collective evidence shows weight loss maintainers comprise only about 20 percent of dieters, and the other 80 percent fail. The reasons for this are complex and under intense investigation. If we had easy answers or simple culprits, then the problem wouldn't be so durable and prevalent. Are we simply wired to fail? Are we doomed to suffer the injustice of biology? I'll do my best to settle that next.

Nature versus nurture: bodyweight set point and "settling" point

Keesey and Boyle[492] deserve credit for pioneering the concept of bodyweight set point a half century ago. They found that lateral hypothalamic lesions in rats result in a tenacious defense of altered bodyweight in the face of attempts at various feeding challenges to disrupt maintenance. These findings spawned the set point theory that bodyweight is genetically predetermined and cannot be altered outside of (unfeasible) changes in hardwired hormonal and neurological circuits.

However, a stiff challenge to set point theory was made in a classic 1977 paper by Wirtshafter and Davis,[493] who were among the first to discuss the concept of a *settling point* determined by habits and environment—which includes sensory stimulation via dietary palatability. These researchers were way ahead of their time. Given a certain degree of control over our environment, the so-called settling point is not entirely out of our control. It doesn't carry the implication of predestiny like set point does. I'll quote the crux of their position, which I find to be eloquent and well reasoned:

"If bodyweight is regulated by an internal set point mechanism, one naturally wonders why it is singularly ineffective in maintaining a constant weight in the face of altered dietary palatability. Rejection of a set point concept of weight regulation would have the additional advantage of resolving the problem of an animal's willingness to ingest highly palatable substances in the absence of deprivation. [...] Since it is widely recognized that input from gustatory, olfactory and other sensory systems play a central role in the control of ingestion, and hence bodyweight, it seems essential that such an input should be an important element of any weight control model."

Wirtshafter and Davis's perspective of the influence of hyperpalatable/ultra-processed foods on eating behavior and obesity didn't come to be fully appreciated until nearly four decades later, when interest in factors influencing food reward and the food environment really started gaining momentum.[494-496]

A contemporary perspective of the set point versus settling point debate was presented in a recent review paper by Müller and colleagues,[497] which discusses what British biologist John Speakman calls the "dual intervention point model." This model does a good job of reconciling the apparent conflict between the set point and settling point paradigms. A simplified interpretation of their view is that biology predetermines upper and lower limits of bodyweight gain and loss. However, the particular *settling point* between those limits is determined by behavioral interaction with environmental factors. (Of course, this includes food and what we do with it on a habitual basis.)

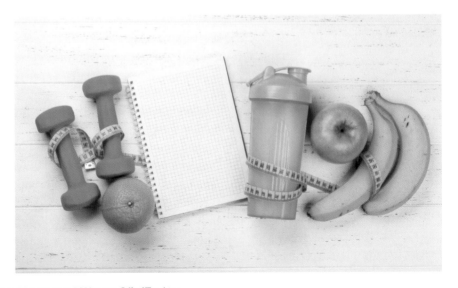

The state of the scientific literature on adherence

After poring through the literature on dietary adherence, I'm amazed at how visionary a classic review by Sherman and colleagues[498] has proven to be based on echoes of its messages through the subsequent literature.[499,500] Despite it being one of the very first peer-reviewed publications on this topic, Sherman's assessment of the issue and potential solutions rings true to current research—with the bonus of being more straightforwardly written than many of its successors. The barriers to changing/improving adverse dietary behaviors are as follows:

- **(Poor) decision-making.** The multitude of food choices and mixed media messages cause confusion and doubt, ultimately adding difficulty to the process of changing habits.

- **Social and cultural forces.** Social, cultural, and religious practices steeped in tradition and inherent pressure to perpetuate these practices can serve as stiff barriers to dietary change.

- **Perceptions and preferences.** The way individuals perceive personal choice or deprivation of food choices can also serve as a barrier to change.

- **Cultural and environmental barriers.** Cost and availability of food are, in many cases, nonnegotiable and insurmountable barriers.

Here are the proposed strategies to breach these barriers to dietary change:

- **Education.** Knowledge of the science-based rationale behind adopting and maintaining certain dietary habits can serve as a motivator to execute and sustain changes.

- **Motivation.** Approaches that empower individuals via helping them identify and "own" the benefits and gains in self-efficacy associated with changed habits can be effective for overcoming barriers to change.

- **Behavioral skills.** Cognitive skills, relapse prevention tactics, and the attainment of social support are helpful in breaking barriers that prevent dietary change. Again, we see social and emotional support implicated as a key player in successful models of habit change.

- **Availability of new/modified foods.** This tactic refers mainly to lower-calorie versions of foods that are deal breakers in typical serving amounts. This paper shows a bit of its age by giving examples of low-fat versions of high-fat foods.

- **Supportive personal interactions.** Social interactions and feedback from others can provide a potent combination of accountability and camaraderie, ultimately facilitating change.

Two decades have flown by since this paper dropped, and the population's collective body composition and health have continued to worsen. Apparently, the wisdom of Sherman and colleagues stayed locked up in the PubMed vault and didn't reverberate loudly enough. A recent ray of hope comes from Spreckley and colleagues,[501] who systematically reviewed qualitative studies on successful long-term weight loss maintenance. Here's a summary of their findings:

- **The effectiveness of continuous monitoring** (divided into self-monitoring and external monitoring) was most consistently mentioned throughout all studies. Subjects consistently stated that having clear monitoring tools for both weight loss and weight loss maintenance helped with focus and accountability.

- **Intrinsic and extrinsic motivators** were important for keeping subjects on track and motivated to sustain weight loss maintenance. Although intrinsic motivators (e.g., the desire to improve health, self-esteem, and self-reinvention) were the primary drivers, extrinsic motivators (e.g., enhancing of social standing and acceptance and career and sports opportunities) also played a critical role.

- **Goal-setting** was most effective for weight loss maintenance when it was clear, personalized, and continuously adjusted. Personalized goals that were self-defined had a greater impact on weight loss maintenance than externally defined goals. Externally defined goals (e.g., sports events and organized challenges involving community or peer accountability) were important but not essential.

- **Enduring/emerging from challenges**—both internal and external—is a constant battle that threatens sustained weight loss maintenance.

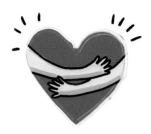

On the intrinsic front, the struggle to keep a focused and productive emotional state in the face of major life events and everyday stresses is an ongoing threat to weight loss maintenance. Extrinsic challenges such as work, relationships, holidays/celebrations, and the obesogenic environment (characterized by high availability of energy-dense, hyperpalatable foods that are easily overconsumed) must be endured while simultaneously managing internal challenges on an ongoing basis for weight loss maintenance to be achieved.

- **The overall experience of weight loss maintainers was diverse,** encompassing encouraging and discouraging elements that varied widely according to individual circumstances. Encouraging experiences included finding a new sense of purpose, new opportunities, and new sense of identity. Discouraging experiences included the nagging fear of weight regain and feelings of deprivation, loneliness, frustration, and fatigue.

- **Lessons and caveats learned from weight regainers** include the motivational challenge of tracking intake (which often gets deprioritized), lack of planning, lack of dedicating time to exercise, difficulty of putting weight loss goals above social/peer pressure, frustration from weight fluctuations, self-esteem drops, and binging.

Ironically, the research literature is rich with understanding of the problems driving a lack of adherence (along with proposed solutions). However, public health messages, which are largely based on the research literature, have not been delivered effectively.

I still think we (health/fitness practitioners and enthusiasts) can cause a large enough ripple in *The Force* to make a real difference. As I mentioned in the initial pages, I would like to think that this book can be the flap of a butterfly's wings described by meteorologist Edward Lorenz, who posited that a minuscule change in the state of the atmosphere could initiate a sequence of events responsible for massive changes in weather across the globe.[502] In the forthcoming sections, I'll discuss various aspects of what I consider to be the "secret" weapon of adherence and program success in general: individualization. Before I dive into the avenues of individualization, though, I'd like to clear up the confusion at the root of the ongoing obesity debate.

There's a never-ending battle of ideas about what to blame for the global obesity problem. Too often, the influence of calories is erroneously eschewed in favor of pointing the finger at food types (e.g., fast food), food groups (e.g., grains and starchy foods), single macronutrients (e.g., carbohydrate), and macronutrient subtypes (e.g., sugar). This reductionism has even gone as far as blaming a single monosaccharide (e.g., fructose) or a single fatty acid type (e.g., linoleic acid). It's frankly ridiculous.

Those familiar with the anti-carb campaign in pop-diet culture are undoubtedly familiar with the scapegoating of a single hormone (insulin) as the driver of obesity—which is yet another erroneous claim.[59,503,504] The thoroughly debunked carbohydrate-insulin hypothesis claims that obesity is a hormonally based condition that has little to do with calories. Of course this is absurd, but it's the default position of folks who have yet to grasp the full picture. I'd guess that roughly 99.9 percent of the debates (online and elsewhere) surrounding the culprits responsible for obesity could be resolved with a simple delineation between the root cause (sustained positive caloric balance) and the *influencing factors* (a multitude). Figure 9a outlines these elements and clarifies this important delineation.

Figure 9a: Resolving the Obesity Blame Game: Root Cause & Influencing Factors

Definition of obesity

- The state of having excess body fat

- The quantitative definition based on BMI (≥30) is a crude measure of adiposity limited to the general population.

- BMI should not be strictly applied to individuals since it tends to overestimate adiposity in athletes, especially those with a high degree of muscle mass.

Root cause of obesity

- Net energy surplus over time. In other words, a positive caloric balance (more energy consumed than expended) sustained over the long term. Obesity is the result of an excessive accumulation of body fat storage.

- A multitude of factors can influence the occurrence and progression of a net energy surplus.

Factors influencing the root cause of obesity

- Physical activity level (exercise and non-exercise physical activity)

- Sleep quality and quantity (influences appetite and energy expenditure)

- Food environment: prevalence and accessibility of energy-dense, highly processed/refined, hyperpalatable foods

- Genetic predisposition (influences the hormonal milieu, which in turn can affect appetite and energy expenditure)

- Socioeconomic status (affects the level of nutrition education and affordability of nutritious foods instead of convenience-driven, energy-dense fast foods or packaged snack foods and beverages)

- Disease state, including chronic, metabolic, orthopedic, and psychological pathologies

- Diet composition and quality (affects satiety, training support, and adherence)

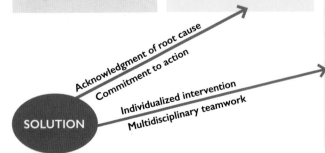

Acknowledgment of root cause
Commitment to action
Individualized intervention
Multidisciplinary teamwork

SOLUTION

INDIVIDUALIZATION: A POWERFUL YET UNDERRATED ADHERENCE DRIVER

If I could boil down the secret ingredient—the most potent weapon in the adherence arsenal—it would be individualization. And not just at the start, but on a continuing basis to support evolving goals and preferences. It's the missing link between doing great on a program for 21 days versus 21 years.

Individualization is the focus of the entire chapter on programming. It's probably easy to miss that while concentrating on the details and flow of the methods/calculations. The reason individualization is so powerful is because it fulfills not just the physical needs of the dieter but also the fundamental psychological needs.

Self-determination theory has fascinated me for a while, especially since I've been able to apply some of its core principles to dietary programming and coaching. According to self-determination theory, humans universally have three basic psychological needs:[505]

- **Competence** refers to the need for attaining mastery over a particular skill or skill set in order to achieve desired outcomes.

- **Relatedness** is the need to coexist harmoniously within a social structure.

- **Autonomy** is the need for a sense of self-direction, self-regulation, and personal agency or control.

Each of these basic needs serendipitously clicks with the tools of program individualization. In the context of health and fitness, individuals gain competence when they progress through the process of learning why certain foods in certain amounts affect their bodies in directions toward or away from the goals at hand. A sense of competence can also come from becoming more adept at eyeballing portions, progressing in exercise performance, or improving aspects of body composition.

The role of relatedness in the success of a program comes from the nurturing and strengthening of intra- and interpersonal accountability. It also comes from the camaraderie and fun of sharing experiences with others along a similar journey. Methods of fulfilling the need for relatedness can be individualized based on one's social proclivities and preferred environments and activities. Purposeful introspective efforts for getting to know oneself can be considered a form of relatedness.

Autonomy shares parallels with competence with the subtle but important distinction that the choices and leadership maneuvers are made by the individual rather than other people or forces in the environment. In the context of dietary programming, giving the individual the power to choose their personally preferred foods in their personally preferred combinations, distribution, and timing throughout the day or week is a tremendous way to nurture a sense of autonomy. When you read the details of Brody's diet plan as well as the notes following it, you'll notice that it strongly facilitates autonomous control. Giving people the tools and knowledge to self-actualize along their journey substantially increases their chances of adherence (and protection from the fabled 80 percent failure rate). So, let's talk more about those tools and tactics.

Individualizing macronutrition

I'll start by discussing research challenging the superiority of permitting dieters to have personal choice. A 48-week trial by Yancy and colleagues[506] reported no significant weight loss advantage between choosing one of two diet options (low-fat versus low-carb) versus being assigned one of those two diets. Weight loss was similar for both the "choice" arm (5.7 kg) and the assigned arm. Importantly, adherence was similar between the groups.

An important detail is that prospective participants with a strong aversion to one of the diets were advised not to enroll in the study. By the admission of the authors themselves (my bolding for emphasis), *"Offering choice among diet options did not improve weight loss, dietary adherence, or weight-related quality of life **in participants who did not have a strong diet preference at baseline.**"* This leaves open questions about the impact of removing the power of choice from folks who do have a strong preference for a particular diet type.

Presenting another potential challenge to the personal choice model, an observational study by McClain and colleagues[507] reported that insulin resistance status might impact adherence to weight loss diets. Lower adherence and lower weight loss were associated with insulin-resistant subjects assigned to low-fat diets. In contrast, no significant differences in adherence or weight loss were associated with the assignment to a low-carbohydrate diet. However, a large, well-controlled, 12-month intervention trial (the DIETFITS study) by Gardner and colleagues[292] found that insulin resistance status had no influence on weight loss from a low-carbohydrate versus a low-fat diet. These findings are highly inconvenient for folks who put a lot of stock in diet typing according to insulin sensitivity. Being far more methodologically sound than McClain's uncontrolled/observational study, Gardner's study strongly supports the flexibility of employing individual preference when seeking optimal macronutrient distribution for long-term weight loss success.

Individualizing food choices within a healthy framework

A diet would not be sustainable over the long term if it consisted of foods that the individual disliked, let alone couldn't stand. This seems like an obvious statement, but it's often overlooked, as evidenced by the general disregard that many coaches and gurus have for their clients' preferences. Cookie-cutter diets are painfully common, and we've all done our share of face-palming upon witnessing them.

A way to avoid this is to develop an awareness of the different food groups, which are separated by the combination of macro- and micronutrition they provide. Once that's learned, personal choice among the multitude of foods within each group can be implemented. If you're familiar with *The Lean Muscle Diet* (which I co-wrote with Lou Schuler—great book, hilarious title), then you're familiar with my mnemonic for the food groups: *"Meg's fabulous figure stopped missing fries."* The first two letters of each word correspond with the first two letters of each food group (meat/protein, fat, fibrous veggies, starch, milk/milk products, fruit).

The choices within each group are nearly endless, and the most sensible recommendation is to choose the foods that you prefer and can consistently access. Consuming a variety of foods within each food group has been a long-standing recommendation in dietetics curriculums. This is not an unreasonable idea, especially when you consider that each species of food has a unique nutrient profile. The broader the range of foods consumed, the fuller the spectrum of nutrient intake.

For example, rather than consuming only lean beef or chicken, including fatty fish in that rotation would retain the benefit of the nutrients in the chicken or beef, along with a greater omega-3 fatty acid intake from the fish. The same principle applies (to varying degrees) to the other food groups.

Let's imagine that someone kicked bananas out of their diet because they saw an online ad saying bananas are "bad" and blueberries are superfoods. Well, a food rotation that includes bananas as well as blueberries allows all the wonderful antioxidants in blueberries plus bananas' high potassium and magnesium content. It's been estimated that 48 percent of the US population consumes less than the recommended amount of magnesium,[508] and more than 98 percent of US adults fail to meet the recommended intake of potassium.[509] Bananas are rich in both, which perhaps makes them a *super duper* food (I hope that sarcasm came through). Anyway, the point is that when variety leads to more complete nutrition, it can be a win-win.

Food variety often gets shot down by the claim that greater variety causes a greater energy intake and thus greater weight/fat gain. This indeed has been shown in research[495] and has been attributed to a phenomenon called sensory-specific satiety, where the presentation of a new, palatable food can stimulate appetite despite a state of satiation. There is also a phenomenon called the monotony effect, where repeated consumption of the same foods results in declining palatability ratings and reduced intake.

Although both of these phenomena would seem to support the recommendation against food variety (if the goal is weight loss), important nuance is missing. A two-year study by Vadiveloo and colleagues[510] found that increased variety of whole foods that are energy-sparse and nutrient-dense (rather than a mix of highly palatable foods and junky snack foods) imparts greater body fat reduction compared with maintaining or reducing variety. The moral of the story is that an increase in variety can actually be an advantage in the context of "healthy" foods. William Cowper called variety the spice of life, and Aphra Behn called variety the soul of pleasure. Yes, variety can be a double-edged sword, but you can learn how to wield the weapon to your advantage.

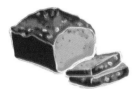

When it comes to individualizing food preferences, there's a common misconception that certain foods are off-limits for dieters. Bread—regardless of type—often gets placed on the "avoid" list. Avoiding any commonly consumed food can work for weight loss. However, the *sustainability* of food avoidance (without a valid clinical/tolerance-based reason) is questionable. With long-term adherence being compromised, food avoidance tactics often backfire.

A great example of this is a 16-week study by Loria-Kohen and colleagues,[511] who compared the hypocaloric effects of a bread-containing diet (averaging 3.7 servings per day) with a bread-free diet. Total calories and macronutrition were equated between the groups. The main findings of this study were threefold:

- There was a lack of significant differences in bodyweight and body fat changes between groups. The bread group lost 4.3 kg (9.5 pounds), while the no-bread group lost 4 kg (8.8 pounds). As for body fat, the bread group lost 2.5 percent, while the no-bread group lost 2.1 percent.

- There were no significant between-group differences in blood lipids, glucose control, or other biochemical measures.

- The bread group showed better dietary adherence. A significant increase in transgressions (which the authors defined as lapses in dietary compliance by 150 kcal) was seen in the no-bread group, while no significant increase in transgressions was seen in the bread group. Furthermore, in the self-reported adherence ratings, the bread group scored higher than the no-bread group (64.3 percent versus 55.6 percent), and dropout was markedly lower in the bread group compared to the no-bread group (6.6 percent versus 21.3 percent). Although the reasons for attrition (dropping out of the study) varied, exclusion of bread was found to be a significant factor.

These findings strongly challenge the anti-bread/anti-grain movement. They also take us back to Chapter 1's discussion of discretionary calorie allowance, which is 10 to 20 percent of total kcal from anything the individual wants, with the remaining 80 to 90 percent being whole and minimally refined foods.

An exception to the "whole and minimally refined" qualification is protein powder. It's an engineered food that's far removed from its original context, yet it's nutrient-dense and conducive to favorable health and body composition outcomes.

This predominance of nutrient-dense foods combined with a moderated allowance for indulgence foods ensures a healthy diet overall that increases the chances of long-term adherence. With that said, it's possible for a minority of the general population to succeed in the long term with an avoidance-based approach to certain foods that they perceive as problematic. However, the risk of this backfiring and sabotaging progress (when feelings of deprivation reach a breaking point) needs to be recognized.

Pyramid schematics in the nutrition and fitness realm aim to convey a hierarchy of importance, but it's impossible to separate the importance of calories and nutrients. My schematic (Figure 9b) preserves a hierarchical theme while establishing the proper ranking of the components. First, note that adherence surrounds the structure, holding it all together. Then, starting from the bottom, notice that calories (energy balance) and nutrients have equal importance in the context of health and are interdependent. Generally speaking, the quality of nutrient sources can be judged based on a food's degree of refinement, processing, or combination with ingredients that are not conducive to health.

With this foundation covered, we can examine the next tier. Over the decades, there have been various incarnations of the food groups (I've seen anywhere from four to nine groups). Striving for a broader intake across the food groups facilitates nutritional completeness, thereby preventing disease and promoting health.[512] The antithesis would be picking a single food group, emotionally attaching yourself to it, and excluding all other groups. The broader the range of foods covered, the broader the spectrum of beneficial nutrients consumed.

An example of diversifying consumption within the food groups would be to shoot for a minimum of three different types of fruit per week, three different types of vegetables, and so on. Much ado is made about the health impact of specific timing of meals (or nutrients) throughout the day, despite this aspect paling in comparison to the overall composition of the diet.

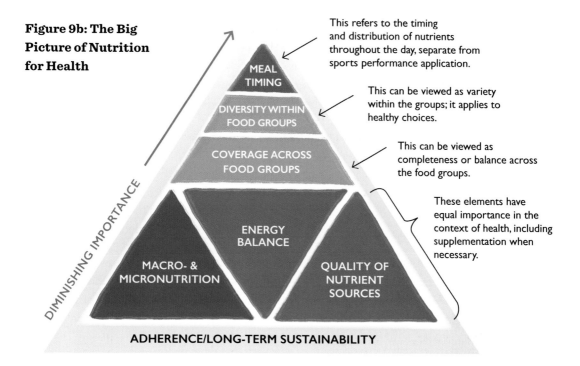

Figure 9b: The Big Picture of Nutrition for Health

MEAL TIMING

This refers to the timing and distribution of nutrients throughout the day, separate from sports performance application.

DIVERSITY WITHIN FOOD GROUPS

This can be viewed as variety within the groups; it applies to healthy choices.

COVERAGE ACROSS FOOD GROUPS

This can be viewed as completeness or balance across the food groups.

ENERGY BALANCE

MACRO- & MICRONUTRITION

QUALITY OF NUTRIENT SOURCES

These elements have equal importance in the context of health, including supplementation when necessary.

ADHERENCE/LONG-TERM SUSTAINABILITY

DIMINISHING IMPORTANCE

Individualizing self-monitoring and accountability

Self-monitoring has been demonstrated as an effective component of program adherence. It doubles as accountability and awareness of progress, regression, or successful maintenance of a given goal. People who are vehemently "anti-scale" would have to endure a degree of cognitive dissonance while reading the research by Steinberg and colleagues[513] showing that daily weighing led to stronger weight control behaviors and greater weight loss. In the same vein, Peterson and colleagues[514] found that frequent and consistent dietary self-monitoring improves long-term weight loss success.[12]

However, the method of self-monitoring should be individualized. Some people do well with a certain degree of micromanagement or quantification, while others don't—especially when it comes to the scale. Remember that research data typically reports mean values (averages) generated from a mixed bag of responses, and plenty of individuals don't fall in the majority for whom daily weighing is a productive (rather than destructive) experience. For some people, daily weighing can be self-sabotaging, particularly when it's difficult to separate their sense of self-worth from daily scale fluctuations. The approach of weighing daily but taking note of the weekly average can lower the potential for anxiety and self-judgment from daily weigh-ins because it keeps the focus on the bigger picture. Nevertheless, I would like to see people wean off of using the scale as a daily crutch or security blanket.

An important finding is that the harmful effects of scale use are potentially gender-specific. Klos and colleagues[515] reported that among women, more frequent self-weighing was associated with greater adverse psychological characteristics related to the preoccupation and concern with bodyweight. Interestingly (and humorously), the opposite was seen among men, where more frequent self-weighing was associated with greater body satisfaction.

Individuals with eating disorders are a prime demographic for whom caution is warranted. Rohde and colleagues[516] reported that frequent self-weighing among young adults (86 percent women) positively correlated with greater weight gain than those with less frequent self-weighing. This association was especially strong among binge-eaters.

Given the aforementioned caveats, it's simply erroneous to assume that daily weighing and vigorous self-monitoring are the ticket to salvation for everyone. It can't be repeated enough—we need to individualize the approach of tracking and self-monitoring. Thankfully, there are several other methods of measuring progress; bodyweight is not the be-all and end-all. Furthermore, the scale's ability to accurately convey what's going on with body composition progressively decreases as an individual gets leaner and/ or gains lean mass.

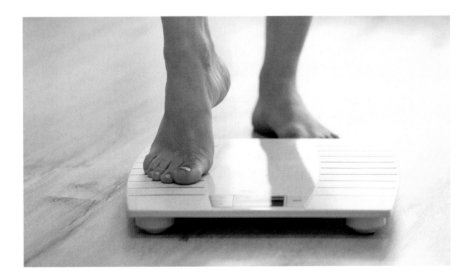

A low-tech, high-value method of tracking body composition

Fortunately, it's possible to track body composition changes with minimal resources and technology. As just discussed, the scale needs to be used with caution since it doesn't suit everyone.

For those who are not averse to using a scale in conjunction with other indicators, I'd like to present a low-tech, high-value method that works well in my remote/online counseling practice, where clients are relegated to doing self-assessments of body composition but don't have access to the traditional assessment devices or the technical skill to use them. Self-assessment can be as simple as tracking weight, waist circumference (I use the navel as a static longitudinal landmark), and lifting strength. Note that circumference measurements throughout the body are all valid indexes of progress, depending on the goal. You don't have to limit your measurements to waist girth if you crave more data to chew on. Waist girth just happens to fit well with this particular method of assessment.

Also, note that lifting strength does not specifically refer to one-rep max strength, but rather lifting volume (sets, reps, load) in general. To simplify this calculation, you can limit your tracking to one or two exercises each for the upper and lower body. If you prefer to keep a detailed/written log of everything, more power to you. Not everyone has the motivation for it, and that's fine; progress can still be made. If you've been lifting for long enough, mentally tracking your progress in key exercises can be easy. It can be done by maintaining an awareness of the number of reps you can complete with the load used in the first work set of the first exercise for each muscle group that's relevant to your push for progress. Give that a try if you've been experiencing logging fatigue and you'd like to see if relying on your memory can suffice; you might be pleasantly surprised.

Keep in mind that when it comes to tracking progress, the body's slow overall rate of change can be deceptive when viewed only in short time frames. Figure 9c presents the "matrix" you can use to interpret your progress without the use of sophisticated equipment.[517] Daily changes and fluctuations tell us very little. Weekly changes provide hints about potential trends. Monthly changes tell the real story.

Figure 9c: The Matrix of Progress

INTERPRETATION	BODY-WEIGHT	WAIST GIRTH	LIFTING STRENGTH
Fat loss only (lean mass stable)	↓	↓	↔
Lean gain only (fat mass stable)	↑	↔	↑
Recomp—in this case, an even rate	↔	↓	↑
Dirty bulking (lean gain with fat gain)	↓	↑	↑
Fading (lean loss with fat loss)	↑	↓	↓
Failing (lean loss, fat gain)—in this case, an even rate	↔	↑	↓

Quick, single-digit adherence ratings instead of detailed records

I've developed and used this simple and effective method with clients for many years but first presented it to seminar and conference audiences in the mid-2010s. The method in its initial form was published in *Girth Control* (my first book) back in 2007. The origins of the method are in my private practice, where I found that a significant proportion of my clients hated writing down everything they ate. The majority were busy businesspeople, busy parents, or both. The time and effort of journaling food intake eventually wore on them.

So, I piloted a system of having them rate their compliance to the program on a scale of 1 to 10. Instead of writing down everything they ate and drank, they simply took a split second to write down a number between 1 and 10, with 10 being what they perceived as perfect compliance. Lo and behold, the method worked! A running average of approximately 8 would consistently yield good progress.

Back in the olden days, I called it the "calendar method" since I had clients buy a physical calendar they could hang on a wall in a prominent location in their home or office and write a number on the calendar, daily. Months filled with mostly 8's and 9's with the occasional slip to a low rating tightly correlated with forward steps toward the client's goals. However, there are a couple of caveats here. Self-reported intake is never perfect. People tend to misreport food intake in general (junk food intake gets disproportionately under-reported, while healthy food intake gets over-reported).[518] So, self-administered performance ratings have an inevitable margin of inaccuracy. In the context of dietary adherence ratings, the tendency is to overrate performance. In order for this single-digit rating system to work, effective education, coaching, and communication were necessary to ensure clients were being as objective and honest as possible.

More rigorous while retaining simplicity: adherence rubrics

Figuring that good things can always be improved, I set out to make the single-digit adherence rating system more rigorous and objective by attaching it to an individualized rubric. Here's how it works. I would develop a 10-point checklist (a rubric) that aligned with the client's goals, preferences, and tolerances. So, instead of a more abstract and arbitrary 1-to-10 rating, it was possible to use a simple checklist of what was and was not accomplished for the day.

The score for the day is based on how many of the assigned program elements were completed. Box 9a presents a sample 10-point adherence rubric (remember that these can and should be tailored to individual requirements and preferences). I was stoked to find that the rubric model was more effective and engaging than the previous version involving a nonspecific 1-to-10 rating. The adherence rubric really pulled the elements together to help people succeed.

Seeing the success of the 10-point rubric, I naturally wanted to see if I could push the envelope of simplicity, so I piloted a 5-point rubric (see Box 9b), and it worked just as well. I used the 5-point rubric for ultra-busy/type-A personalities whose attention would wander halfway through the 10-point checklist. Again, employing the 10-point versus 5-point rubric comes down to assessing which approach would work better according to the characteristics of the individual. The beauty of this approach is that it can serve as a graduation point after succeeding on a detailed/scripted diet plan. In other words, the adherence rubrics can serve as a step toward weaning off of the micromanagement of tracking intake (and other program variables).

With that said, I've initiated client programs by skipping the building of a diet plan and going straight to building the rubric. Clients were excited about the novel, simple, and objective nature of the approach—and of course, they were happy with its effectiveness. Not to mention, journaling was whittled down to writing a single number (or crossing off completed elements), and this thrilled folks who felt time-pressed and overwhelmed by traditional tracking methods that felt like a chore. Another cool thing about the rubric method is that troubleshooting is as simple as assessing which specific elements show a pattern of nonadherence and then making the necessary modifications to either the rubric or the priorities and lifestyle variables of the dieter.

BOX 9A: 10-POINT ADHERENCE RUBRIC (THIS NEEDS TO BE TAILORED TO INDIVIDUAL GOALS, PREFERENCES, AND TOLERANCES)

1. Get a minimum of 7 hours of high-quality sleep.

2. Do your scheduled physical activity (or scheduled rest).

3. Drink a minimum of 1 liter of plain water in addition to other fluid intake.

4. Eat only when physically hungry (no snacking out of boredom or ritual).

5. Stop eating when satisfied but not stuffed.

6. At each meal, start with the least calorie-dense items (beginning with water) and progress toward the most calorie-dense items.

7. Eat 2 to 4 servings of fresh fruit.

8. Eat at least 3 servings of fibrous vegetables.

9. Have at least 20 grams of protein with each meal.

10. Optional: Drink a maximum of 2 glasses of wine (or) eat a maximum of 1 small serving of dessert.

Circling back to self-determination theory,[505] the adherence rubric is an effective tool for building the basic human psychological needs (autonomy, competence, and relatedness) while reaching physical goals. Collaborating with the client on tweaking/adjusting the terms of the rubric, such as serving ranges and physical activity dosing, would nurture autonomy. Including the client in the building and adjustment of the rubric would facilitate a sense of self-direction and self-regulation. A sense of competence would be nurtured as a default of ongoing progress by successfully using the adherence rubric to get results. A sense of relatedness would be fostered through practitioner-client communication, as well as community interaction on the client's end, outside of counseling sessions.

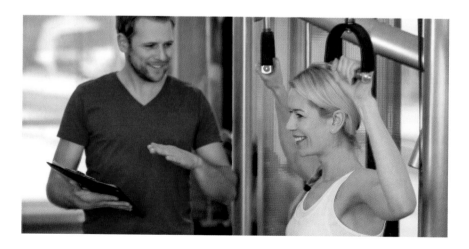

Individualizing daily (and weekly) meal frequency and distribution

Daily meal frequency

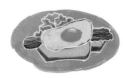

This is a contentious subject because people tend to be emotionally attached to and defensive about their eating routines. However, the reality is that there is no universally superior distribution pattern of meals or nutrients throughout the day or week. What matters is that it fits the individual's goals, preferences, and tolerances. Meal frequency (number of meals per day) can be individually tailored. Whether you prefer to eat one or ten meals a day does not matter, as long as your mind state, mood, performance, and progress are consistently good and you're hitting the appropriate daily totals.

My colleagues and I conducted a 15-study meta-analysis that examined the effect of meal frequency on body composition.[135] Overall, meal frequency had no significant effect on bodyweight. Higher meal frequency showed a greater advantage for lean mass retention and fat loss, but this was due to a single study with a particularly large effect, skewing the overall results. When we removed that study from the analysis, the influence of meal frequency on body composition was gone. Our interpretation and the practical implication of these findings is that a wide range of meal frequencies can be tailored to individual preference.

Of course, there are limits of practicality on the extreme ends of high and low meal frequency. For example, someone trying to gain weight while eating one or two meals per day would likely experience gastrointestinal challenges. There are also limits of effectiveness for optimizing athletic performance if meal frequency is insufficient to support acute fueling needs.

Another consideration is that maximizing muscle growth involves a minimum of four meals with protein dosed at 0.4 g/kg per meal.[37] However, those considerations don't apply to everyone. You can still grow muscle with a lower meal frequency; you just might not be maximizing the rate of growth. In hypocaloric/dieting conditions, low meal frequencies—including intermittent fasting (IF)—have repeatedly been shown to support the retention of lean mass comparably to conventional meal frequencies.[59] IF is not conducive to maximizing muscle hypertrophy,[111] but once again, that's not everyone's goal. Be aware of your total daily targets and adopt the meal frequency that best suits your goals and preferences.

Intermittent fasting

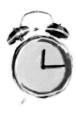

It might disappoint or even anger you to hear me say that IF has trivial benefits beyond being an optional tool in the shed for controlling caloric intake. But that function shouldn't be dismissed as unimportant or insignificant. After all, controlling caloric intake is one of the cornerstone requirements for preventing and mitigating the cardiometabolic diseases plaguing the modern world.

Before I qualify my nonzealous opinion about IF, let's do a quick rundown of its variants, which boil down to two main types: time-restricted feeding (TRF) and whole-day fasting. Each of those variants has subvariants, and the relevant ones will be discussed.

TRF aims to shorten the daily feeding window, typically to six to eight hours. Whole-day fasting is self-descriptive, with further subvariants that include alternate-day fasting (ADF) and the 5:2 model, which involves two fasting days per week, usually but not limited to nonconsecutive days. IF is often referred to as "intermittent energy restriction" since the fasting protocols tested don't always involve zero-calorie days unless explicitly specified. Instead, restricting intake to about 25 percent of maintenance calories (roughly 500 kcal) constitutes a fasting day, as in the case of the majority of ADF and 5:2 research. The most commonly studied IF variants are ADF, TRF, and 5:2.

Due to the tendency of IF to cause spontaneous reductions in total energy intake, it's not surprising that there's a consistency of research showing IF causing weight loss and favorable clinical outcomes compared to non-dieting control conditions in subjects with overweight and obesity.[519] Ad libitum (unrestricted) eating during the feeding time frames of the full range of IF regimens (ADF, TRF, and 5:2) consistently leads to lower total energy intake by the end of the day/week, and thus weight loss.[520-524]

To me, this is the most attractive aspect of IF, as it involves less restriction (during feeding times) and less micromanagement. However, an important point to recognize is that systematic reviews and meta-analyses find that, on the whole, IF regimens perform similarly to daily caloric restriction for weight/fat loss and improving cardiovascular risk factors.[525-531] Die-hard fans of IF tend to get disgruntled about this lack of difference, but I see it as a win from the standpoint of individualizing programs.

It's worth mentioning that of all the IF variants, TRF has the potential for superior effects on glucose control, even in isocaloric comparisons.[532] Superior effects in this regard have mostly been observed in early time-restricted feeding (eTRF), which typically involves a six- to eight-hour feeding window that begins at breakfast and ends in the mid- to late afternoon.

However, there's a lot of fawning over eTRF without consideration of its drawbacks. First of all, a lifestyle that omits conventionally scheduled dinners can present sociocultural conflicts that compromise long-term sustainability.[533] Secondly, the premise of eTRF's clinical utility (better improvements in glucose control) has limited relevance to healthy populations engaged in regular exercise—and even less relevance to such populations who are lean (or progressing in leanness).

Consuming more calories in the later part of the day has shown advantages in the presence of exercise. A 12-week hypocaloric trial by Keim and colleagues[217] compared the effects of consuming 70 percent of total calories during the day versus the evening. Exercise (a combination of aerobic and resistance) occurred between 9 a.m. and 2:30 p.m. No significant differences in fat loss were seen, but the group consuming the bulk of their calories in the evening preserved more lean mass.

Even in the absence of training, it's possible that shunting carbohydrate calories toward the last meal may have inherent benefits. This was illustrated by a hypocaloric trial by Sofer and colleagues,[218] who compared the bulk of the day's carbs concentrated at dinner (making it the day's highest-calorie meal) with carbs spread evenly across all meals. The late-shifted carb intake was superior for body fat loss, glycemic control, hunger control, reducing markers of inflammation, and improving blood lipids. A major strength of this trial, aside from its generally sound methodology, was its long duration (six months).

Speaking of which, an important limitation of the current body of IF research is the lack of long-term trials. In the only meta-analysis addressing it thus far, Headland and colleagues[528] reported that in trials lasting a minimum of six months, IF did not alter blood lipids, glucose, and insulin to a greater degree than daily caloric restriction. A more recent 12-month study by Headland and colleagues[523] compared three diets: 1) continuous energy restriction: 1,000 kcal per day for women and 1,200 kcal per day for men, 2) week-on-week-off energy restriction: alternating 1,000 to 1,200 one week with one week of habitual diet, and 3) the 5:2 IF variant: five days of unrestricted eating and two days at 500 kcal per day for women and 600 kcal per day for men. By the end of the yearlong trial, there were no significant differences among the groups in any of the parameters tested. Weight loss was 6.6 kilograms in the continuous dieting group, 5.1 kilograms in the week-on-week-off group, and 5 kilograms in the 5:2 group. All groups showed improvements in blood lipids with no significant changes in blood glucose.

A follow-up study of the same subjects was conducted 12 months later,[534] and two-year weight loss across the groups was 4.5, 2.8, and 3.5 kilograms, respectively, with differences among the groups failing to reach statistical significance. No differences were seen in glucose and blood lipids. The authors concluded that all three groups were able to achieve "modest" and similar weight loss. Despite this study's limitations (including highly aggressive caloric restriction and a 70 percent dropout rate that was similar across groups), it's yet another mark against the claimed superiority of IF—and this was seen in the longest study to date on this topic.

With such a big focus on weight loss and improvement of clinical parameters via IF, it's easy to forget that it's not the right tool for every job. For the goal of maximizing muscle gain or retention, purposeful fasting is antagonistic at all levels, from anabolic signaling to MPS.[111] This applies to both early-shifted and late-shifted TRF regimens. Individuals shortening their feeding window by skipping breakfast risk compromising resistance exercise capacity.[203] On the other side of the coin, there are lost opportunities for pre-sleep protein feedings, which can benefit athletes and older adults seeking to maximize or preserve muscle protein balance.[106]

Despite the limitations of IF, the collective evidence shows that it's a valid, effective option that has performed similarly overall compared to linear energy restriction. Although the pervasive claims of universal superiority are false, IF is still a viable tool for practitioners and enthusiasts.

Individualizing the degree of dietary nonlinearity

IF variants technically fall under the larger umbrella of nonlinear dieting. The nonlinearity I'll be discussing encompasses carbohydrate and protein distribution across the week, diet breaks across periods of weeks or months, and, finally, hedonic allotment strategies ("cheat" days and meals). Many different permutations of and justifications for specific nonlinear carbohydrate intake schemes have floated through the fitness space for nearly three decades. A common theme among these protocols is to prevent or mitigate the "metabolic slowing" as a result of prolonged dieting— especially carbohydrate restriction. However, despite the long-standing interest in carbohydrate manipulation in fitness communities, nonlinear carb intake within the context of resistance training found its way into the peer-reviewed research only within the past two years.[535-537]

FLEXIBLE VOCAB

Nonlinear dieting

Nonlinear dieting, also called intermittent energy restriction, involves intermittent bouts of energy or calorie maintenance throughout the dieting period, the goal being to mitigate metabolic adaptation, or the process by which your body adjusts to more efficiently turn the food you consume into energy. This typically involves specific "refeed" or high-carb days. In many cases, nonlinear dieting serves as a tool for strengthening adherence and preserving exercise capacity rather than stimulating metabolism.

Prior to this, a notable trial by Byrne and colleagues (the MATADOR study)[538] reported that an intermittent energy restriction protocol alternating two hypocaloric weeks with two weeks at non-maintenance calories for eight cycles (30 weeks total, 16 of which were hypocaloric) resulted in more fat loss and a lesser proportional drop in resting energy expenditure (REE) than the control diet, which was 16 consecutive weeks of caloric restriction. The differences in REE were mysterious since both groups lost an equal amount of lean mass. This study sparked further interest in the investigation of how nonlinear diets might positively affect body composition and REE in protocols more reflective of those in the real world, among the fitness community.

Enter Campbell and colleagues,[535] who conducted a realistically designed nonlinear versus linear carbohydrate intake protocol in resistance trainees. A refeed group involving a 35 percent deficit (via carbohydrate restriction) on five days followed by two days at maintenance calories (via refeeding carbs), carried out for seven weeks. The continuous group maintained a daily 25 percent deficit. Carbohydrate intake in the refeed and continuous groups were equivalent when averaged by the end of the week. The refeed group lost less FFM and experienced a lower drop in REE than the continuous group, with no significant difference in fat loss between groups.

In my personal communication with lead author Bill Campbell, he candidly conceded to a few key limitations. REE was measured using a different device in a small portion of the subjects due to an equipment malfunction in the primary device. High participant dropout rate was due to the study being done in two phases, one phase at the start of the semester with good retention, and another later in the semester where retention was low. Finally, it's possible that there was not enough time (two days) after the carbohydrate refeed to allow sufficient glycogen reduction via exercise before assessing body composition. This potentially gave an unfair advantage to the refeed group when assessing lean mass.

A subsequent study by Kysel and colleagues[537] compared the moderately hypocaloric effects of a linear, high-carbohydrate (55 percent), low-fat (30 percent) "reduction" diet (RD) with a cyclical ketogenic diet (CKD) involving weekend carb-ups (8 to 10 g/kg of lean mass) in young resistance-trained men. Training was a mix of strength and endurance work. Protein was set at 15 percent of total calories in the RD and 1.6 g/kg in the CKD on ketogenic days (carb-up days brought protein down to 15 percent of total calories). Unfortunately, absolute values of macronutrient intakes were not specified, which makes it difficult to speculate why the RD outperformed the CKD in lean mass retention, fat loss (not significantly), aerobic performance, and strength in the lat pull-down and leg press. Without any additional data such as hunger/appetite or psychological parameters such as mood state or motivation level, the absence of dietary intake data leaves unresolved questions about this trial's results.

The latest in this saga is Peos and colleagues' ICECAP study.[536] The main finding of this study on resistance trainees was a general lack of metabolic magic or body composition advantage from monthly, weeklong diet breaks (at maintenance, via increased carbohydrate) between three weeks of hypocaloric conditions. Both groups lost fat mass, with no significant difference between groups, and both similarly retained lean mass.

Advantages of Peos's trial over Campbell's were the low dropout rate and assessments that weren't potentially compromised by inconsistencies in the measuring instrument. Both nonlinear dieting protocols resemble what has been engaged in the real world, with one being a weekly carb-up model and the other being a monthly diet break model. Although Peos and colleagues didn't observe any metabolic or body composition advantages in the nonlinear dieting group, the subjects in that group did report less hunger and desire to eat—which is a potentially profound advantage for long-term success.

Takeaways from the emerging nonlinear dieting research on resistance trainees is that it's largely been superior to linear caloric restriction for a range of outcomes, including hunger control, lean mass retention, and fat loss. However, the study with the least threats to internal validity while retaining real-world applicability is the ICECAP trial by Peos and colleagues, and the differences they found between linear and nonlinear dieting were not nearly as dramatic or mysterious as the other studies discussed.

At this point, there are not nearly enough studies from which to form strong opinions about what the optimal nonlinear dieting structure would be. However, in practice, nonlinear carbohydrate intake is a mainstay of trainees who are pushing the limits of leanness for various purposes, including physique contests, photo shoots, and just to satisfy personal goals. In my field observations, nonlinear carbohydrate intake is best suited for hypocaloric conditions with low carbohydrate levels. Purposeful nonlinear carb intakes have minimal utility in chronic hypercaloric conditions with a large daily carb allotment.

Protein hyperfeeds

"Protein hyperfeed" is a cool-sounding term and a concept I came up with. It's the protein equivalent of a carb-up without the low intake part of the cycle. In contrast to carb refeeds (high carb intakes alternated with carb restriction of varying severity), protein hyperfeeds are high-protein days (2 to 2.5 times the normal intake) placed strategically through the week, in the midst of normal protein intake. Whereas "normal" protein intake would be defined as what's optimal in typical circumstances (≥1.6 g/kg/day), hyperfeeds would put protein at ~3.2 to 4.5 g/kg (1.45 to 2 g/lb) for the day. For example, a 75-kilogram (165-pound) person might consume 135 grams of protein on a normal day. A hyperfeed day would provide 2 to 2.5 times this amount, which would be 270 to 337 grams.

There are three main uses/objectives for protein hyperfeeds, which can be pursued separately or in combination, depending on the individual's goals and training status:

- To maximize satiety and minimize cravings in general, and especially on carb-restricted days

- To allow bouts of unrestricted eating for the purpose of alleviating psychological "diet fatigue" with minimal risk for undue fat gain

- To push toward recomposition in higher-intermediates and advanced trainees

This third point is more of a dice-roll than the others. In my observations, even when protein hyperfeeds are calculated as surplus calories (beyond maintenance needs), there is still a "disappearance" of the extra protein, as seen in multiple studies by Antonio and colleagues.[51-53,539] No significant or favorable changes in body composition (fat loss and/or muscle gain) occurred in resistance-trained subjects as a result of increasing protein intakes to ≥3 g/kg from baseline intakes ranging from 2 to 2.2 g/kg.

Potential explanations for Antonio et al.'s "disappearing" protein surpluses include increased thermogenesis (dietary, exercise-based, and non-exercise-based), increased satiety driving down intake of the other macronutrients, misreporting of intake, and increased excretory energy losses.

I witnessed this type of protein-induced recomp in clients several years before Antonio et al.'s protein overfeeding studies were published, so, while some viewed the findings with skepticism, they actually reflected my notes from the trenches. In eucaloric (maintenance) conditions, and even in purposefully targeted net weekly surplus conditions, I have observed recomp in clients on regular protein hyperfeeds.

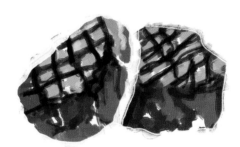

A multitude of variables make recomp possible,[44] but in my observations, experimenting with protein hyperfeeds throughout the week is a tool worth trying out for this purpose. In my experience with clients, two to three protein hyperfeeds per week is what most people can tolerate (and enjoy). Protein hyperfeeds should ideally be positioned on or immediately before days when cravings are historically highest for the individual. Or choose any day(s) when carbohydrate intake is not elevated for refeeding or carbing up. An interesting phenomenon I've observed repeatedly is that the satiating effects of the protein hyperfeed can last through the entire following day. Individual responses vary here.

To sum up protein hyperfeeds:

- Rather than lowballing protein on days off, it's better to keep protein at levels known to optimize adaptations to resistance training. Protein turnover and heightened muscular sensitivity to protein feeding can last 24 to 48 hours after a training bout.

- Protein hyperfeeds are a tool I've used with dieters seeking novel tactics to increase satiety and minimize the psychological fatigue of dieting. It has also worked for intermediate and advanced trainees seeking recomposition.

- My field experience with protein hyperfeeds reflects the intriguing results of Antonio et al.'s protein overfeeding studies,[51-53,539] as well as Barakat and colleagues' recent review reporting that a protein intake of 2.6 to 3.5 g/kg of FFM is associated with recomposition.[125]

- The protein hyperfeed protocol I've found success with involves 2 to 2.5 times normal protein intake, two to three days per week. Protein choices should be kept lean for the most part.

- Protein hyperfeeds make protein lovers extremely excited about their diets—especially those who prefer savory foods to sweet foods. Those with more of a sweet tooth can still engage in protein hyperfeeds, since endless dessert variants can be derived from protein powder.

- It's unknown whether the apparent "magic" of protein hyperfeeds is behavioral, metabolic, or both, but the bottom line is that I (and others with whom I've shared the protocols) have seen the positive effects of the approach in the field. This is at least partially due to it being a dietary control tactic that involves increasing intake rather than restricting it. This makes protein hyperfeeds a potent weapon against the feelings of deprivation that are common to the dieting process.

Diet breaks

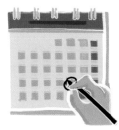

Studies on diet breaks are surprisingly scarce. Back in 2003, Wing and Jeffery[540] compared the effect of a six-week continuous break from dieting, three two-week breaks, and a control condition with no diet breaks. All three conditions were in the context of a weight loss program involving 14 weekly group sessions. This was a relatively large and diverse sample (142 subjects ranging in age from 25 to 60 years, 15 to 70 percent over ideal bodyweight).

Interestingly, weight loss in both groups during the breaks was not significantly different from the control group without breaks, and overall weight loss within the same time frame did not differ between conditions. These findings show that even extensive time off from dieting does not necessarily sabotage progress.

The diet break model that has worked well in my field observations involves a weeklong break every four to eight weeks, autoregulated according to the physical and psychological fatigue level of the dieter. A diet break is a return to pre-dieting intake levels—without purposeful restriction, but also without purposeful abandonment of discretion (technically known as YOLO-ing). On the note of diet breaks adding a layer of protection against physical fatigue in the face of dieting, Peos and colleagues[541] conducted a secondary analysis of the ICECAP trial[536] and reported significant increases in muscular endurance in the legs, demonstrated by improvements in 25-rep max sets for the quads and hamstrings.

It should be noted that if an individual is not dieting aggressively or for a long period, then full-blown breaks may not be needed, especially if the person's profession, hobbies, or lifestyle don't involve pushing the limits of leanness. I've developed *nonlinearizing* tactics for folks who want to enjoy periodic high-carbohydrate intakes (carb-ups) throughout the week but still net a low to moderate average daily amount. These tactics work their magic by mitigating the psychological fatigue (and, to a degree, the physical fatigue) of dieting. I created the Nonlinear Dieting Matrix (Figure 9d) for nonlinearizing any given daily nutrient allotment. The vast majority of the time, it's used for planning carb-ups.

Figure 9d: Nonlinear Dieting Matrix

AVERAGE DAILY TARGET ➡	X 1.5	X 2	X 2.5	X 3	X 3.5	X 4
1 carb-up per week	0.91	0.83	0.75	0.66	0.58	0.5
2 carb-ups per week	0.8	0.6	0.4	0.2	0	N/A
3 carb-ups per week	0.62	0.25	N/A	N/A	N/A	N/A
4 carb-ups per week	0.33	N/A	N/A	N/A	N/A	N/A

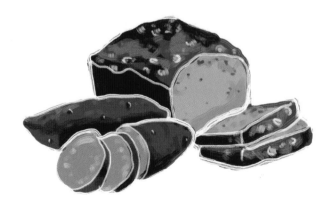

Here's how to use the Nonlinear Dieting Matrix:

1. Figure out your daily carb target (see Chapter 5).

2. Decide how many carb-up days you want per week (first column).

3. Decide how big the carb-ups are going to be (top row), then multiply your daily carb allotment by this number to get your carb-up grams.

4. Just follow those two conditions to where they perpendicularly intersect on the grid.

5. Multiply your daily carb allotment by the value that's intersected by the conditions you chose. This calculation gives you the amount of carbs you'll have on carb-restricted days. I gave a blue background to the most common values used.

This is much easier done than explained. I'll use 100 grams of carbs as an example of a daily carb target. Here are the steps:

1. This is easy; we've already established it's 100 grams.

2. Twice a week (see the first column, third row down).

3. I'll be a wild man and do a carb-up that's 2.5 times the size of my daily carb allotment (see the first row, fourth column). $100 \times 2.5 = 250$ grams of carbs on my carb-up days.

4. These two conditions (values) intersect at 0.4. See how that works?

5. $0.4 \times 100 = 40$ grams of carbs on my low days, which are five days per week since I chose two carb-up days per week.

In this example, two days a week you consume 250 grams of carbs, and the other five days you consume 40 grams of carbs. For the week, it still ends up averaging 100 grams per day. It's like magic!

Individualizing hedonic strategy

The term "cheat meal" is polarizing in the fitness field. Some practitioners hate its negative connotations, and some don't think anything of it at all. Dwayne "The Rock" Johnson revels in it. He's famous for his "cheat" meals that range from gigantic stacks of pancakes to multiple plates of sushi chased down with dessert (and whatever adult beverage he's selling).

The funny thing about him labeling these meals as "cheats" is that they are the furthest thing from it. They are a regular, precisely planned part of his program; they're obviously carb-ups between periods of substantially lower carb intake. These meals don't even qualify as what do Vale and colleagues refer to as "planned hedonic deviations,"[542] which are characterized by actual deviations from a structured path to goal achievement. The Rock's cheat meals are quite literally part of the structure. Nevertheless, do Vale and colleagues concluded that hedonic deviations, or periodic bouts of "being bad," can actually enhance goal achievement as long as these indulgences are systematically integrated in the program from the outset.

The concept of *discretionary* calories is discussed in chapter 1 of this book. Briefly, discretionary calories are a margin of intake that you can fill with basically whatever you want, given that the strong majority (80 to 90 percent) of your diet is composed of nutrient-dense foods conducive to your health and your goals. The discretionary 10 to 20 percent is the optional territory of "cheating"—but of course it's not actually cheating.

Using a 2,000-kcal diet as an example, discretionary calories amount to 200 to 400 kcal per day from anything you want. The 10 to 20 percent rule is not confined to a linear daily model. As in the case of nonlinear carbohydrate intake, discretionary calories (in this case, 1,400 to 2,800 kcal) can be consumed flexibly over the course of the week. It's a pretty substantial amount of calories to work with if you decide to allot all of it to stuff you'd consider indulgent or worthy of the "cheat meal" designation. The discretionary calorie allotment also takes care of the question of cheat *meal* versus cheat *day* when you consider that you have control over the decision to consume it in larger or smaller installments.

Individuals differ in their response to indulgence intake. I've tried all different permutations of cheat meal allowances with clients. Like everyone else in the late 1990s, I was influenced by Bill Phillips's once-a-week "free day" allowance, where you could eat whatever you wanted for the whole day.

I found out very quickly that my clients had highly disparate responses to that allowance. One client admitted to me that he ate from morning to night, stuffing himself all day, to the point of pain, with the junkiest possible foods. It was instantly clear that he was the wrong candidate for that approach. I then experimented with prescribing optional "junk meals," a maximum of two per week. A junk meal can be defined as a high-calorie entrée such as a burger, pizza (a few slices, not the whole thing), pasta, casserole, or large dessert. What typically qualifies is any restaurant or fast food meal that has saucy, creamy, greasy, or fried elements (sounds like most meals out, doesn't it?). These meals are not easily decipherable nutritionally, and it's virtually guaranteed that they are loaded with ingredients that will, at best, impede your progress. At worst, they'll set you back a step or two if not consumed judiciously.

With that said, it's entirely possible to prepare burgers, pizza, and pasta at home and exempt them from the "junk" status that's inevitable when they're prepared by establishments whose aim is to put flavor over nutrition and health by loading up dishes with at least double the butter, oil, salt, and/ or sugar of homemade meals. The "two junk meals max" strategy worked surprisingly well for clients who preferred to go hard with their plans during the week, leaving room for a junk meal on the weekend. Although the option to have two junk meals was there, the tendency was to circle back into focus after one junk meal. In order to keep a strong safety net in place, I imposed the following junk meal rules:

- A junk meal should be eaten in place of a main meal, not in addition to the meals on the plan.

- On a day when a junk meal is consumed, omit all floating snacks from the plan in order to counterbalance the caloric overload (especially for a client seeking weight loss).

- The magnitude of the junk meal should be clear in the client's mind: a single dish/entrée for a single person. A dinner with appetizers, drinks, and dessert is beyond a junk meal; it's more like two meals, and you're done for the week.

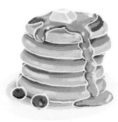

- Fill up on plain water (at least two tall glasses) immediately before starting the junk meal. This simple trick will greatly reduce the tendency to finish a massive entrée *and* order dessert.

A quick note about the "water trick": I call it that because it works like magic, and it indeed is conducive to bodyweight control by initiating satiety signals as well as displacing stomach space and ultimately curbing the amount of calories you would have eaten. It works on all meals to varying degrees. It's especially useful if you arrive really hungry to a restaurant. It's also comforting to know that this tactic is supported by research.[543-545]

My "two junk meals max" guideline was a tool I kept in the toolbox and used occasionally, even as I developed the starch bullet "wildcard" optional substitution tactic, which I found to work even better for minimizing and actually eliminating junk food cravings in most clients. That tactic gives the client up to 20 percent of total daily calories as *discretionary* calories, which often takes away the desire for full-blown junk meals. Combining the two tactics (optional two junk meals/week max, as well as optional daily wildcard calories) has worked just as well as either tactic in isolation. As you can see, there are several possibilities for fitting in indulgences. Ultimately, you would coach the individual toward developing a steady routine that is predominated by healthy habits: one that's proactive instead of reactive and haphazard. This comes with maintaining a clear week-ahead (minimum) view of the personal, professional, and social events on the calendar.

Notes about alcohol

For those who want to fit alcohol into their diet, alcohol can take the place of fat and/or carbohydrate calories. It wouldn't be wise to sacrifice protein to fit in alcohol. Alcohol falls under the discretionary calorie allotment (10–20% of total calories from essentially anything you want). However, it has a more complicated and cautionary story than the other "junk" or "indulgence" foods. Whereas the latter foods (including sugar-sweetened beverages) don't attempt to masquerade as healthy, alcoholic beverages enjoy a fair amount of positive press for being healthy in moderation. Before we get to that claim and its caveats, let's first establish some important definitions.

A standard drink serving in US terms is defined as containing 14 grams of alcohol. Examples include the following:[546]

- 12 ounces of regular beer (about 5% alcohol)

- 5 ounces of wine (about 12% alcohol)

- 1.5 ounces of distilled spirits (about 40% alcohol)

Although there's no formal or standardized definition of moderation, the literature indicates a range of roughly one to two drinks per day for women, and two to three drinks per day for men.[547] Note that the latter dosing exceeds limits recommended by major health agencies. The National Institute on Alcohol Abuse and Alcoholism (NIAAA), an agency under the National Institutes of Health (NIH), shares the same definition of "moderation" as the Dietary Guidelines for Americans, jointly authored by the US Department of Health and Human Services and the US Department of Agriculture.[284] These agencies define moderation as one and two drinks per day for women and men, respectively. The NIAA defines binge drinking as any amount resulting in a blood alcohol level of 0.08 percent or higher, which translates to more than five drinks in two hours for men and more than four drinks in two hours for women. Heavy alcohol use is defined as more than four drinks on any day or more than 14 drinks per week (men), and more than three drinks on any day or more than seven drinks per week (women).

The health implications of alcohol consumption have been studied extensively over the past several decades. Observational/epidemiological research tends to show that low-to-moderate alcohol intakes are protective against cardiovascular disease (CVD).[548] It's possible that the polyphenol content—especially in red wine—can impart cardiovascular benefits.[549] A recent systematic review by Estruch and Hendriks[550] compared the associations of the three main beverages (wine, beer, and spirits), consumed at low to moderate levels, on various health outcomes (cancer, CVD, and T2D) and all-cause mortality. Overall, the findings were mixed, with no consistent advantage or disadvantage among the types of beverages in terms of impact on health outcomes. However, wine was associated with a decreased risk for T2D and all-cause mortality. The authors speculated that these benefits of wine may be confounded by surrounding factors, since wine drinkers tend to have healthier diets and lifestyles than drinkers of beer and spirits.

It's important to keep in mind that alcohol consumption is a double-edged sword, showing protective potential at low-to-moderate intakes[551] but adverse-to-catastrophic potential at high intakes. Widespread media glamorization and marketing/commercialization of alcohol can distract the public's awareness of the risks of excess consumption. Disease conditions whose primary cause is alcohol include dependence syndrome, alcoholic polyneuropathy, alcoholic myopathy, alcoholic gastritis, alcoholic fatty liver disease, alcoholic cirrhosis of the liver, alcohol-induced pancreatitis, and fetal alcohol syndrome. Disease conditions with alcohol as a component include infectious disease, cancer, diabetes, neuropsychiatric disease, cardiovascular disease, liver disease, pancreas disease, unintentional injury, and intentional injury.[552]

The potential for collateral damage (to individuals other than the drinker) is an overlooked consideration. Alcohol-driven social harms include family disruptions, employment/financial disruptions, and criminal convictions. Given these potentially life-altering consequences (not the least of which are addiction and abuse), the decision to even begin drinking must be carefully contemplated. Individuals differ in the potential for alcohol at any level of consumption to be good, bad, or neutral. An excerpt from a recent review by Chiva-Blanch and Badimon[548] is relevant to conclude this topic:

> *"It is worth mentioning that, despite the cardioprotective effects derived from low/moderate alcohol consumption, these benefits may be weighed against the potential harms from an individual perspective and addressing serious issues such as the propensity to alcohol dependence and collateral social harms, genetic vulnerability, pregnancy or even the family history of cancer. On the other hand, heavy and binge alcohol consumption should be categorically discouraged without any exception or pretext."*

How I personally manage hedonic intake

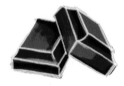

Fitting "indulgence" foods into an overall healthy diet is a matter of controlling their dose and/or frequency throughout the day, week, or month. Every day, I have about an ounce (28 grams) of dark chocolate, which amounts to two squares of chocolate that I have at one or two points in the day (after lunch and/or dinner) with a handful of almonds or a spoonful of peanut butter. I love this combo, and it satisfies my "indulgence" itch.

I limit junk meals like burgers and fries to a maximum of once a week, and I don't worry about it. On days when I eat a junk meal, I almost automatically skip the meal before or after it and have a small protein-based snack instead. Out of my 100 to 120 meals per month, a maximum of about four to six are truly naughty. This flexible allowance for imperfection and indulgence keeps my social life, sanity, and sense of rebellion intact. Individuals vary in their personal level of dietary hedonic requirements. Finding that sweet spot is a powerful tool for long-term adherence to an overall healthy diet.

Clearing up misconceptions about carbohydrate refeeds

If I may shift gears from practitioner mode to researcher mode, let's discuss the claim that carbohydrate refeeds (what most people call cheat meals) help dieters by raising leptin energy expenditure to stoke the metabolism. This idea is not completely imaginary, but it's a misleading oversimplification.

Classic research by Dirlewanger and colleagues[553] compared the effects of three days of a carbohydrate overfeeding diet (2,460 kcal with 394 grams of carb and 60 grams of fat) and a fat overfeeding diet (2,508 kcal with 219 grams of carb and 153 grams of fat), both of which were 40 percent above maintenance caloric requirements. The carbohydrate treatment showed a 28 percent increase in leptin and a 7 percent increase in 24-hour energy expenditure. No such increases were seen with fat overfeeding. While these phenomena sound like solid support for the link between carbohydrate, leptin, and hikes in metabolism, we can't overlook that the actual increase in 24-hour energy expenditure was only 7 percent. Since the diets imposed a 40 percent caloric surplus, this leaves us with a 33 percent net increase in energy intake. We're still looking at a substantial caloric surplus when all is said and done, which effectively nullifies the possibility of direct fat loss from the presumed metabolic effects of carbohydrate refeeds.

Now, just because there might not be a metabolic or thermic advantage to carbohydrate-focused targeting of leptin increases doesn't mean that carb-based refeeds are not beneficial to the dieter. They can be beneficial through increasing exercise energy expenditure as well as non-exercise energy expenditure. A concerted effort can be made to utilize the transient periods of greater carb (and total energy) intake to fuel greater exercise output. Greater storage of glycogen can facilitate greater training capacity in the face of dieting conditions, as recently demonstrated by Peos and colleagues.[541] Finally, there's the potential for cyclic higher-carbohydrate periods to facilitate adherence given the psychological fatigue of dieting. As previously discussed, diet breaks or carb-ups can be customized at a frequency and magnitude that suits the individual's goals and circumstances.

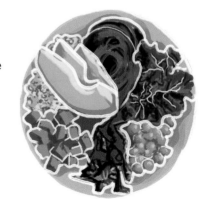

REDEFINING MAINTENANCE

Maintenance is a term that's perpetually thrown around but rarely gets the deeper consideration it deserves. Before addressing that, let's start with the widely accepted definition of "successful" or "healthy" weight loss within the academic and professional literature, which is a 5 to 10 percent reduction of initial bodyweight.[554,555] In cases of overweight and obesity, even a modest weight reduction of 3 to 5 percent can cause clinically relevant improvements in blood lipid profile and glucose control,[555] which can lower the risk for an array of chronic diseases.

Defining weight loss maintenance is inevitably as subjective as defining the designation of "long term." A classic review by Wing and Hill[556] proposed the definition of long-term weight loss maintenance as losing a minimum of 10 percent of initial bodyweight and sustaining that reduction for a minimum of one year.

So, weight loss maintenance definitions vary, but rarely is maintenance discussed as anything beyond an unmoving state. In reality, maintenance can be a winding road and even quite an adventure, depending on what goals the individual chooses to pursue once a state of overweight or obesity is overcome.

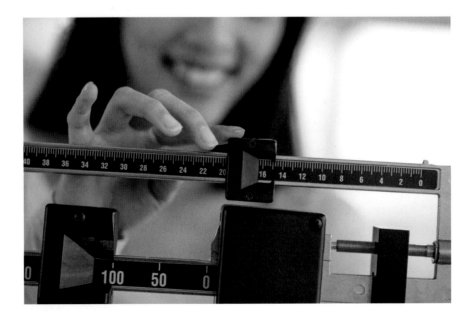

Maintenance as a dynamic target

Bodyweight or body composition maintenance doesn't have to be rigid and static to be considered successful or healthy. Maintenance can be viewed as a seasonal or cyclical ebb and flow.

For example, sports typically have off-season, preseason, and in-season phases, with the length of a season varying widely from sport to sport. Each season involves different energetic demands, thus spawning different bodyweights. Whereas bodyweight for competitive athletes is dynamic by default due to different training seasons, recreational athletes and the general public can opt for *periodizing* or implementing a degree of seasonality to bodyweight or body composition. It's different from the adverse effects of yo-yo dieting or insidiously accumulating holiday weight gain from periodic bingelike behavior. Rather, these bidirectional shifts in body fat are planned and purposeful.

A classic example with origins in fitness/physique circles is getting leaner for warm weather and less clothing while donning more of a "winter coat" for colder weather and more clothing. But, in my observations, this largely vanity-based model is (ironically) effective for freeing people from the anxiety of rigidly static maintenance goals, where even minuscule weight changes are a source of psychological stress.

Instead of becoming emotionally attached to a very specific bodyweight target, I suggest a more flexible approach that allows a margin of weight fluctuation. I also recommend an allowance for change and evolution of individual goals that might preclude a rigid/static bodyweight. Once weight goals are hit, I've found that a roughly 2 to 3 percent bodyweight fluctuation across "seasons" is a reasonable amount of wiggle room for living life and pursuing different physical goals but still successfully maintaining or progressing.

Those who engage in dedicated bulking and cutting cycles have the potential for larger weight fluctuations over the course of various time periods, and we'll discuss that. My point for now is that some folks have a tendency toward very static bodyweight while they maintain, and others "maintain" with a wider margin of fluctuation. There's nothing inherently wrong with the latter as long as there's purpose and awareness behind the fluctuation.

Recomp, cutting, bulking, gaintaining

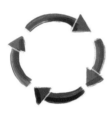

Recomposition, or "recomp" (simultaneous muscle gain and fat reduction), is discussed at various points throughout this book, and I've reiterated the point that recomp is mainly a default result of being far from your potential in terms of muscular size and leanness. It's also worth reiterating that the literature has several studies of recomp occurring in trained/athletic subjects who are relatively lean.[125]

However, a common thread among these studies is the implementation of supervised, hypertrophy-focused, periodized, progressive resistance training programs and/or protein supplementation in subjects who weren't necessarily training progressively for hypertrophy or optimizing their nutrition and supplementation for hypertrophy prior to the trials. Another common detail among these studies is the use of young adults (several studies were on college students) who weren't even close to the limits of leanness. Men had body fat percentages ranging in the mid to high teens, and women were in the low twenties.

To recap, the subjects were put through novel/progressive training stimuli that included optimized nutrition and/or supplementation in conditions highly conducive to elevated levels of effort and consistency compared to pre-trial routines. It wouldn't be fair to wave around this body of research as a green light for all lean, well-trained lifters to chase the goal of recomp as opposed to focusing on one goal at a time. On the positive side, the current body of evidence shows that recomp is still possible for trainees who are significantly past newbie status.

The cycling (alternating) of bulking and cutting phases is the classic model employed by bodybuilders and fitness/physique enthusiasts, but it has always garnered criticism for being an alternation of looking good (but feeling horrible) and looking horrible (but feeling good). The common "dirty bulking" approach, where aggressive caloric surpluses are employed—and substantial amounts of fat are gained—has cast a somewhat negative light on the practice of cycling cutting and bulking phases. However, dedicated cutting and bulking cycles are still the best option for individuals who are advanced in their muscular development and leanness and are still seeking to push the envelope with dietary manipulations.

It's the magnitude of the caloric surplus that needs more careful consideration for more advanced trainees. A 10 to 20 percent surplus above caloric maintenance needs is recommended for intermediate and more advanced trainees, who have a greater tendency toward fat gain with more aggressive surpluses.[57] A recent illustration of this is Ribeiro and colleagues' study[557] comparing the four-week effects of 4,501 versus 6,087 kcal per day on elite-level male bodybuilding competitors. Despite these massive intakes, lean mass gains were minimal in both groups. The higher-kcal group gained more lean mass (1 versus 0.4 kg), but fat mass gains were also greater (7 versus 0.8 percent). The time frames for bulking vary with the individual and the goal. However, considering the slow rate of muscle gain in intermediate trainees even in best-case scenarios (1 to 2 pounds per month at best; half this rate in advanced folks), bulking phases should last at least six months to allow sufficient time for meaningful/measurable gains before shifting gears.

Cutting phases would not be necessary if fat were never gained during bulking, but life is not that fair, and mother nature is not always kind. In intermediates and up, a lean-to-fat ratio of 1:1 during bulking is common, but 1:0.5-ish is not unheard of if the bulk is slow/subtle enough. Purely fat-free muscle gains are a possibility for beginners ripe for the recomp train, but beyond the newbie stage, concurrent gains of fat and muscle during hypercaloric conditions get progressively unavoidable.

Cutting cycles should facilitate a rate of fat loss that doesn't put lean mass gains at risk and defeat the whole purpose of the process (a 0.5 to 1 percent weekly decrease in bodyweight).[489] As explained in the programming chapter, the time frame is determined by the goal and its associated benchmarks of change: 1 to 2 pounds per month for muscle gain in beginners and intermediates, and 1 to 2 pounds per week for fat loss regardless of training status.

Because muscle gain is a much slower process than fat loss, it makes sense for bulking phases to be much longer than cutting phases. For natural trainees, I wouldn't recommend less than a 3:1 to 4:1 ratio of time spent bulking versus cutting. There are various claims and practices surrounding "mini-cuts," which are short cutting phases that essentially interrupt bulking phases. While I've heard positive anecdotes from folks who swear by incorporating "mini-cuts," I usually hear them from folks who bulked too aggressively in the first place!

And that brings us to one of my favorite terms, "gaintaining"—and I'd give the term's creator credit, but no one seems to know who it is. Gaintaining is nothing more than a very slow and linear state of gains targeted by a very small net daily or weekly surplus. Unlike bulking cycles that commonly last a few months, gaintainers are proud to be looking ahead a few years.

The benefit of this approach is that no time is spent in "off-season" body fat levels. The drawback is that it's not ideal for trainees who are still far from their desired level of muscle hypertrophy. Constantly courting a vanishingly small net caloric surplus can compromise anabolic signaling and MPS in addition to compromising the fueling of increases in training volume that drive progressive overload and muscle growth.[57]

Now, with all of that said, gaintaining can be an attractive option for trainees who are further along in their journey and are satisfied with their degree of muscular development, although not quite at their ultimate goal. These individuals likely have undergone years of cycling through conventional bulking phases (fat gains and all) and have reaped the benefits of more efficient anabolic leveraging before transitioning to the slow but scenic road of gaintaining.

Putting progress plateaus into the proper perspective

A weight loss plateau can be defined as an extended period—about a month or more—of no change in bodyweight (or, more accurately, body composition). There are only two possible causes for a weight loss plateau. Either 1) there's a lack of adherence to the program, or 2) a new point of equilibrium in energy balance has been reached—a new point of maintenance where energy intake and output are equal on an ongoing basis. It's difficult to pinpoint the factors driving an individual's lack of program compliance. It's also difficult to isolate what occurs physiologically (and behaviorally) when the body is seemingly resistant to program changes. Let's start by looking at the primary culprit, nonadherence.

Reason #1: Nonadherence

There are two types of nonadherence: conscious and unconscious. Nonadherence (synonymous with noncompliance) is automatically thought of as a premeditated rebellion against the prescribed diet and/or exercise protocol, but that's not always the case. People often fail to adhere without realizing it. Unconscious or unintentional nonadherence is likely a more common problem than purposeful nonadherence. And intermittent lapses in adherence are more likely to occur than consistent/complete lack of adherence.

Unconscious nonadherence is seen in a great multitude of diet studies that track self-reported intake (as opposed to lab-provided intake). A "regression to the mean" or "drift toward the middle" occurs over time, regardless of the diet treatment. This is due to a gradual decrease in adherence. It even happens in clinical populations with a lot at stake, such as subjects with T2D. It's typical in long-term trials for subjects assigned to ketogenic diets to begin the trial with a carbohydrate intake of less than 50 grams per day to be consuming ~130 to 160 grams per day at the 12-month mark.[209]

A related phenomenon to nonadherence is the misreporting of dietary intake (and physical activity). In classic research by Lichtman and colleagues,[558] obese subjects with a self-proclaimed history of "diet resistance" have been shown to under-report food intake by an average of 47 percent and over-report physical activity by 51 percent.

Thomas and colleagues[559] aimed to investigate the factors related to weight loss plateaus in diet trials that commonly occur at the six-month point despite validated mathematical models showing weight plateaus between one and two years. In order to do so, they developed separate mathematical models that were validated with four large-scale, long-term studies. They determined that weight loss plateaus were due to intermittent lack of adherence rather than metabolic adaptation (metabolic slowing).

Reason #2: Arrival at equilibrium

An unfortunate yet familiar scenario is when uninformed dieters seek the next fad once they run into their first weight loss plateau. Reaching a point where an imposed energy deficit has finally diminished or closed up entirely is something that people mistakenly consider to be some sort of failure. On the contrary, this is merely a "landing" on the way down the nonlinear staircase of weight loss. Weight loss plateaus are supposed to happen, and when the weight loss goal is large enough, plateaus are unavoidable.

In the field, I've advised clients with substantial weight loss goals to be aware that several plateaus will occur before they reach their goal. Each new plateau will likely be longer than the previous one, but here's the punch line: this is a good thing. After all, the end goal is indeed a plateau of some sort. Plateaus are typically placed in a negative light, but I've found that it's much more productive to frame them as opportunities to test the sustainability of the progress made up to that point. Therefore, I encourage dieters to view plateaus as "maintenance practice."

The tendency is to keep pushing forward under the illusion that plateaus are something to immediately flee from. When a plateau has been reached, I routinely challenge clients to sustain the plateau (that is, maintain and not regain any significant weight/fat) for another few weeks, and in some cases months, depending on the individual situation.

A final point is that monthly water weight fluctuations associated with the menstrual cycle need to be carefully considered when judging whether or not a plateau has been reached. People who menstruate should be wary of falsely identifying a weight loss plateau that is shorter than the approximate four-week cycle.

Breaking through plateaus

Tackling weight loss plateaus requires an understanding of the root cause of weight/fat gain. The fundamental mechanism is a sustained surplus of unused calories that accumulate in adipose (fat) tissue storage. In other words, fat gain is the result of chronically consuming more calories than you burn (or use for gains in lean mass).

While the mechanism/root cause of fat gain is relatively straightforward (excess energy intake and/or insufficient energy output), the many factors contributing to chronic hypercaloric conditions are difficult to account for. Obesity is a multifactorial condition whose pathogenesis involves the complex interaction between genetic predisposition, psychological/behavioral state, social parameters, economic constraints, physical limitations, and concurrent states of disease. All of these factors can influence an individual's state of energy balance either directly or indirectly.

This is why telling the public to just eat less and move more is an oversimplification that fails to solve the obesity problem, even though it's technically correct. Unfortunately, "Eat less, move more!" is far catchier than saying, "Maintain an energy deficit with appropriate macronutrient targets and personally preferred foods within a healthy diet pattern while engaged in regular physical activity that includes resistance training with properly individualized programming and progression."

Within this multifactorial framework is an overlooked but important obstacle to weight loss and weight loss maintenance: the food environment. The so-called *obesogenic environment* is characterized by an abundance of highly refined/processed food products that are calorie-dense, hyperpalatable, easily accessible, affordable, and effectively marketed.[496,560] This environment facilitates passive/unintentional overconsumption.

The good news is that the food environment is modifiable to a certain degree. For example, you can do a bit of legwork to make nutrient-dense/calorie-sparse foods (like fresh fruit) highly visible and easily available in the home or the workplace. In addition, you can keep junk foods (e.g., packaged snacks, desserts, and sugar-sweetened beverages) out of the home/workplace, or at least away from areas of high visibility and easy accessibility. Another tactic is to avoid snacking while watching television or movies or mindlessly browsing the internet. And when you do snack, do not eat straight out of the package or bag—this can lead to consuming the whole package. Eating foods on smaller plates and bowls can help, as can pre-portioning foods and snacks before storing them.

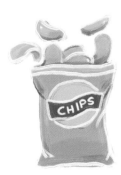

It's appropriate to plan on breaking plateaus that occur en route to the end-goal. But before that, an honest, diligent assessment of adherence should be done. If good compliance to the program is confirmed, then you must decide how to reopen the caloric deficit, and there are only three options: 1) decrease energy intake, 2) increase energy output, or 3) some combination of the two.

The program adjustment you make depends on what's most realistic for the individual, as well as how urgent the time frame is. If calories are already low and hunger/appetite control is already a persistent challenge, then reducing intake even further is probably not the best move. In this scenario, options for increasing energy expenditure through exercise or non-exercise means should be considered. On the other hand, if energy output is already high, with little room for pushing exercise volume further, then decreasing energy intake is a viable option. This should be done in cautious increments; 10 percent of total calories is a safe benchmark.

It's understood that the urgency of the time frames for hitting goals varies from individual to individual. Ratcheting up the aggressiveness of the program adjustment past the 10 percent benchmark (up to 20 percent) is sometimes warranted with a tight deadline to achieve a certain weight or look. There are also individuals who have a stronger adaptive response (subconscious changes in NEAT) and thus are "resistant" to changes in energy intake and output, requiring more aggressive caloric adjustments (toward 20 percent up or down).

However, keep in mind that the risk of nonadherence increases alongside the degree of restriction. Plateaus in weight gain should be dealt with in a similarly methodical manner, with 10 percent increments in caloric intake being my preference as a safe benchmark. As discussed earlier, an alternative solution would be to back away from the fire and simply maintain for a period of time, realizing that weight loss maintenance is a legitimate goal—and a challenging one.

In sum, the program must be scrutinized to determine the most realistic and prudent plan of action. How much room does the individual have for increasing the intensity, duration, or frequency of training or non-exercise activity? How much room is there for reducing or increasing caloric intake? How aggressive, urgent, or time-sensitive is the goal? The answers to these questions will vary widely from person to person, making it impossible to issue a universal prescription.

One thing is certain, however—the protocol must match the individual's physical and psychological tolerance, or it will end up being a recipe for either conscious or unconscious nonadherence. I'll also reiterate that "breaking" plateaus should be attempted only when an actual plateau is detected, which is no less than four weeks of progress stagnation. Figure 9e guides the decision process for managing fat loss plateaus.

Figure 9e: Plateau Flow Chart: Big-Picture Decision Guide

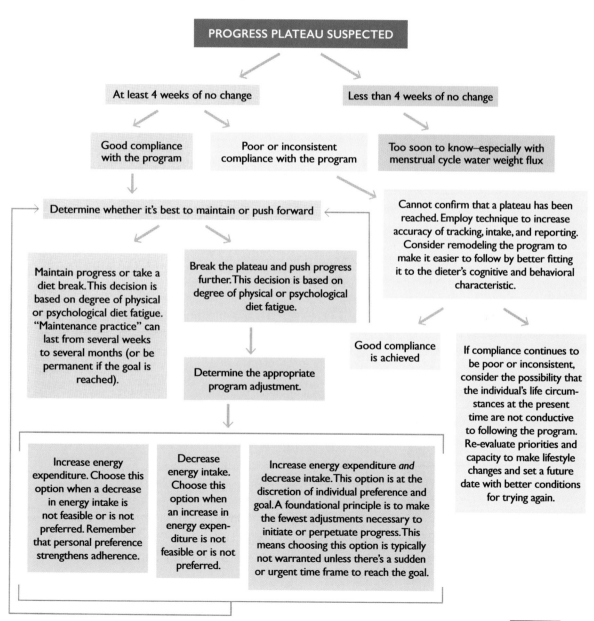

The underrated yet crucial impact of NEAT

It's important to be aware of the body's homeostatic drive—in other words, its hardwired aim to survive and preserve the status quo. The body has many tricks up its sleeve for foiling dieting efforts. One of the greatest impacts on drops in energy expenditure alongside dieting is a subconscious drop in NEAT.[59]

As mentioned earlier, NEAT includes any movement outside of formal exercise, such as occupational physical activity, subconscious and non-purposeful movement such as fidgeting, and movement during sleep. It also includes lifestyle habits such as choosing the stairs versus the elevator. NEAT is the most widely variable component of total daily energy expenditure across individuals; it can differ by as much as 500 to 1,000 kcal between people of the same body mass.[59]

Decreased NEAT is a major component of metabolic adaptation, but it's often overlooked and difficult to track. Most post–weight loss decreases in total daily energy expenditure are not attributable to decreased RMR. This is a false presumption called "starvation mode" in uninformed fitness circles.

It's true that there's a small margin of the decrease in RMR (10 to 15 percent at most) that can be attributed to *adaptive thermogenesis*, which is defined as a decrease in RMR that's not attributable to a decrease in lean mass. However, it's been estimated that 85 to 90 percent of the drop in total daily energy expenditure that can't be accounted for by drops in LBM can be attributed to a drop in NEAT.[561] Essentially, what people commonly blame on a "slowed metabolism" is actually an insidious decrease in subconscious and non-exercise movement.

So, one of the possible solutions to weight loss plateaus is to take an inventory of the person's lifestyle and daily routine and estimate where the drops in NEAT could have occurred. Then you can form potential strategies on how to reverse some of those drops in NEAT.

The untapped power of shifting the focus off of weight loss

An underappreciated and underutilized weight loss tactic is—ironically—taking the focus off of weight loss. This concept isn't just a cool-sounding idea; it's been shown to be effective in relatively recent literature.

Clark[562] performed a two-year study on subjects with an average eight-year history of being overweight and chronically yo-yo dieting. The assigned caloric deficit was relatively aggressive (just under their RMR). Protein was abundantly set at 2.2 g/kg per day, Carbohydrate was set at a low but flexible and not necessarily ketogenic target (50 to 100 grams per day). The remainder of calories targeted a majority from unsaturated fat (a 3:1 ratio of unsaturated:saturated fat was prescribed). The resistance training program was progressive and periodized, with sessions done a minimum of three times per week. Endurance training was done at least twice a week. Total training was a maximum of six days per week. The subjects were highly engaged in a dynamic and challenging protocol that allowed them to self-select exercises (which likely bolstered adherence through an increased sense of autonomy).

So far so good, and nothing particularly special (aside from the boldly high-end assignment of protein intake). What separates this program from others in the literature is how the subjects were instructed to focus on making progress in exercise performance—and not focus on weight loss. Ultimately, this was a highly effective long-term approach; subjects lost 35 percent of their starting bodyweight, almost exclusively from body fat. Average body fat reduction was 41.2 kilograms (90.6 pounds) in men and 21.4 kilograms (47.1 pounds) in women.

Unfortunately, the manuscript doesn't delve into the specifics of counseling subjects toward the mindset of focusing on performance improvements rather than weight loss. I hope that future research can better elucidate protocol guidelines in this vein, since it may be a viable alternative to the conventional approach. For the time being, the success of Clark's protocol (high-protein, non-keto low-carb, focus on performance instead of weight loss) makes a compelling case for further investigation.

The big-picture perspective

Figure 9f is an aerial view of the big picture. It's what I call the Cycle of Progress,[563] depicting the succession of progress curves that surge, slow, and stop as a plateau is reached. Each progress curve is initiated by adjusting program variables to create a new set of challenges that force the body to change and adapt. This is conceptually what the road to the goal looks like. The progress phases become progressively less robust and the plateau periods become progressively longer until the goal is attained. Let me reiterate that, yes, the goal itself is a plateau.

Figure 9f: The Cycle of Progress

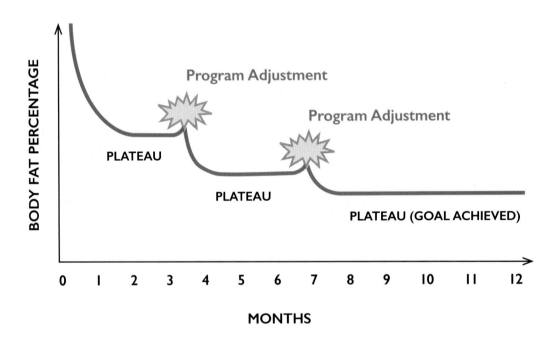

WEANING OFF OF TRACKING

It's easy to read the title of this section and automatically think that I'm denouncing the concept or practice of tracking dietary intake. I'm not. My aim is to provide guidance for those who have been tracking for a while (typically via an app) and feel trapped by or dependent on it. This is for folks who want to abandon tracking but fear they will lose a critical degree of control and awareness and then slip from their goals.

I fully acknowledge that there are individuals who don't want (and don't need) to stop tracking. I personally know several who actually *enjoy* it, and that's fine—different strokes for different folks. Successful program individualization means acknowledging that everyone is different. A recent trial by Hahn and colleagues[564] found that in women at low risk for eating disorders (ED), four weeks of diet tracking app use did not affect ED risk. So, preliminary data suggest that people with a low risk for ED are more appropriate candidates for app use, whereas those at higher risk for ED could find that using an app triggers or worsens ED symptoms. Any way you slice it, caution is warranted since there's an unsurprisingly high prevalence of eating disorders among athletes (especially in the physique competition realm) and fitness coaches/instructors.

Some folks simply dislike tracking their intake, or they used to be OK with it but have grown to detest it. They see it at as a chore or a source of anxiety. For some people, tracking every detail strengthens an unhealthy degree of perfectionism and micromanagement. At worst, using diet tracking apps can become a means of contributing to or exacerbating eating disorders.[565-567] Furthermore, there are validity and reliability limits to tracking energy and nutrient consumption, just as there are limits to accurately tracking energy expenditure. Griffiths and colleagues[568] examined the accuracy of five of the most popular free nutrition tracking apps and found that each had a tendency to report lower values than the Nutrition Data System for Research.

On a related note, activity tracking devices can be prone to inaccuracy. Passler and colleagues[569] compared five popular wrist-worn activity tracking devices with indirect calorimetry. Quoting their conclusion:

> *"The tested trackers could not show valid results. Hence, it is concluded that current commercially available activity trackers are most likely not*

accurate enough to be used for neither purposes in sports, nor in health care and rehabilitative applications."

A systematic review by Evenson and colleagues[561] found that wearable devices had higher validity for tracking steps but lower validity for tracking energy expenditure.

Good candidates for transitioning away from tracking

People who have been tracking for a while (typically a number of years) are the group most commonly asking how to stop. The good news is, this group is in a perfect position to stop tracking because they've been doing it long enough to have gained a sufficiently accurate perspective of the caloric and nutritive values of various foods and beverages, in the various serving sizes that they consume. This is a very useful skill, and, in my observations, it takes roughly two to four weeks to become adept at it.

Individuals whose goal is to maintain their progress are good candidates for taking the steps to let go of the reins. Keep in mind that it doesn't have to be a permanent commitment. Taking an extended break (several weeks at least) from tracking, while setting a goal of maintenance during this break, is a good setup for weaning off of tracking. In contrast, those who are proactively trying to lose or gain weight under time-constrained deadlines are not ideal for attempts to wean off of tracking.

Changing false perceptions

A common perception is that meticulous tracking is what led to results, so stopping tracking will lead to a lack of progress. While this unfavorable scenario is not impossible, it shouldn't automatically be presumed as inevitable (or even probable). The act of tracking adds a layer of accountability and awareness. However, it also tends to reduce flexibility and openness to impromptu adjustments based on internal hunger and satiety cues. Now, the kicker is this—accountability and awareness are entirely possible without the meticulous quantification of dietary intake.

Proactively building awareness of internal cues: ICAN

It's ironic that many people who track everything to the gram do not have an awareness of when they are actually satiated or hungry. This is partially due to the pressure of fulfilling the plan (hitting the nutrient targets per meal or per day). This gets combined with avoiding the shame of a breached contract or broken promise with ourselves or our coaches. These distractions hinder the ability to build awareness of internal cues, which is an extremely important skill. Building awareness of internal hunger and satiety cues involves purposely not sticking to a predetermined diet script.

For those seeking an effective way to approach awareness building, here's a technique inspired by Los Angeles–based dietitian Toby Levine. I've successfully used my own adaptation of Toby's methods with clients who had varying degrees of psychological challenges with traditional tracking. I used to call it internal cue awareness training (ICAT) but changed it recently when I realized that calling it internal cue awareness nurturing makes the acronym even better (ICAN). Figure 9g provides a form that you can use as a template or guide.

Figure 9g: Internal Cue Awareness Nurturing (ICAN)

TIME	HUNGER LEVEL	MEAL	FULLNESS LEVEL	THOUGHTS / FEELINGS / NOTES

How to use the ICAN form:

- Before each meal, note the time of the meal, and then give yourself a hunger rating. I use a five-point scale, as follows:

    1. Not hungry at all

    2. Slightly hungry

    3. Moderately hungry

    4. Very hungry

    5. Fricking HANGRY

- Write down what you ate, estimating the quantities to the best of your ability (without actually measuring them), and give yourself a fullness rating. I use a five-point scale, as follows:

    1. Barely feel like I ate anything

    2. Slightly satisfied

    3. Moderately full

    4. Very full

    5. Stuffed and uncomfortable

- Write down objective as well as subjective feelings and thoughts after each meal. Don't hold back; be very honest and raw.

And that's it. That's the journaling method for ICAN. Over time, you'll notice patterns, and you'll be able to draw correlations between your hunger and fullness levels to mood, time of day, and surrounding events. You'll notice patterns of how the types of foods you choose correlate with hunger and fullness levels. Depending on the goal (not everyone wants to lose weight), you'll be more conscious of hunger and fullness levels and better able to proactively make moves that align with your goal.

After one to two weeks of ICAN, it's far more common for people to either lose or maintain weight than to gain. And at the end of the one to two weeks, your perception of hunger and fullnes, and your overall awareness of how your emotional state affects your eating behavior will be much keener. If you decide to try ICAN, run it for an entire month in order to subject it to a full range of experiences.

A note to practitioners: the ICAN method works very well with clients who are struggling with their "relationship" with food and have tried conventional routes without much success. ICAN provides a glimpse into the minds of clients (or patients). In addition to getting in touch with hunger and satiety cues, it's a way to stay mindful of how eating habits affect the mind state and behavior patterns that keep people on the path toward their goals.

Taking off the training wheels

It bears repeating that awareness of body composition progress (or maintenance of progress) is relatively simple when you just open your eyes a little. What works well as a mental safety net for those who are afraid of regaining weight while not tracking their diet intake is to focus on two main elements: exercise performance and total bodyweight.

If the scale is stable (weekly bodyweight averages are what to keep an eye on) and training performance is maintained, these are reliable indicators that body composition is being maintained. If lifting performance is maintained while bodyweight remains stable, that's a good indicator that muscle is not being lost. Of course, there could be the welcome scenario of lifting performance improving while bodyweight is stable, which could indicate recomposition. What I just described is the minimalist version of the low-tech body composition tracking method that I talked about earlier in this chapter.

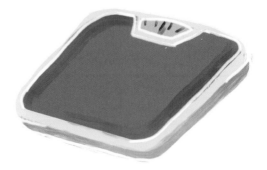

Protein tracking as the last step of graduation

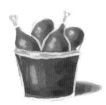

Another strategy for those who aren't ready to let go of formal tracking is to track only protein and total kcals while keeping all else flexible. If you're not a competitive athlete with very specific carb requirements, the beauty of tracking just protein and calories is that you're not boxed into a fixed proportion of carbs and fat. If you're in the mood for a carby day, have at it. If you're in the mood for a fatty day after that, have at it. The carb-fat proportion of the diet has been shown time and again to have minimal influence on body composition changes. It blows people's minds to know that they can go full keto one day and high-carb/low-fat the next and get virtually the same body fat results as they do when sticking to only one of those approaches. Using this approach while staying mindful of hunger and satiety cues is effective and significantly less tedious than tracking all three macros.

The next step in the graduation process would be tracking only protein while putting your newly attuned sense of hunger and satiety to use once you've completed the ICAN exercise for roughly a month. From that point, you can abandon weighing and measuring protein foods once you're comfortable. Instead of tracking protein to the gram, you can simply target "significant" protein servings, which for most folks average three to four per day, depending on your personal preference (and how much lean mass you plan to carry). A significant protein serving would be about a quarter to a third of your protein allotment for the day (30 to 60 grams per day for most individuals). Examples of a significant protein serving would be a palm-sized piece of meat/fish/poultry, two scoops of protein powder (either animal- or plant-based), or two cups of a high-protein dairy food such as Greek yogurt. Protein tracking by eyeballing portions of foods you routinely consume gets easier with time.

Once you're comfortable, you can stop taking formal/written/app-accounted records of your protein intake and just maintain a mental awareness of it while paying attention to hunger and satiety cues to manage general dietary intake levels. Assess your progress monthly as you journey through this process.

Note that a major objective is to establish an effective eating pattern that involves meals you enjoy and even look forward to. Every time someone asks me how to achieve lasting results without counting calories or grams,

I tell them that the "secret" is in locking in a consistent dietary routine with the foods you love in amounts that satisfy you. This is the opposite of eating reactively and haphazardly. When you lock in an ironclad routine, then changing your body—if/when you decide to do so, either seasonally or permanently—becomes a simple matter of adjusting your intake or output levels up or down.

Headfirst into deep water

When someone asks how to stop tracking, I'm tempted to answer, "Just stop tracking." The vast majority of people who ask me that question have simply never tried it! Stopping cold turkey is indeed one of the options. I've issued 30-day "stop tracking and just live your life" challenges many times. I'm not talking about YOLO-ing for a month; I'm talking about maintaining mindful eating patterns and choices conducive to your goals—just don't track or obsess over the details. If you have enough courage, don't weigh yourself for the full month. The overwhelming majority brave enough to try this approach are pleasantly surprised to see that any changes are minimal, and well within the small margin of fluctuation in hydration levels and gastrointestinal content. Our bodies are wired toward preserving the status quo, and the 30-day no-tracking challenge demonstrates this time and again. After you've made it past the first month without tracking, you can reassess your goals and plan your next moves. I dare you to try it.

CHAPTER 9 IN A NUTSHELL

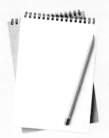

- Adherence is everything. A program or plan is only as good as its ability to be followed for the length of time it's intended to work.

- Weight loss maintainers comprise only about 20 percent of dieters; the other 80 percent fail. While this statistic is disheartening, there's still hope to make a dent in it.

- Bodyweight set point is better regarded as a "settling point" determined by behavioral interaction with environmental and genetic factors. Settling points can be shifted up or down depending on conscious and strategic building of habits.

- A multitude of factors influence our ability to adhere to programs. Strategies to breach barriers to dietary adherence and counterproductive habits include education, social support, continual resetting/reassessment of goals, and modification of the food environment.

- Individualization is perhaps the most powerful facilitator of successful programs that result in long-term adherence, yet individualization is lacking in most programs.

- My approach aims at fulfilling the fundamental psychological needs (autonomy, competence, and relatedness) to strengthen adherence and progress.

- All program elements should be individualized. These elements include macronutrition, food choices within a healthy framework, self-monitoring and accountability, meal frequency and distribution, degree of dietary nonlinearity, and hedonic ("cheat" meal) strategy.

- Bodyweight maintenance doesn't have to be rigid and static to be considered successful or healthy. Maintenance can be viewed as a seasonal or cyclical ebb and flow.

- Recomp, cutting, bulking, and gaintaining have unique indexes of progress that vary with individual training status. Recomp capacity is determined by your proximity to your potential for muscle size and leanness.

- Cutting cycles should facilitate a rate of weight/fat loss that doesn't put lean mass gains at risk (0.5 to 1 percent weekly). Bulking phases should last at least six months to allow sufficient time for meaningful/measurable gains. For natural trainees, I wouldn't recommend less than a 3:1 to 4:1 ratio of time spent bulking versus cutting.

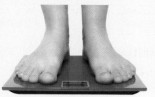

- Weight loss plateaus can be defined as a stasis of body composition lasting a month or more. There are only two possible causes for a plateau: 1) lack of adherence to the program, or 2) a new point of equilibrium in energy balance.

- Plateaus are always placed in a negative light, but I've found that it's much more productive to frame them as opportunities to test the sustainability of progress. Therefore, I encourage dieters to view plateaus as "maintenance practice." It blows people's minds (in a good way) when they gain that perspective.

- Non-exercise activity thermogenesis (NEAT) is perhaps the most widely variable component of energy expenditure across individuals. The "metabolic slowing" phenomenon that accompanies weight loss is due in large part to drops in NEAT rather than resting metabolic rate (RMR).

- Shifting the focus off of weight loss and onto improvements in exercise performance ironically can result in substantial weight loss. This approach is a viable option to explore, especially for individuals who are burnt out from years of fruitless focus on scale weight.

- Tracking program variables can be a double-edged sword. On one hand, it's important for objectively knowing the nature of changes occurring. On the other hand, it can foster obsessiveness and perfectionism. In some individuals, it has the potential to cause or exacerbate eating disorders.

- Weaning off of tracking is a delicate process that can be assisted by developing a keener awareness of hunger and satiety cues (you now have the ICAN form in your arsenal if you need it; see Figure 9g). A stepwise weaning process from tracking all macros involves first tracking just protein and total daily calories and then tracking only protein—first in grams, then by significant protein servings. The final step is staying in the ballpark of an effective eating pattern that you enjoy and can sustain.

REVIEWING THE KEY CONCEPTS & TAMING THE BEAST

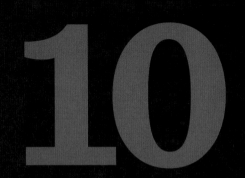

Speaking candidly, this book is more like a certification textbook than a stroll through the park (whereas the latter describes many other popular diet books). I pulled no punches while covering an exhausting number of details. Nutrition is incredibly complex, and this book does not shy away from that complexity. Throughout this journey, we've delved into the theory and application of nutrition for not only multiple goals (muscle gain, fat loss, and athletic performance) but also different aspects within each goal (total daily dose, timing relative to training, etc.).

The aim of this chapter is to tame this beast of a book, reinforce the key takeaways of each chapter, and make the messages more digestible. Please note that while this chapter attempts to distill the key concepts, it is far from a worthy substitute for the fine details and nuances within the individual chapters.

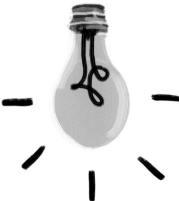

Chapter 1: The origin & evolution of flexible dieting

The heart of flexible dieting is the individualization of the dietary approach. Some folks love tracking macro grams, while others do best maintaining a general awareness of portion targets or simply eating more of certain types of foods and less of others. It's not possible to define *flexible dieting* by a single approach—whether that be tracking macro gram targets or changing general eating habits. Flexible dieting is the umbrella that encompasses all of these approaches.

In peer-reviewed literature dating back to the early 1990s, flexible dieting was originally defined as a style of cognitive restraint characterized by flexible rather than rigid dietary control. Instead of viewing foods and dieting in a dichotomous (good-or-bad, all-or-nothing) light, flexible dieting allows for shades of gray within the bigger picture of long-term success.

One such shade of gray is the option to let roughly 10 to 20 percent of total caloric intake consist of whatever you want (including junk foods and beverages), which can strengthen long-term sustainability and protect against the common cycle of self-sabotaging perfectionism.

The literature favors flexible dieting over rigid dieting for controlling bodyweight and mitigating the risk of eating disorders, which is the big revelation of this book: it's not about a singular, universally applicable protocol that emphasizes a set of "special" foods while banning others. The key to long-term success is individualizing the dietary program, which includes the flexibility or rigidity of the approach as well as accountability and tracking. The individual decides based on personal goals and preferences, which can change over time.

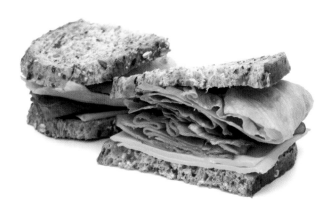

Chapter 2: The big picture of science

To understand flexible dieting, you must understand nutritional science. Science is a set of principles that guide the process of determining how the natural world works. It can also be viewed as a road map to uncovering the truth.

Research is the vehicle for carrying out the aims of science. Since research is carried out by humans, it's inevitably subject to human error and bias. Good research has multiple safeguards that maximize transparency and minimize bias. The process of peer review provides an important layer of quality control for published research.

As imperfect as peer-reviewed research often is, it still provides higher-quality information than what pervades the mass media, which ultimately boils down to unchecked opinion. The landscape is littered with bold speculations and false claims. Scientific research serves as a lighthouse in a sea of misinformation, but there is a sprawling expanse of unknowns.

This is where evidence-based practice (EBP) comes in. EBP in the context of nutrition and fitness recognizes that there's plenty of gray area in our knowledge of what improves health and performance. It uses scientific research as a basis for programming and fills in the knowledge gaps with what has been consistently observed in practice (aka, *the trenches*).

Chapter 3: Demystifying scientific research

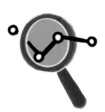

The next step is learning what strengthens or weakens a study in terms of methodology and, perhaps more importantly, relevance to the topic/question at hand.

The different types of research exist on a continuum from descriptive to experimental. The main types common to nutrition and fitness are observational and experimental (also called interventional). These types differ in their basic methodological structure. Observational research does not intervene with the variables under examination. In contrast, experimental research involves the comparison of a control group (or control condition) with a treatment group (also called the experimental group) that receives the intervention (i.e., the drug, nutrient, or exercise protocol being tested). This fundamental difference in methodology allows experimental research to determine causation, whereas observational research can only draw potential correlations.

Randomized controlled trials (RCTs) are known as the gold standard of study designs because they can determine whether a given agent or protocol can directly cause a given outcome, which can investigate the potential for cause and effect. RCTs can examine intermediate end points such as changes in blood lipids in shorter trial durations and carry a higher degree of rigor but also higher costs and more logistical challenges.

It's generally infeasible (and sometimes unethical) to design RCTs that compare experimental versus control conditions to examine "hard" end points such as heart disease and mortality (death rate), which can take years or decades to manifest. This is the job of epidemiology, which falls under observational research. We depend on epidemiology to study large populations over long periods of time to track disease-related outcomes and mortality. In this sense, observational and interventional research complement each other. We need both; observational studies can provide hints and hypotheses, and controlled interventions can provide answers to the questions raised by observational findings.

On the hierarchy of evidence, anecdotes are the weakest. The next level up is observational research, which is useful for generating hypotheses but limited in its ability to show causation. RCTs are the next level up because they can demonstrate causation.

However, all research designs, including RCTs, can have flaws and limitations that compromise their validity. Summational research such as systematic reviews and meta-analyses attempts to convey the evidence as a whole by accounting for the data of multiple studies that meet the inclusion criteria to satisfy a given question or topic. Systematic reviews and meta-analyses of RCTs are perched at the top of the evidence hierarchy and represent what's referred to as the *weight of the evidence.* Position stands are narrative summations of the state of the evidence, which include the experience of the authors (usually the most prolific or decorated researchers on the topic). They provide practical applications of the research, whereas systematic reviews and meta-analyses typically fall short of arriving at actionable guidelines, making position stands a great place to start when seeking out the scientific consensus.

Chapter 4: Protein

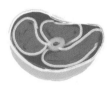

Now let's review the macronutrients. Protein is an essential one, meaning it's necessary for human survival, facilitating a wide range of physiological processes and playing a multitude of roles in the body. Essential nutrients must be derived from the diet because the body is incapable of sufficiently biosynthesizing them to meet basic needs. Protein contains 4 kcal per gram of energy.

Skeletal muscle is the single largest store of protein in the body. As such, maintaining a healthy degree of muscle mass is crucial to innumerable metabolic aspects that preserve strength and mobility and protect against disease related to the loss of lean body mass.

Protein quality is determined by the essential amino acid content and the digestibility of a given source. Animal-based proteins are generally of higher quality than plant-based proteins and are more efficient in their anabolic effect. However, advancing food technology (particularly isolated plant-based proteins and protein blends) is narrowing that gap.

For a typical mixed diet that includes a variety of protein sources, getting enough total daily protein is the most important objective. The distribution and timing of protein doses throughout the day are secondary concerns for those with specialized athletic or aesthetic goals. For most healthy individuals engaged in regular exercise, an appropriate protein intake range is 1.6 to 2.2 g/kg (0.7 to 1.0 g/lb) of total bodyweight. Observational data indicate that lean, exercise-trained individuals who are pushing the competitive envelope under hypocaloric (dieting) conditions can benefit from higher intakes of 2.3 to 3.1 g/kg of fat-free mass. Recomposition, which is the simultaneous loss of fat and gain of muscle, has been observed with protein intakes ranging from 2.6 to 3.5 g/kg of fat-free mass. Further observational data indicate that athletes pushing the envelope of leanness, such as physique competitors in prolonged caloric deficits, can use the guideline of 2.2 to 3.3 g/kg (1 to 1.5 g/lb) of total bodyweight.

There is a false idea that protein intake needs to be minimized to avoid triggering molecular mechanisms that shorten life span. This idea is based primarily on research involving worms, flies, and rodents. For humans, the most sensible approach is to optimize musculoskeletal functionality, which in turn optimizes cardiometabolic health. This muscle-centric approach best supports the metabolic engine of the body and translates to improved health, longevity, and overall quality of life. This is simply not achievable with protein intake at the RDA level of 0.8 g/kg. Most people need about 50 to 100 percent more protein (i.e., 1.2 to 1.6 g/kg) to prevent and mitigate age-related muscle loss and the chronic and degenerative diseases that can accompany it.

These figures assume normal bodyweight. You can accurately set protein intake by basing it on goal bodyweight (or target bodyweight). If your current bodyweight is your target bodyweight, use that figure when establishing protein intake.

Chapter 5: Carbohydrate

Carbohydrate is also a macronutrient, and its primary role is to provide energy for the myriad physiological processes of the body. Carbohydrate is unique among the macronutrients in that it is not considered essential because the body can derive all its carbohydrate needs from non-carbohydrate sources, thus rendering dietary carbohydrate unnecessary for survival.

However, there is an important distinction between preventing death and optimizing health and athletic performance. You could choose to avoid consuming carbohydrate and survive, but you would kiss goodbye any goal of maximizing athletic performance potential. Just because it's possible to steer a car with your feet doesn't make it the optimal way to drive. Furthermore, high-quality (whole and minimally refined) carbohydrate sources provide fiber and nutrients that promote good health and prevent chronic disease. Added sugars (as opposed to intrinsic sugars in milk and fruit) should be limited to a maximum of 10 percent of total caloric intake.

Programming for the goal of fat loss can accommodate very low carbohydrate intakes, including ketogenic intakes (50 grams per day or less), or high intakes if a net caloric deficit is sustained throughout the day or week. The hype surrounding the superior fat loss of ketogenic diets is based on comparisons that fail to equate protein and total caloric intake between the diets in question. When those variables are properly controlled, there's no

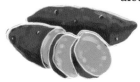

difference in fat loss between ketogenic and non-ketogenic diets, regardless of differences in carbohydrate–fat proportion. Most studies on this topic suggest that carbohydrate restriction to ketogenic levels is not sustainable in the long term; carb intake gradually creeps up, reaching double or even triple the originally assigned intake at the 12-month mark. So, for the goal of fat loss, a wide range of carbohydrate intakes are fair game and should be dictated by personal preference.

Performance-related goals in strength- and power-oriented sports are best supported by a daily carbohydrate intake ranging from 3 to 8 g/kg of total bodyweight. This is the same dosing range that optimally supports muscle growth. Compared to higher-carb control diets, ketogenic diets have consistently resulted in less gains or greater losses in lean body mass in resistance trainees. So, while keto is a legitimate option for fat loss, it's not optimal for muscle gain or retention.

For maximizing competitive endurance performance, an appropriate daily carbohydrate intake range is 6 to 12 g/kg. Implementing a ketogenic diet to become "fat-adapted" or "keto-adapted" to maximize endurance capacity has repeatedly failed to pan out in research with properly controlled variables. From a performance perspective, ketogenic diets can be maladaptive because they impair glycogen breakdown. This is a bad thing when the goal is to win competitive endurance events, where *race-winning moves* (characterized by strategic bursts of high-intensity muscular work) depend on carbohydrate availability.

The timing and distribution of carbohydrate intake for maximizing athletic performance can't be summed up in a sound bite, so refer to the details in Chapter 5.

Chapter 6: Fat

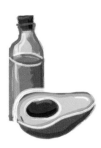

Fat is the most energy-dense macronutrient, providing 9 kcal per gram, as opposed to protein and carbohydrate, which both provide 4 kcal per gram. (Alcohol provides 7 kcal per gram, and although it can technically be called a macronutrient because it provides energy, it's not essential and is a health hazard when consumed in excess.)

Fat is considered an essential macronutrient and plays multiple physiological roles. As such, sufficient fat must be derived from the diet to preserve health and ensure survival. The practical minimum intake of dietary fat is about 20 percent of total calories; underconsumption is not necessarily conducive to essential fatty acid deficiency but tends to be unsustainable and can compromise hormone production. Fat intake recommendations are usually listed as a percentage of total calories out of tradition and convenience, but this leaves absolute amounts at the mercy of the wide variation in individual energy intake requirements. So, in the vein of carbohydrate and protein recommendations, an appropriate fat intake range that encompasses most goals and preferences is 0.7 to 2.2 g/kg (0.32 to 1 g/lb).

Higher fat intakes are typically the result of purposeful carbohydrate restriction and require greater awareness of the types of fat-rich foods consumed. The weight of the evidence points to lower cardiovascular disease risk when dietary fat intake is predominantly from unsaturated fat. Plant-based fat sources (e.g., olive oil, nuts, seeds, and avocados) are conducive to good health, while land animal–based fats warrant more careful moderation of intake. Fatty fish are a significant source of omega-3 fatty acids, which are a healthy yet widely underconsumed nutrient, especially in Westernized countries.

An exception to the plant-based "healthy" fat rule are hydrogenated vegetable oils, which are engineered to be more spreadable and shelf-stable but adversely affect blood lipids and increase cardiovascular risk. While the major health agencies push for a saturated fat intake of no more than 10 percent of total calories, a focus on individual fatty acids might be less productive than assessing whether food choices are whole or minimally processed versus highly refined and processed. The concept of the "food matrix" is important, since foods contain multiple nutritive components that can offer net benefits to health despite the presence of cholesterol or saturated fat.

One interesting twist in the dietary fat story is the consistency of neutral-to-beneficial effects on blood lipids from the intake of dark chocolate and cheese, both of which are rich sources of saturated fat. Another twist in the saga is that whole eggs, once vilified for their cholesterol content, have been repeatedly shown in the research to lack health concerns with moderate intakes of one to three eggs per day, depending on how cautious you want to be. Getting regular checkups and keeping an eye on blood lipids (and heeding your doctor's advice) is prudent, since individual response varies widely.

Then there is the fringe alarmism against vegetable oils—more specifically, seed oils and linoleic acid (an omega-6 fatty acid). The evidence shows that although the general population can benefit from more omega-3 fatty acids, omega-6 fatty acid alarmism is first-world mythology.

Chapter 7: Exercise performance–enhancing supplements

The supplement realm is just as packed with misinformation as the diet world, but only a handful of compounds have enough scientific support to warrant consideration for use. This makes it relatively simple to choose what you might want to add to your nutritional arsenal.

It's worth mentioning the folly of seeking optimization in this area while neglecting to cover potential gaps in essential micronutrition. The risk of nutrient shortfalls can be simply and economically reduced with a daily multivitamin mineral (MVM) supplement. MVMs benefit individuals whose diets lack completeness across the food groups and diversity of food selection within the food groups (this describes most of the population). Adding hypocaloric/dieting conditions to the mix exacerbates the micronutrient shortcomings of consuming a narrow range of nutrient-sparse, energy-dense foods that characterize typical diet patterns.

On the note of hypocaloric conditions, "fat-burners" are a class of supplements that you can safely skip. You'll save money, lower the risk of adverse effects, and won't be missing out on any magic, since the weight/fat loss effects are not clinically meaningful in the long term. The win-win combination for effective fat loss is proper diet and exercise, which unfortunately takes a lot more discipline than taking a fat-burner pill.

Conversely, safe and effective supplementation exists for gaining muscle mass, strength, and power—thanks to creatine. The body biosynthesizes roughly 1 gram of creatine per day and derives another gram per day from diet (given omnivorous conditions). Creatine naturally occurs both in the body and in animal-based foods. Supplementation works by saturating muscle phosphocreatine stores, increasing the bioavailability of ATP, the body's energy currency. In addition, creatine is effective at increasing mean mass. The performance benefits of creatine are mainly confined to the strength/power end of the strength-endurance continuum, which includes lifting, sprinting, and mixed sports with intermittent high-intensity demands.

On the endurance side, the best research-supported supplements are beta-alanine, sodium bicarbonate (baking soda), and nitrate (derived from root vegetables and green leafy vegetables). Beta-alanine and sodium bicarbonate have similar mechanisms of action; they act as buffering agents that counteract exercise-induced acidosis, thereby staving off fatigue and increasing work capacity. Beta-alanine augments the performance of activities ranging from one to four minutes (possibly up to 10 minutes), and sodium bicarbonate enhances bouts lasting 30 seconds to 12 minutes. Nitrate (often called *dietary nitrate*) increases endurance capacity by increasing nitric oxide production and is most effective for bouts lasting 12 to 40 minutes.

Despite technically being a drug rather than a supplement, caffeine needs to be included in the discussion of ergogenic (performance-enhancing) compounds since it's been demonstrated as effective across the strength-endurance continuum. Caffeine is naturally occurring in a multitude of plant species and works by blocking adenosine receptors and stimulating the central nervous system. Of all the ergogenic agents discussed here, caffeine has the most serious adverse potential if abused. The harmful effects of excessive caffeine dosing are well known and should be respected. Dosing protocols and caveats for these agents are outlined in Chapter 7.

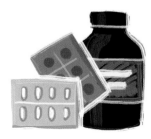

Chapter 8: Dietary programming

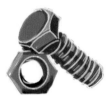

This is a nuts-and-bolts "workshop" chapter, where we walk through the steps of setting body composition goals, establishing macronutrient targets, and building a meal plan (which is more like a framework or template) for two case examples. This is the one chapter where you need to engage your quantitative capabilities. An online calculator (alanaragon.com/calculator) is available if needed. Here are the five steps for establishing macronutrient targets for the primary goal of altering body composition:

1. Set the goal and time frame.

2. Set calories.

3. Set protein.

4. Set fat.

5. Fill in the remainder with carbohydrate.

For the primary goal of athletic performance, steps 4 and 5 are switched; you set carbohydrate first and then fill in the remainder with fat.

Setting the goal and time frame requires an awareness of realistic rates of muscle gain and fat loss, depending on the starting status of the individual. Rates in beginners or deconditioned/formerly fit folks are significantly greater than in intermediate and advanced trainees, who are closer to their potential for either (or both) goals.

My method of setting macronutrient targets is based on the maintenance needs of the targeted body composition and physical activity level. There are two ways to establish a target bodyweight (TBW); one is quick and dirty, and the other is a methodical set of calculations. Whichever method you choose, the difference between your current weight and your target weight determines the time frame you can expect to set your sights on. When you've established your TBW, the next step is factoring in your average weekly exercise and non-exercise activity level. Like magic, the formula then spits out a theoretical total daily caloric intake target.

My calorie formula is most useful for folks who do not have a grasp of what daily caloric intake level maintains their current weight. This unawareness is common and perpetuated by haphazard eating habits or a lack of consistent focus on a given goal. For individuals who know how many calories maintains their bodyweight, the usefulness of my formula is limited to providing an idea of the caloric intake that's required to maintain their targeted body composition and activity level. While this is a helpful figure to have in mind, it's still hypothetical.

Those who know their maintenance calories (and have no interest in knowing the theoretical daily caloric need of their "goal self") are free to skip the calculations and go the traditional route. This involves imposing a reasonable caloric deficit or surplus (10 to 20 percent below or above maintenance in most cases) depending on whether the goal is weight loss or weight gain. In cases of obesity, a deficit of 20 to 30 percent below maintenance may be safely targeted. If the goal is weight maintenance, then current caloric intake should be kept the same.

One of the most important ingredients in any program is patience. In most cases, programs should be put to trial for a full month before making any adjustments. Sufficient progress at the four-week mark indicates that the program can continue unmodified. Speaking very generally, muscle gain of 1 to 2 pounds per month is realistic in intermediate and beginning male trainees, while more advanced trainees can expect half of that. Expectations for muscle gain in women are about 30 percent less. Realistic rates of fat loss (1 to 2 pounds per week) are the same for men and women.

If progress is insufficient, make sure you're at a bona fide progress plateau before making any program adjustments. A plateau is defined as four full weeks of no change. At this point, you can strategize the next move, which is discussed in Chapter 9.

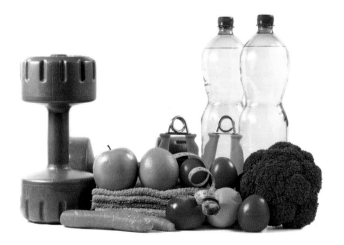

Chapter 9: Adherence, maintenance & weaning off of tracking

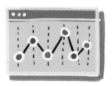

Adherence to a diet or exercise program is everything. After all, what good is a program if it's only effective for a few weeks or months, when the goal was to achieve and sustain lifelong improvements?

Dietary adherence has been studied extensively over the past two decades, and the wisdom gleaned from this research lays the groundwork for effective applications. Barriers to dietary adherence include poor decision-making, socio-cultural forces, environmental and economic forces, a lack of planning, and a lack of physical activity. Solutions to overcoming these barriers include education, motivation, cognitive/behavioral skills, improved food environment, social support, and better goal-setting/adjustment, monitoring/accountability, and individualized programming. Individualization is perhaps the most potent yet underrated driver of program adherence. Every program element, from macronutrient targets to food choices to accountability tactics, should be individualized to meet personal preferences, tolerances, and goals.

Bodyweight maintenance has been given various definitions. For example, successful weight loss maintenance has been proposed to be a 10 percent decrease sustained for a minimum of one year. While this definition is arbitrary, it's a decent initial benchmark for an obese or overweight starting status. But people's goals can evolve over time within a healthy framework, and bodyweight/composition does not need to be static to indicate success. There can be a cyclical ebb and flow of bodyweight/fat levels throughout the year. Classic examples include the cycle of cutting and bulking in fitness/physique circles and a similar cycle of off-, pre-, and in-season in competitive sports. So, maintenance can be viewed as a dynamic target.

A progress plateau can be defined as a four-week period of stagnation. The two possible reasons for arriving at a plateau are nonadherence to the program and the attainment of energy equilibrium—in other words, a new maintenance point. Nonadherence isn't always intentional, as it's common for people to misestimate their energy intake and output.

Dieters must understand the nature of progress at the outset of their endeavor to improve body composition. A "surge, slow, stop" cycle of progress repeats itself, with each cycle being less dramatic and with the "stop" or plateau phase getting longer each time. Picture progressively shortening stairways with progressively lengthening landings. The success of reaching a given goal is largely determined by how long you can sustain it, which is the equivalent of maintaining a plateau. Therefore, an effective psychological tactic is to frame progress plateaus as "maintenance practice."

Overcoming plateaus involves a careful assessment of the program variables to arrive at the most prudent strategy to re-establish an energy deficit for weight loss or energy surplus for weight gain. My preference is to impose caloric changes of 10 to 20 percent, depending on individual circumstances and response. I tend to be more careful and gradual, so 10 percent increments are more common, especially when there's no significant time crunch. An underutilized but powerful way to manage the plateaus and psychological fatigue caused by a constant focus on body composition changes is to shift the focus from the weight displayed on the scale to the improvement of exercise performance.

Tracking calories and macronutrient grams has become so popular that it's nearly thought of as a mandatory practice for those who are serious about their health and fitness goals. However, the reality is that not everyone benefits from this form of micromanagement, and not everyone is unharmed by it. Macronutrient gram targets can be beneficial for building awareness of the nutritive values of the foods and the servings an individual consumes. However, they can also trigger or exacerbate eating disorders in predisposed individuals. Some people just don't like doing tracking or grow to depend on it too much. Abandoning the micromanagement of dietary intake is a legitimate goal for those who want out. Those who love tracking every detail should go for it. But for those who want to wean off of tracking, it can be done in a step-wise manner while building a keener perception of hunger and satiety cues.

Congratulations; you've reached the end of the book! Now that you've gained a deeper understanding of the research, how nutrition affects your body composition and athletic performance, and how to program your diet, I hope this will be the beginning of a new adventure toward a better, healthier you.

REFERENCES

1. Herman CP, Mack D. Restrained and unrestrained eating. *J Pers.* Dec 1975;43(4):647–60. doi:10.1111/j.1467-6494.1975.tb00727.x

2. Westenhoefer J. Dietary restraint and disinhibition: is restraint a homogeneous construct? *Appetite.* Feb 1991;16(1):45–55. doi:10.1016/0195-6663(91)90110-e

3. Westenhoefer J, Stunkard AJ, Pudel V. Validation of the flexible and rigid control dimensions of dietary restraint. *Int J Eat Disord.* Jul 1999; 26(1):53–64. doi:10.1002/(sici)1098-108x(199907)26:1<53::aid-eat7>3.0.co;2-n

4. Shearin EN, Russ MJ, Hull JW, Clarkin JF, Smith GP. Construct validity of the Three-Factor Eating Questionnaire: flexible and rigid control subscales. *Int J Eat Disord.* Sep 1994;16(2):187–98. doi:10.1002/1098-108x(199409)16:2<187::aid-eat2260160210>3.0.co;2-u

5. Williamson DA, Lawson OJ, Brooks ER, et al. Association of body mass with dietary restraint and disinhibition. *Appetite.* Aug 1995;25(1):31–41. doi:10.1006/appe.1995.0039

6. Smith CF, Williamson DA, Bray GA, Ryan DH. Flexible vs. rigid dieting strategies: relationship with adverse behavioral outcomes. *Appetite.* Jun 1999;32(3):295–305. doi:10.1006/appe.1998.0204

7. Stewart TM, Williamson DA, White MA. Rigid vs. flexible dieting: association with eating disorder symptoms in nonobese women. *Appetite.* Feb 2002;38(1):39–44. doi:10.1006/appe.2001.0445

8. Conlin LA, Aguilar DT, Rogers GE, Campbell BI. Flexible vs. rigid dieting in resistance-trained individuals seeking to optimize their physiques: a randomized controlled trial. *J Int Soc Sports Nutr.* Jun 29 2021;18(1):52. doi:10.1186/s12970-021-00452-2

9. Tiggemann M. Dieting and cognitive style: the role of current and past dieting behaviour and cognitions. *J Health Psychol.* Jan 2000;5(1):17–24. doi:10.1177/135910530000500106

10. Byrne S, Cooper Z, Fairburn C. Weight maintenance and relapse in obesity: a qualitative study. *Int J Obes Relat Metab Disord.* Aug 2003;27(8):955–62. doi:10.1038/sj.ijo.0802305

11. Ramacciotti CE, Coli E, Bondi E, Burgalassi A, Massimetti G, Dell'osso L. Shared psychopathology in obese subjects with and without binge-eating disorder. *Int J Eat Disord.* Nov 2008;41(7):643–9. doi:10.1002/eat.20544

12. Lethbridge J, Watson HJ, Egan SJ, Street H, Nathan PR. The role of perfectionism, dichotomous thinking, shape and weight overvaluation, and conditional goal setting in eating disorders. *Eat Behav.* Aug 2011;12(3):200–6. doi:10.1016/j.eatbeh.2011.04.003

13. Palascha A, van Kleef E, van Trijp HC. How does thinking in black and white terms relate to eating behavior and weight regain? *J Health Psychol.* May 2015;20(5):638–48. doi:10.1177/1359105315573440

14. Berg AC, Johnson KB, Straight CR, et al. Flexible eating behavior predicts greater weight loss following a diet and exercise intervention in older women. *J Nutr Gerontol Geriatr.* 2018 Jan–Mar 2018;37(1):14–29. doi:10.1080/21551197.2018.1435433

15. Fredricks SC. Is the word getting out? *J Acad Nutr Dietet.* 1997;Sep;97 (9):A113. doi:10.1016/S0002-8223(97)00708-6

16. Freeland-Graves J, Nitzke S. Position of the American Dietetic Association: total diet approach to communicating food and nutrition information. *J Am Diet Assoc.* Jan 2002;102(1):100–8. doi:10.1016/s0002-8223(02)90030-1

17. HHS, USDA. Dietary Guidelines for Americans, 2005. 6th Edition. Washington, DC: US Government Printing Office 2005.

18. Marton R. Science, advocacy, and quackery in nutritional books: an analysis of conflicting advice and purported claims of nutritional best-sellers. *Palgrave Communications.* 2020;6(43): 1–6. doi:10.1057/s41599-020-0415-6

19. Mogre V, Stevens FCJ, Aryee PA, Amalba A, Scherpbier AJJA. Why nutrition education is inadequate in the medical curriculum: a qualitative study of students' perspectives on barriers and strategies. *BMC Med Educ.* Feb 2018; 18(1):26. doi:10.1186/s12909-018-1130-5

20. National Research Council (US). *National science education standards: observe, interact, change, learn.* National Academy Press; 1996:ix, 262 pp.

21. National Academy of Sciences. *Science, evolution, and creationism.* National Academies Press; 2008:xv, 70 pp.

22. Gormally C, Brickman P, Lutz M. Developing a Test of Scientific Literacy Skills (TOSLS): measuring undergraduates' evaluation of scientific information and arguments. *CBE Life Sci Educ.* 2012;11(4):364–77. doi:10.1187/cbe.12-03-0026

23. Kreider RB, Kalman DS, Antonio J, et al. International Society of Sports Nutrition position stand: safety and efficacy of creatine supplementation in exercise, sport, and medicine. *J Int Soc Sports Nutr.* 2017;14:18. doi:10.1186/s12970-017-0173-z

24. Onakpoya IJ, Posadzki PP, Watson LK, Davies LA, Ernst E. The efficacy of long-term conjugated linoleic acid (CLA) supplementation on body composition in overweight and obese individuals: a systematic review and meta-analysis of randomized clinical trials. *Eur J Nutr.* Mar 2012;51(2):127–34. doi:10.1007/s00394-011-0253-9

25. National Academies of Sciences Engineering and Medicine (US). Committee on Reproducibility and Replicability in Science, National Academies of Sciences Engineering and Medicine (US). Committee on National Statistics, National Academies of Sciences Engineering and Medicine (US). Nuclear and Radiation Studies Board, National Academies of Sciences Engineering and Medicine (US). Committee on Applied and Theoretical Statistics, Committee on Science Engineering Medicine and Public Policy (US). *Reproducibility and replicability in science.* National Academies Press; 2019:1 online resource (1 PDF file (xxi, 234 pp.)). www.ncbi.nlm.nih.gov/books/NBK547537/ NLM Bookshelf Books

26. Shaughnessy JJ, Zechmeister EB. *Research Methods in Psychology.* McGraw-Hill; 1990.

27. Sackett DL, Rosenberg WM, Gray JA, Haynes RB, Richardson WS. Evidence based medicine: what it is and what it isn't. *BMJ.* Jan 1996;312(7023):71–2. doi:10.1136/bmj.312.7023.71

28. Hill AB. The environment and disease: association or causation? 1965. *J R Soc Med.* Jan 2015;108(1):32–7. doi:10.1177/0141076814562718

29. Sylvetsky AC, Rother KI. Nonnutritive sweeteners in weight management and chronic disease: a review. *Obesity* (Silver Spring). Apr 2018;26(4):635–40. doi:10.1002/oby.22139

30. Laviada-Molina H, Molina-Segui F, Pérez-Gaxiola G, et al. Effects of nonnutritive sweeteners on body weight and BMI in diverse clinical contexts: systematic review and meta-analysis. *Obes Rev.* Jul 2020;21(7):e13020. doi:10.1111/obr.13020

31. Aragon AA, Schoenfeld BJ. Nutrient timing revisited: is there a post-exercise anabolic window? *J Int Soc Sports Nutr.* Jan 2013;10(1):5. doi:10.1186/1550-2783-10-5

32. Liberati A, Altman DG, Tetzlaff J, et al. The PRISMA statement for reporting systematic reviews and meta-analyses of studies that evaluate health care interventions: explanation and elaboration. *J Clin Epidemiol.* Oct 2009;62(10):e1–34. doi:10.1016/j.jclinepi.2009.06.006

33. Taubes G. Treat obesity as physiology, not physics. *Nature.* Dec 2012;492(7428):155. doi:10.1038/492155a

34. Taubes G. The science of obesity: what do we really know about what makes us fat? An essay by Gary Taubes. *BMJ.* Apr 2013;346:f1050. doi:10.1136/bmj.f1050

35. Witard OC, Wardle SL, Macnaughton LS, Hodgson AB, Tipton KD. Protein considerations for optimising skeletal muscle mass in healthy young and older adults. *Nutrients.* Mar 2016;8(4):181. doi:10.3390/nu8040181

36. Burke LM, Hawley JA, Jeukendrup A, Morton JP, Stellingwerff T, Maughan RJ. Toward a common understanding of diet-exercise strategies to manipulate fuel availability for training and competition preparation in endurance sport. *Int J Sport Nutr Exerc Metab.* Sep 2018;28(5):451–63. doi:10.1123/ijsnem.2018-0289

37. Schoenfeld BJ, Aragon AA. How much protein can the body use in a single meal for muscle-building? Implications for daily protein distribution. *J Int Soc Sports Nutr.* 2018;15:10. doi:10.1186/s12970-018-0215-1

38. Schardt C, Adams MB, Owens T, Keitz S, Fontelo P. Utilization of the PICO framework to improve searching PubMed for clinical questions. *BMC Med Inform Decis Mak.* Jun 2007;7:16. doi:10.1186/1472-6947-7-16

39. Methley AM, Campbell S, Chew-Graham C, McNally R, Cheraghi-Sohi S. PICO, PICOS and SPIDER: a comparison study of specificity and sensitivity in three search tools for qualitative systematic reviews. *BMC Health Serv Res.* Nov 2014;14:579. doi:10.1186/s12913-014-0579-0

40. Moore DR, Churchward-Venne TA, Witard O, et al. Protein ingestion to stimulate myofibrillar protein synthesis requires greater relative protein intakes in healthy older versus younger

men. *J Gerontol A Biol Sci Med Sci.* Jan 2015;70(1):57–62. doi:10.1093/gerona/glu103

41. Jornayvaz FR, Jurczak MJ, Lee HY, et al. A high-fat, ketogenic diet causes hepatic insulin resistance in mice, despite increasing energy expenditure and preventing weight gain. *Am J Physiol Endocrinol Metab.* Nov 2010;299(5):E808–15. doi:10.1152/ajpendo.00361.2010

42. Nilsson J, Ericsson M, Joibari MM, et al. A low-carbohydrate high-fat diet decreases lean mass and impairs cardiac function in pair-fed female C57BL/6J mice. *Nutr Metab* (Lond). 2016;13:79. doi:10.1186/s12986-016-0132-8

43. Borghjid S, Feinman RD. Response of C57Bl/6 mice to a carbohydrate-free diet. *Nutr Metab* (Lond). Jul 2012;9(1):69. doi:10.1186/1743-7075-9-69

44. Jonas DE, Ferrari RM, Wines RC, Vuong KT, Cotter A, Harris RP. Evaluating evidence on intermediate outcomes: considerations for groups making healthcare recommendations. *Am J Prev Med.* Jan 2018;54(1S1):S38–52. doi:10.1016/j.amepre.2017.08.033

45. Ecker ED, Skelly AC. Conducting a winning literature search. *Evid Based Spine Care J.* May 2010;1(1):9–14. doi:10.1055/s-0028-1100887

46. Institute of Medicine (US). Committee on Military Nutrition Research. The role of protein and amino acids in sustaining and enhancing performance. National Academy Press; 1999:xv, 429 pp.

47. Liu Z, Long W, Fryburg DA, Barrett EJ. The regulation of body and skeletal muscle protein metabolism by hormones and amino acids. *J Nutr.* Jan 2006;136(1 Suppl):212S–7S. doi:10.1093/jn/136.1.212S

48. Berryman CE, Lieberman HR, Fulgoni VL, Pasiakos SM. Protein intake trends and conformity with the dietary reference intakes in the United States: analysis of the National Health and Nutrition Examination Survey, 2001–2014. *Am J Clin Nutr.* Aug 2018;108(2):405–13. doi:10.1093/ajcn/nqy088

49. Manore M. Exercise and the Institute of Medicine recommendations for nutrition. *Curr Sports Med Rep.* 2005;4(4):193–8. doi: 10.1097/01.csmr.0000306206.72186.00

50. Devries MC, Sithamparapillai A, Brimble KS, Banfield L, Morton RW, Phillips SM. Changes in kidney function do not differ between healthy adults consuming higher- compared with lower- or normal-protein diets: a systematic review and meta-analysis. *J Nutr.* Nov 2018;148(11):1760–75. doi:10.1093/jn/nxy197

51. Antonio J, Ellerbroek A, Silver T, et al. A high protein diet (3.4 g/kg/d) combined with a heavy resistance training program improves body composition in healthy trained men and women—a follow-up investigation. *J Int Soc Sports Nutr.* 2015;12:39.

52. Antonio J, Ellerbroek A, Silver T, Vargas L, Peacock C. The effects of a high protein diet on indices of health and body composition—a crossover trial in resistance-trained men. *J Int Soc Sports Nutr.* 2016;13:3. doi:10.1186/s12970-016-0114-2

53. Antonio J, Ellerbroek A, Silver T, et al. A high protein diet has no harmful effects: a one-year crossover study in resistance-trained males. *J Nutr Metab.* 2016;2016:9104792. doi:10.1155/2016/9104792

54. Antonio J, Ellerbroek A, Evans C, Silver T, Peacock CA. High protein consumption in trained women: bad to the bone? *J Int Soc Sports Nutr.* 2018;15:6. doi:10.1186/s12970-018-0210-6

55. Groenendijk I, den Boeft L, van Loon LJC, de Groot LCPG. High versus low dietary protein intake and bone health in older adults: a systematic review and meta-analysis. *Comput Struct Biotechnol J.* 2019;17:1101–12. doi:10.1016/j.csbj.2019.07.005

56. Hevia-Larraín V, Gualano B, Longobardi I, et al. High-protein plant-based diet versus a protein-matched omnivorous diet to support resistance training adaptations: a comparison between habitual vegans and omnivores. *Sports Med.* Feb 2021;doi:10.1007/s40279-021-01434-9

57. Schoenfeld B, Aragon A. Magnitude and composition of the energy surplus for maximizing muscle hypertrophy: implications for bodybuilding and physique athletes. *Strength and Conditioning Journal.* 2020;42(5):79–86. doi:10.1519/SSC.0000000000000539

58. Phillips SM, Chevalier S, Leidy HJ. Protein "requirements" beyond the RDA: implications for optimizing health. *Appl Physiol Nutr Metab.* May 2016;41(5):565–72. doi:10.1139/apnm-2015-0550

59. Aragon AA, Schoenfeld BJ, Wildman R, et al. International Society of Sports Nutrition position stand: diets and body composition. *J Int Soc Sports Nutr.* 2017;14:16. doi:10.1186/s12970-017-0174-y

60. Nowson C, O'Connell S. Protein requirements and recommendations for older people: a

review. *Nutrients.* Aug 14 2015;7(8):6874–99. doi:10.3390/nu7085311

61. Xue QL. The frailty syndrome: definition and natural history. *Clin Geriatr Med.* Feb 2011;27(1):1–15. doi:10.1016/j.cger.2010.08.009

62. Cederholm T. Overlaps between frailty and sarcopenia definitions. *Nestle Nutr Inst Workshop Ser.* 2015;83:65–9. doi:10.1159/000382063

63. Tipton KD, Hamilton DL, Gallagher IJ. Assessing the role of muscle protein breakdown in response to nutrition and exercise in humans. *Sports Med.* Mar 2018;48(Suppl 1):53–64. doi:10.1007/s40279-017-0845-5

64. Rudrappa SS, Wilkinson DJ, Greenhaff PL, Smith K, Idris I, Atherton PJ. Human skeletal muscle disuse atrophy: effects on muscle protein synthesis, breakdown, and insulin resistance—a qualitative review. *Front Physiol.* 2016;7:361. doi:10.3389/fphys.2016.00361

65. Bauer J, Biolo G, Cederholm T, et al. Evidence-based recommendations for optimal dietary protein intake in older people: a position paper from the PROT-AGE Study Group. *J Am Med Dir Assoc.* Aug 2013;14(8):542–59. doi:10.1016/j.jamda.2013.05.021

66. Morton RW, Murphy KT, McKellar SR, et al. A systematic review, meta-analysis and meta-regression of the effect of protein supplementation on resistance training-induced gains in muscle mass and strength in healthy adults. *Br J Sports Med.* Mar 2018;52(6):376–84. doi:10.1136/bjsports-2017-097608

67. Nunes EA, Currier BS, Lim C, Phillips SM. Nutrient-dense protein as a primary dietary strategy in healthy ageing: please sir, may we have more? *Proc Nutr Soc.* Oct 2020:1–14. doi:10.1017/S0029665120007892

68. Burd NA, McKenna CF, Salvador AF, Paulussen KJM, Moore DR. Dietary protein quantity, quality, and exercise are key to healthy living: a muscle-centric perspective across the lifespan. *Front Nutr.* 2019;6:83. doi:10.3389/fnut.2019.00083

69. Tang JE, Moore DR, Kujbida GW, Tarnopolsky MA, Phillips SM. Ingestion of whey hydrolysate, casein, or soy protein isolate: effects on mixed muscle protein synthesis at rest and following resistance exercise in young men. *J Appl Physiol* (1985). Sep 2009;107(3):987–92. doi:10.1152/japplphysiol.00076.2009

70. Yang Y, Churchward-Venne TA, Burd NA, Breen L, Tarnopolsky MA, Phillips SM. Myofibrillar protein synthesis following ingestion of soy protein isolate at rest and after resistance exercise in elderly men. *Nutr Metab* (Lond). Jun 2012;9(1):57. doi:10.1186/1743-7075-9-57

71. Gorissen SH, Horstman AM, Franssen R, et al. Ingestion of wheat protein increases in vivo muscle protein synthesis rates in healthy older men in a randomized trial. *J Nutr.* Sept 2016;146(9):1651–9. doi:10.3945/jn.116.231340

72. van Vliet S, Burd NA, van Loon LJ. The skeletal muscle anabolic response to plant- versus animal-based protein consumption. *J Nutr.* Sep 2015;145(9):1981–91. doi:10.3945/jn.114.204305

73. Duan Y, Li F, Li Y, et al. The role of leucine and its metabolites in protein and energy metabolism. *Amino Acids.* Jan 2016;48(1):41–51. doi:10.1007/s00726-015-2067-1

74. Gorissen SHM, Witard OC. Characterising the muscle anabolic potential of dairy, meat and plant-based protein sources in older adults. *Proc Nutr Soc.* Feb 2018;77(1):20–31. doi:10.1017/S002966511700194X

75. Berrazaga I, Micard V, Gueugneau M, Walrand S. The role of the anabolic properties of plant- versus animal-based protein sources in supporting muscle mass maintenance: a critical review. *Nutrients.* Aug 2019;11(8):1825. doi:10.3390/nu11081825

76. Brennan JL, Keerati-U-Rai M, Yin H, et al. Differential responses of blood essential amino acid levels following ingestion of high-quality plant-based protein blends compared to whey protein—a double-blind randomized, cross-over, clinical trial. *Nutrients.* Dec 2019;11(12):2987. doi:10.3390/nu11122987

77. Babault N, Païzis C, Deley G, et al. Pea proteins oral supplementation promotes muscle thickness gains during resistance training: a double-blind, randomized, placebo-controlled clinical trial vs. whey protein. *J Int Soc Sports Nutr.* 2015;12(1):3. doi:10.1186/s12970-014-0064-5

78. Banaszek A, Townsend JR, Bender D, Vantrease WC, Marshall AC, Johnson KD. The effects of whey vs. pea protein on physical adaptations following 8-weeks of high-intensity functional training (HIFT): a pilot study. *Sports* (Basel). Jan 2019;7(1):12. doi:10.3390/sports7010012

79. Nieman DC, Zwetsloot KA, Simonson AJ, et al. Effects of whey and pea protein supplementation on post-eccentric exercise muscle damage: a randomized trial. *Nutrients.* Aug 2020;12(8):2382. doi:10.3390/nu12082382

80. Messina M, Lynch H, Dickinson JM, Reed KE. No difference between the effects of supplementing

with soy protein versus animal protein on gains in muscle mass and strength in response to resistance exercise. *Int J Sport Nutr Exerc Metab.* Nov 2018;28(6):674–85. doi:10.1123/ijsnem.2018-0071

81. Lim MT, Pan BJ, Toh DWK, Sutanto CN, Kim JE. Animal protein versus plant protein in supporting lean mass and muscle strength: a systematic review and meta-analysis of randomized controlled trials. *Nutrients.* Feb 2021;13(2):661. doi:10.3390/nu13020661

82. Wu G. Important roles of dietary taurine, creatine, carnosine, anserine and 4-hydroxyproline in human nutrition and health. *Amino Acids.* Mar 2020;52(3):329–60. doi:10.1007/s00726-020-02823-6

83. Kerksick CM, Wilborn CD, Roberts MD, et al. ISSN exercise & sports nutrition review update: research & recommendations. *J Int Soc Sports Nutr.* Aug 2018;15(1):38. doi:10.1186/s12970-018-0242-y

84. Zdzieblik D, Oesser S, Baumstark MW, Gollhofer A, König D. Collagen peptide supplementation in combination with resistance training improves body composition and increases muscle strength in elderly sarcopenic men: a randomised controlled trial. *Br J Nutr.* Oct 2015;114(8):1237–45. doi:10.1017/S0007114515002810

85. Jendricke P, Centner C, Zdzieblik D, Gollhofer A, König D. Specific collagen peptides in combination with resistance training improve body composition and regional muscle strength in premenopausal women: a randomized controlled trial. *Nutrients.* Apr 2019;11(4):892. doi:10.3390/nu11040892

86. Kirmse M, Oertzen-Hagemann V, de Marées M, Bloch W, Platen P. Prolonged collagen peptide supplementation and resistance exercise training affects body composition in recreationally active men. *Nutrients.* May 2019;11(5):1154. doi:10.3390/nu11051154

87. Bagheri R, Hooshmand Moghadam B, Ashtary-Larky D, et al. Whole egg vs. egg white ingestion during 12 weeks of resistance training in trained young males: a randomized controlled trial. *J Strength Cond Res.* Feb 2021;35(2):411–9. doi:10.1519/JSC.0000000000003922

88. Riechman SE, Andrews RD, Maclean DA, Sheather S. Statins and dietary and serum cholesterol are associated with increased lean mass following resistance training. *J Gerontol A Biol Sci Med Sci.* Oct 2007;62(10):1164–71. doi:10.1093/gerona/62.10.1164

89. Dinu M, Abbate R, Gensini GF, Casini A, Sofi F. Vegetarian, vegan diets and multiple health outcomes: a systematic review with meta-analysis of observational studies. *Crit Rev Food Sci Nutr.* Nov 2017;57(17):3640–9. doi:10.1080/10408398.2016.1138447

90. Rogerson D. Vegan diets: practical advice for athletes and exercisers. *J Int Soc Sports Nutr.* 2017;14:36. doi:10.1186/s12970-017-0192-9

91. Schüpbach R, Wegmüller R, Berguerand C, Bui M, Herter-Aeberli I. Micronutrient status and intake in omnivores, vegetarians and vegans in Switzerland. *Eur J Nutr.* Feb 2017;56(1):283–93. doi:10.1007/s00394-015-1079-7

92. Pinckaers P, Trommelen J, Snijders T, van Loo L. The anabolic response to plant-based protein ingestion. *Sports Med.* Sept 2021;51(Suppl 1):59–74. doi: 10.1007/s40279-021-01540-8

93. Rondanelli M, Nichetti M, Peroni G, et al. Where to find leucine in food and how to feed elderly with sarcopenia in order to counteract loss of muscle mass: practical advice. *Front Nutr.* 2020;7:622391. doi:10.3389/fnut.2020.622391

94. Kraemer WJ, Solomon-Hill G, Volk BM, et al. The effects of soy and whey protein supplementation on acute hormonal reponses to resistance exercise in men. *J Am Coll Nutr.* 2013;32(1):66–74. doi:10.1080/07315724.2013.770648

95. Goodin S, Shen F, Shih WJ, et al. Clinical and biological activity of soy protein powder supplementation in healthy male volunteers. *Cancer Epidemiol Biomarkers Prev.* Apr 2007;16(4):829–33. doi:10.1158/1055-9965.EPI-06-0882

96. Reed KE, Camargo J, Hamilton-Reeves J, Kurzer M, Messina M. Neither soy nor isoflavone intake affects male reproductive hormones: an expanded and updated meta-analysis of clinical studies. *Reprod Toxicol.* Mar 2021;100:60–7. doi:10.1016/j.reprotox.2020.12.019

97. Messina M, Nagata C, Wu AH. Estimated Asian adult soy protein and isoflavone intakes. *Nutr Cancer.* 2006;55(1):1–12. doi:10.1207/s15327914nc5501_1

98. Siepmann T, Roofeh J, Kiefer FW, Edelson DG. Hypogonadism and erectile dysfunction associated with soy product consumption. *Nutrition.* 2011 Jul–Aug 2011;27(7–8):859–62. doi:10.1016/j.nut.2010.10.018

99. Tipton KD. Gender differences in protein metabolism. *Curr Opin Clin Nutr Metab Care.* Nov 2001;4(6):493–8. doi:10.1097/00075197-200111000-00005

100. Smith GI, Atherton P, Reeds DN, et al. No major sex differences in muscle protein synthesis rates in the postabsorptive state and during hyperinsulinemia-hyperaminoacidemia in middle-aged adults. *J Appl Physiol* (1985). Oct 2009;107(4):1308–15. doi:10.1152/japplphysiol.00348.2009

101. Dreyer HC, Fujita S, Glynn EL, Drummond MJ, Volpi E, Rasmussen BB. Resistance exercise increases leg muscle protein synthesis and mTOR signalling independent of sex. *Acta Physiol* (Oxf). May 2010;199(1):71–81. doi:10.1111/j.1748-1716.2010.02074.x

102. Smith GI, Atherton P, Villareal DT, et al. Differences in muscle protein synthesis and anabolic signaling in the postabsorptive state and in response to food in 65–80 year old men and women. *PLoS One*. Mar 26 2008;3(3):e1875. doi:10.1371/journal.pone.0001875

103. Phillips SM, Atkinson SA, Tarnopolsky MA, MacDougall JD. Gender differences in leucine kinetics and nitrogen balance in endurance athletes. *J Appl Physiol* (1985). Nov 1993;75(5):2134–41. doi:10.1152/jappl.1993.75.5.2134

104. Tarnopolsky LJ, MacDougall JD, Atkinson SA, Tarnopolsky MA, Sutton JR. Gender differences in substrate for endurance exercise. *J Appl Physiol* (1985). Jan 1990;68(1):302–8. doi:10.1152/jappl.1990.68.1.302

105. McKenzie S, Phillips SM, Carter SL, Lowther S, Gibala MJ, Tarnopolsky MA. Endurance exercise training attenuates leucine oxidation and BCOAD activation during exercise in humans. *Am J Physiol Endocrinol Metab*. Apr 2000;278(4):E580–7. doi:10.1152/ajpendo.2000.278.4.E580

106. Snijders T, Trommelen J, Kouw IWK, Holwerda AM, Verdijk LB, van Loon LJC. The impact of pre-sleep protein ingestion on the skeletal muscle adaptive response to exercise in humans: an update. *Front Nutr*. 2019;6:17. doi:10.3389/fnut.2019.00017

107. Macnaughton LS, Wardle SL, Witard OC, et al. The response of muscle protein synthesis following whole-body resistance exercise is greater following 40 g than 20 g of ingested whey protein. *Physiol Rep*. Aug 2016;4(15):e12893. doi:10.14814/phy2.12893

108. Park S, Jang J, Choi MD, et al. The anabolic response to dietary protein is not limited by the maximal stimulation of protein synthesis in healthy older adults: a randomized crossover trial. *Nutrients*. Oct 2020;12(11):3276. doi:10.3390/nu12113276

109. Burd NA, Beals JW, Martinez IG, Salvador AF, Skinner SK. Food-first approach to enhance the regulation of post-exercise skeletal muscle protein synthesis and remodeling. *Sports Med*. Feb 2019;49(Suppl 1):59–68. doi:10.1007/s40279-018-1009-y

110. Rynders CA, Thomas EA, Zaman A, Pan Z, Catenacci VA, Melanson EL. Effectiveness of intermittent fasting and time-restricted feeding compared to continuous energy restriction for weight loss. *Nutrients*. Oct 2019;11(10):2442. doi:10.3390/nu11102442

111. Williamson E, Moore DR. A muscle-centric perspective on intermittent fasting: a suboptimal dietary strategy for supporting muscle protein remodeling and muscle mass? *Front Nutr*. 2021;8:640621. doi:10.3389/fnut.2021.640621

112. Schoenfeld BJ, Aragon A, Wilborn C, Urbina SL, Hayward SE, Krieger J. Pre- versus post-exercise protein intake has similar effects on muscular adaptations. *PeerJ*. 2017;5:e2825. doi:10.7717/peerj.2825

113. Candow DG, Chilibeck PD, Facci M, Abeysekara S, Zello GA. Protein supplementation before and after resistance training in older men. *Eur J Appl Physiol*. Jul 2006;97(5):548–56. doi:10.1007/s00421-006-0223-8

114. Bird SP, Tarpenning KM, Marino FE. Liquid carbohydrate/essential amino acid ingestion during a short-term bout of resistance exercise suppresses myofibrillar protein degradation. *Metabolism*. May 2006;55(5):570–7. doi:10.1016/j.metabol.2005.11.011

115. Beelen M, Koopman R, Gijsen AP, et al. Protein coingestion stimulates muscle protein synthesis during resistance-type exercise. *Am J Physiol Endocrinol Metab*. Jul 2008;295(1):E70–7. doi:10.1152/ajpendo.00774.2007

116. Deldicque L, De Bock K, Maris M, et al. Increased p70s6k phosphorylation during intake of a protein-carbohydrate drink following resistance exercise in the fasted state. *Eur J Appl Physiol*. Mar 2010;108(4):791–800. doi:10.1007/s00421-009-1289-x

117. Ivy J, Portman R. *Nutrient Timing: The Future of Sports Nutrition*. Basic Health Publications; 2004.

118. Schoenfeld BJ, Aragon AA, Krieger JW. The effect of protein timing on muscle strength and hypertrophy: a meta-analysis. *J Int Soc Sports Nutr*. Dec 2013;10(1):53. doi:10.1186/1550-2783-10-53

119. Martens EA, Gonnissen HK, Gatta-Cherifi B, Janssens PL, Westerterp-Plantenga MS. Maintenance of energy expenditure on high-protein vs. high-carbohydrate diets at a constant body weight may prevent a positive energy balance. *Clin Nutr.* Oct 2015;34(5):968–75. doi:10.1016/j.clnu.2014.10.007

120. Bray GA, Redman LM, de Jonge L, et al. Effect of protein overfeeding on energy expenditure measured in a metabolic chamber. *Am J Clin Nutr.* Mar 2015;101(3):496–505. doi:10.3945/ajcn.114.091769

121. Hector AJ, Phillips SM. Protein recommendations for weight loss in elite athletes: a focus on body composition and performance. *Int J Sport Nutr Exerc Metab.* Mar 2018;28(2):170–7. doi:10.1123/ijsnem.2017-0273

122. Helms E, Zinn C, Rowlands D, Brown S. A systematic review of dietary protein during caloric restriction in resistance trained lean athletes: a case for higher intakes. *Int J Sport Nutr Exerc Metab.* 2014;24(2):127–38.

123. Mäestu J, Eliakim A, Jürimäe J, Valter I, Jürimäe T. Anabolic and catabolic hormones and energy balance of the male bodybuilders during the preparation for the competition. *J Strength Cond Res.* Apr 2010;24(4):1074–81. doi:10.1519/JSC.0b013e3181cb6fd3

124. Chappell AJ, Simper T, Barker ME. Nutritional strategies of high level natural bodybuilders during competition preparation. *J Int Soc Sports Nutr.* 2018;15:4. doi:10.1186/s12970-018-0209-z

125. Barakat C, Pearson J, Escalante G, Campbell B, De Souza E. Body recomposition: can trained individuals build muscle and lose fat at the same time? *Strength and Conditioning Journal.* Oct 2020;42(5):7–21. doi:10.1519/SSC.0000000000000584

126. Lee H, Kim K, Kim B, et al. A cellular mechanism of muscle memory facilitates mitochondrial remodelling following resistance training. *J Physiol.* Sept 2018;596(18):4413–26. doi:10.1113/JP275308

127. Bruusgaard JC, Johansen IB, Egner IM, Rana ZA, Gundersen K. Myonuclei acquired by overload exercise precede hypertrophy and are not lost on detraining. *Proc Natl Acad Sci USA.* Aug 2010;107(34):15111–6. doi:10.1073/pnas.0913935107

128. Leuchtmann AB, Mueller SM, Aguayo D, et al. Resistance training preserves high-intensity interval training induced improvements in skeletal muscle capillarization of healthy old men: a randomized controlled trial.

Sci Rep. Apr 2020;10(1):6578. doi:10.1038/s41598-020-63490-x

129. Khan MA, Gannon MC, Nuttall FQ. Glucose appearance rate following protein ingestion in normal subjects. *J Am Coll Nutr.* Dec 1992;11(6):701–6. doi:10.1080/07315724.1992.10718270

130. Fromentin C, Tomé D, Nau F, et al. Dietary proteins contribute little to glucose production, even under optimal gluconeogenic conditions in healthy humans. *Diabetes.* May 2013;62(5):1435–42. doi:10.2337/db12-1208

131. Volek J, Phinney S. *The Art and Science of Low Carbohydrate Performance.* Beyond Obesity LLC; 2012.

132. Wilson JM, Lowery RP, Roberts MD, et al. Effects of ketogenic dieting on body composition, strength, power, and hormonal profiles in resistance training men. *J Strength Cond Res.* Dec 2020;34(12):3463–74. doi:10.1519/JSC.0000000000001935

133. Burke L, Ross M, Garvican-Lewis L, et al. Low carbohydrate, high fat diet impairs exercise economy and negates the performance benefit from intensified training in elite race walkers. *J Physiol.* May 2017;595(9):2785–807. doi:10.1113/JP273230

134. Volek JS, Freidenreich DJ, Saenz C, et al. Metabolic characteristics of keto-adapted ultra-endurance runners. *Metabolism.* Mar 2016;65(3):100–10. doi:10.1016/j.metabol.2015.10.028

135. Schoenfeld BJ, Aragon AA, Krieger JW. Effects of meal frequency on weight loss and body composition: a meta-analysis. *Nutr Rev.* Feb 2015;73(2):69–82. doi:10.1093/nutrit/nuu017

136. Iwao S, Mori K, Sato Y. Effects of meal frequency on body composition during weight control in boxers. *Scand J Med Sci Sports.* Oct 1996;6(5):265–72. doi:10.1111/j.1600-0838.1996.tb00469.x

137. Arnal MA, Mosoni L, Boirie Y, et al. Protein feeding pattern does not affect protein retention in young women. *J Nutr.* Jul 2000;130(7):1700–4. doi:10.1093/jn/130.7.1700

138. Arnal MA, Mosoni L, Boirie Y, et al. Protein pulse feeding improves protein retention in elderly women. *Am J Clin Nutr.* Jun 1999;69(6):1202–8. doi:10.1093/ajcn/69.6.1202

139. Moro T, Tinsley G, Bianco A, et al. Effects of eight weeks of time-restricted feeding (16/8) on basal metabolism, maximal strength, body composition, inflammation, and cardiovascular risk factors in resistance-trained males. *J Transl Med.* 2016;14(1):290.

140. Tinsley GM, Moore ML, Graybeal AJ, et al. Time-restricted feeding plus resistance training in active females: a randomized trial. *Am J Clin Nutr*. Sept 2019;110(3):628–40. doi:10.1093/ajcn/nqz126

141. Stratton MT, Tinsley GM, Alesi MG, et al. Four weeks of time-restricted feeding combined with resistance training does not differentially influence measures of body composition, muscle performance, resting energy expenditure, and blood biomarkers. *Nutrients*. Apr 2020;12(4):1126. doi:10.3390/nu12041126

142. Schoenfeld BJ, Aragon AA, Wilborn CD, Krieger JW, Sonmez GT. Body composition changes associated with fasted versus non-fasted aerobic exercise. *J Int Soc Sports Nutr*. 2014;11(1):54. doi:10.1186/s12970-014-0054-7

143. Hackett D, Hagstrom A. Effect of overnight fasted exercise on weight loss and body composition: a systematic review and meta-analysis. *J Funct Morphol Kinesiol*. 2017;2(4):43. https://doi.org/10.3390/jfmk2040043

144. Hackney KJ, Bruenger AJ, Lemmer JT. Timing protein intake increases energy expenditure 24 h after resistance training. *Med Sci Sports Exerc*. May 2010;42(5):998–1003. doi:10.1249/MSS.0b013e3181c12976

145. Wingfield HL, Smith-Ryan AE, Melvin MN, et al. The acute effect of exercise modality and nutrition manipulations on post-exercise resting energy expenditure and respiratory exchange ratio in women: a randomized trial. *Sports Med Open*. Jun 2015;11. doi:10.1186/s40798-015-0010-3

146. Jäger R, Kerksick CM, Campbell BI, et al. International Society of Sports Nutrition position stand: protein and exercise. *J Int Soc Sports Nutr*. 2017;14:20. doi:10.1186/s12970-017-0177-8

147. Thomas DT, Erdman KA, Burke LM. Position of the Academy of Nutrition and Dietetics, Dietitians of Canada, and the American College of Sports Medicine: nutrition and athletic performance. *J Acad Nutr Diet*. Mar 2016;116(3):501–28. doi:10.1016/j.jand.2015.12.006

148. Elango R, Ball RO, Pencharz PB. Recent advances in determining protein and amino acid requirements in humans. *Br J Nutr*. Aug 2012;108 (Suppl 2):S22–30. doi:10.1017/S0007114512002504

149. Kato H, Suzuki K, Bannai M, Moore DR. Protein requirements are elevated in endurance athletes after exercise as determined by the indicator amino acid oxidation method. *PLoS One*. Jun 2016;11(6):e0157406. doi:10.1371/journal.pone.0157406

150. Bandegan A, Courtney-Martin G, Rafii M, Pencharz PB, Lemon PWR. Indicator amino acid oxidation protein requirement estimate in endurance-trained men 24 h postexercise exceeds both the EAR and current athlete guidelines. *Am J Physiol Endocrinol Metab*. May 2019;316(5):E741–8. doi:10.1152/ajpendo.00174.2018

151. Rowlands DS, Hopkins WG. Effect of high-fat, high-carbohydrate, and high-protein meals on metabolism and performance during endurance cycling. *Int J Sport Nutr Exerc Metab*. Sep 2002;12(3):318–35. doi:10.1123/ijsnem.12.3.318

152. Kloby Nielsen LL, Tandrup Lambert MN, Jeppesen PB. The effect of ingesting carbohydrate and proteins on athletic performance: a systematic review and meta-analysis of randomized controlled trials. *Nutrients*. May 2020;12(5):1483. doi:10.3390/nu12051483

153. Saunders MJ, Kane MD, Todd MK. Effects of a carbohydrate-protein beverage on cycling endurance and muscle damage. *Med Sci Sports Exerc*. Jul 2004;36(7):1233–8. doi:10.1249/01.mss.0000132377.66177.9f

154. Saunders MJ, Luden ND, Herrick JE. Consumption of an oral carbohydrate-protein gel improves cycling endurance and prevents postexercise muscle damage. *J Strength Cond Res*. Aug 2007;21(3):678–84. doi:10.1519/R-20506.1

155. Power O, Hallihan A, Jakeman P. Human insulinotropic response to oral ingestion of native and hydrolysed whey protein. *Amino Acids*. Jul 2009;37(2):333–9. doi:10.1007/s00726-008-0156-0

156. Craven J, Desbrow B, Sabapathy S, Bellinger P, McCartney D, Irwin C. The effect of consuming carbohydrate with and without protein on the rate of muscle glycogen re-synthesis during short-term post-exercise recovery: a systematic review and meta-analysis. *Sports Med Open*. Jan 2021;7(1):9. doi:10.1186/s40798-020-00297-0

157. Kerksick CM, Arent S, Schoenfeld BJ, et al. International Society of Sports Nutrition position stand: nutrient timing. *J Int Soc Sports Nutr*. 2017;14:33. doi:10.1186/s12970-017-0189-4

158. Holesh J, Aslam S, Martin A. Physiology, Carbohydrates. [Updated 2020 Aug 25]. In: StatPearls [Internet]. Treasure Island (FL): StatPearls Publishing; 2021 Jan–. Available

from: https://www.ncbi.nlm.nih.gov/books/
NBK459280/

159. Reynolds A, Mann J, Cummings J, Winter N, Mete E, Te Morenga L. Carbohydrate quality and human health: a series of systematic reviews and meta-analyses. *Lancet*. Feb 2019;393(10170):434–45. doi:10.1016/S0140-6736(18)31809-9

160. Anderson JW, Baird P, Davis RH, et al. Health benefits of dietary fiber. *Nutr Rev*. Apr 2009;67(4):188–205. doi:10.1111/j.1753-4887.2009.00189.x

161. Dahl WJ, Stewart ML. Position of the Academy of Nutrition and Dietetics: health implications of dietary fiber. *J Acad Nutr Diet*. Nov 2015;115(11):1861–70. doi:10.1016/j.jand.2015.09.003

162. Behall KM, Howe JC. Contribution of fiber and resistant starch to metabolizable energy. *Am J Clin Nutr*. Nov 1995;62(5 Suppl):1158S–60S. doi:10.1093/ajcn/62.5.1158S

163. Miketinas DC, Bray GA, Beyl RA, Ryan DH, Sacks FM, Champagne CM. Fiber intake predicts weight loss and dietary adherence in adults consuming calorie-restricted diets: the POUNDS Lost (Preventing Overweight Using Novel Dietary Strategies) study. *J Nutr*. Oct 2019;149(10):1742–8. doi:10.1093/jn/nxz117

164. Jovanovski E, Mazhar N, Komishon A, et al. Can dietary viscous fiber affect body weight independently of an energy-restrictive diet? A systematic review and meta-analysis of randomized controlled trials. *Am J Clin Nutr*. Feb 2020;111(2):471–85. doi:10.1093/ajcn/nqz292

165. Barr S, Wright J. Postprandial energy expenditure in whole-food and processed-food meals: implications for daily energy expenditure. *Food Nutr Res*. Jul 2010;54. doi:10.3402/fnr.v54i0.5144

166. Ordonio RL, Matsuoka M. Increasing resistant starch content in rice for better consumer health. *Proc Natl Acad Sci USA*. Nov 2016;113(45):12616–8. doi:10.1073/pnas.1616053113

167. Sonia S, Witjaksono F, Ridwan R. Effect of cooling of cooked white rice on resistant starch content and glycemic response. *Asia Pac J Clin Nutr*. 2015;24(4):620–5. doi:10.6133/apjcn.2015.24.4.13

168. Yang CZ, Shu XL, Zhang LL, et al. Starch properties of mutant rice high in resistant starch. *J Agric Food Chem*. Jan 2006;54(2):523–8. doi:10.1021/jf0524123

169. White U, Peterson CM, Beyl RA, Martin CK, Ravussin E. Resistant starch has

no effect on appetite and food intake in individuals with prediabetes. *J Acad Nutr Diet*. Jun 2020;120(6):1034–41. doi:10.1016/j.jand.2020.01.017

170. Guo J, Tan L, Kong L. Impact of dietary intake of resistant starch on obesity and associated metabolic profiles in human: a systematic review of the literature. *Crit Rev Food Sci Nutr*. 2021;61(6):889–905. doi:10.1080/10408398.2020.1747391

171. Knuiman P, Hopman MT, Mensink M. Glycogen availability and skeletal muscle adaptations with endurance and resistance exercise. *Nutr Metab* (Lond). 2015;12:59. doi:10.1186/s12986-015-0055-9

172. Olsson KE, Saltin B. Variation in total body water with muscle glycogen changes in man. *Acta Physiol Scand*. Sep 1970;80(1):11–8. doi:10.1111/j.1748-1716.1970.tb04764.x

173. Spriet LL. Regulation of skeletal muscle fat oxidation during exercise in humans. *Med Sci Sports Exerc*. Sep 2002;34(9):1477–84. doi:10.1097/00005768-200209000-00013

174. Spriet LL, Watt MJ. Regulatory mechanisms in the interaction between carbohydrate and lipid oxidation during exercise. *Acta Physiol Scand*. Aug 2003;178(4):443–52. doi:10.1046/j.1365-201X.2003.01152.x

175. Murray B, Rosenbloom C. Fundamentals of glycogen metabolism for coaches and athletes. *Nutr Rev*. Apr 2018;76(4):243–59. doi:10.1093/nutrit/nuy001

176. Jenkins DJ, Wolever TM, Taylor RH, et al. Glycemic index of foods: a physiological basis for carbohydrate exchange. *Am J Clin Nutr*. Mar 1981;34(3):362–6. doi:10.1093/ajcn/34.3.362

177. Hermansen ML, Eriksen NM, Mortensen LS, Holm L, Hermansen K. Can the glycemic index (GI) be used as a tool in the prevention and management of type 2 diabetes? *Rev Diabet Stud*. 2006;3(2):61–71. doi:10.1900/RDS.2006.3.61

178. Sacks FM, Carey VJ, Anderson CA, et al. Effects of high vs low glycemic index of dietary carbohydrate on cardiovascular disease risk factors and insulin sensitivity: the OmniCarb randomized clinical trial. *JAMA*. Dec 2014;312(23):2531–41. doi:10.1001/jama.2014.16658

179. Karl JP, Roberts SB, Schaefer EJ, et al. Effects of carbohydrate quantity and glycemic index on resting metabolic rate and body composition during weight loss. *Obesity* (Silver Spring). Nov 2015;23(11):2190–8. doi:10.1002/oby.21268

180. Clar C, Al-Khudairy L, Loveman E, et al. Low glycaemic index diets for the prevention of cardiovascular disease. *Cochrane Database Syst Rev.* Jul 2017;7:CD004467. doi:10.1002/14651858. CD004467.pub3

181. Khan TA, Sievenpiper JL. Controversies about sugars: results from systematic reviews and meta-analyses on obesity, cardiometabolic disease and diabetes. *Eur J Nutr.* Nov 2016;55(Suppl 2):25–43. doi:10.1007/s00394-016-1345-3

182. Khan TA, Tayyiba M, Agarwal A, et al. Relation of total sugars, sucrose, fructose, and added sugars with the risk of cardiovascular disease: a systematic review and dose-response meta-analysis of prospective cohort studies. *Mayo Clin Proc.* Dec 2019;94(12):2399–414. doi:10.1016/j. mayocp.2019.05.034

183. Yang Q, Zhang Z, Gregg EW, Flanders WD, Merritt R, Hu FB. Added sugar intake and cardiovascular diseases mortality among US adults. *JAMA Intern Med.* Apr 2014;174(4):516–24. doi:10.1001/jamainternmed.2013.13563

184. Erickson J, Sadeghirad B, Lytvyn L, Slavin J, Johnston BC. The scientific basis of guideline recommendations on sugar intake: a systematic review. *Ann Intern Med.* Feb 2017;166(4):257–67. doi:10.7326/M16-2020

185. Stellingwerff T, Cox GR. Systematic review: carbohydrate supplementation on exercise performance or capacity of varying durations. *Appl Physiol Nutr Metab.* Sep 2014;39(9):998–1011. doi:10.1139/apnm-2014-0027

186. Krogh A, Lindhard J. The relative value of fat and carbohydrate as sources of muscular energy: with appendices on the correlation between standard metabolism and the respiratory quotient during rest and work. *Biochem J.* Jul 1920;14(3–4):290–363. doi:10.1042/bj0140290

187. Jeukendrup A. A step towards personalized sports nutrition: carbohydrate intake during exercise. *Sports Med.* May 2014;44 (Suppl 1): S25–33. doi:10.1007/s40279-014-0148-z

188. Tarnopolsky MA. Sex differences in exercise metabolism and the role of 17-beta estradiol. *Med Sci Sports Exerc.* Apr 2008;40(4):648–54. doi:10.1249/MSS.0b013e31816212ff

189. Hausswirth C, Le Meur Y. Physiological and nutritional aspects of post-exercise recovery: specific recommendations for female athletes. *Sports Med.* Oct 2011;41(10):861–82. doi:10.2165/11593180-000000000-00000

190. Wismann J, Willoughby D. Gender differences in carbohydrate metabolism and carbohydrate loading. *J Int Soc Sports Nutr.* Jun 2006;3:28–34. doi:10.1186/1550-2783-3-1-28

191. Grgic J, McIlvenna LC, Fyfe JJ, et al. Does aerobic training promote the same skeletal muscle hypertrophy as resistance training? A systematic review and meta-analysis. *Sports Med.* Feb 2019;49(2):233–54. doi:10.1007/s40279-018-1008-z

192. Vargas S, Romance R, Petro JL, et al. Efficacy of ketogenic diet on body composition during resistance training in trained men: a randomized controlled trial. *J Int Soc Sports Nutr.* Jul 2018;15(1):31. doi:10.1186/s12970-018-0236-9

193. Greene DA, Varley BJ, Hartwig TB, Chapman P, Rigney M. A low-carbohydrate ketogenic diet reduces body mass without compromising performance in powerlifting and Olympic weightlifting athletes. *J Strength Cond Res.* Dec 2018;32(12):3373–82. doi:10.1519/JSC.0000000000002904

194. Kephart WC, Pledge CD, Roberson PA, et al. The three-month effects of a ketogenic diet on body composition, blood parameters, and performance metrics in CrossFit trainees: a pilot study. *Sports* (Basel). Jan 2018;6(1):1. doi:10.3390/sports6010001

195. Vargas-Molina S, Petro JL, Romance R, et al. Effects of a ketogenic diet on body composition and strength in trained women. *J Int Soc Sports Nutr.* Apr 2020;17(1):19. doi:10.1186/s12970-020-00348-7

196. Paoli A, Cenci L, Pompei P, et al. Effects of two months of very low carbohydrate ketogenic diet on body composition, muscle strength, muscle area, and blood parameters in competitive natural body builders. *Nutrients.* Jan 2021;13(2):374. doi:10.3390/nu13020374

197. Ashtary-Larky D, Bagheri R, Bavi H, et al. Ketogenic diets, physical activity, and body composition: a review. *Br J Nutr.* Jul 2021:1–68. doi:10.1017/S0007114521002609

198. Ashtary-Larky D, Bagheri R, Asbaghi O, et al. Effects of resistance training combined with a ketogenic diet on body composition: a systematic review and meta-analysis. *Crit Rev Food Sci Nutr.* Feb 2021:1–16. doi:10.1080/10408398.2021.1890689

199. Lambert CP, Frank LL, Evans WJ. Macronutrient considerations for the sport of bodybuilding. *Sports Med.* 2004;34(5):317–27. doi:10.2165/00007256-200434050-00004

200. Slater G, Phillips SM. Nutrition guidelines for strength sports: sprinting, weightlifting, throwing

events, and bodybuilding. *J Sports Sci.* 2011;29 (Suppl 1):S67–77. doi:10.1080/02640414.2011.5 74722

201. Spendlove J, Mitchell L, Gifford J, et al. Dietary intake of competitive bodybuilders. *Sports Med.* Jul 2015;45(7):1041–63. doi:10.1007/ s40279-015-0329-4

202. Cholewa JM, Newmire DE, Zanchi NE. Carbohydrate restriction: friend or foe of resistance-based exercise performance? *Nutrition.* Apr 2019;60:136–46. doi:10.1016/j. nut.2018.09.026

203. Bin Naharudin MN, Yusof A, Shaw H, Stockton M, Clayton DJ, James LJ. Breakfast omission reduces subsequent resistance exercise performance. *J Strength Cond Res.* Jul 2019;33(7):1766–72. doi:10.1519/ JSC.0000000000003054

204. Schoenfeld B, Aragon A. Is there a postworkout anabolic window of opportunity for nutrient consumption? Clearing up controversies. *J Orthop Sports Phys Ther.* 2018;48(12):911–4. doi:10.2519/jospt.2018.0615

205. Morton RW, McGlory C, Phillips SM. Nutritional interventions to augment resistance training-induced skeletal muscle hypertrophy. *Front Physiol.* 2015;6:245. doi:10.3389/ fphys.2015.00245

206. Glynn EL, Fry CS, Drummond MJ, et al. Muscle protein breakdown has a minor role in the protein anabolic response to essential amino acid and carbohydrate intake following resistance exercise. *Am J Physiol Regul Integr Comp Physiol.* Aug 2010;299(2):R533–40. doi:10.1152/ ajpregu.00077.2010

207. Greenhaff PL, Karagounis LG, Peirce N, et al. Disassociation between the effects of amino acids and insulin on signaling, ubiquitin ligases, and protein turnover in human muscle. *Am J Physiol Endocrinol Metab.* Sep 2008;295(3):E595–604. doi:10.1152/ajpendo.90411.2008

208. Hulmi JJ, Laakso M, Mero AA, Häkkinen K, Ahtiainen JP, Peltonen H. The effects of whey protein with or without carbohydrates on resistance training adaptations. *J Int Soc Sports Nutr.* 2015;12:48. doi:10.1186/s12970-015-0109-4

209. van Wyk HJ, Davis RE, Davies JS. A critical review of low-carbohydrate diets in people with type 2 diabetes. *Diabet Med.* Feb 2016;33(2):148–57. doi:10.1111/dme.12964

210. Huntriss R, Campbell M, Bedwell C. The interpretation and effect of a low-carbohydrate diet in the management of type 2 diabetes:

a systematic review and meta-analysis of randomised controlled trials. *Eur J Clin Nutr.* Mar 2018;72(3):311–25. doi:10.1038/ s41430-017-0019-4

211. Goldenberg JZ, Day A, Brinkworth GD, et al. Efficacy and safety of low and very low carbohydrate diets for type 2 diabetes remission: systematic review and meta-analysis of published and unpublished randomized trial data. *BMJ.* Jan 2021;372:m4743. doi:10.1136/bmj.m4743

212. Hall K, Guo J. Obesity energetics: body weight regulation and the effects of diet composition. *Gastroenterology.* Feb 2017:pii: S0016–5085(17)30152-X. doi: 10.1053/j. gastro.2017.01.052

213. Buga A, Kackley ML, Crabtree CD, et al. The effects of a 6-week controlled, hypocaloric ketogenic diet, with and without exogenous ketone salts, on body composition responses. *Front Nutr.* Mar 2021;8:618520. doi:10.3389/ fnut.2021.618520

214. Crabtree CD, Kackley ML, Buga A, et al. Comparison of ketogenic diets with and without ketone salts versus a low-fat diet: liver fat responses in overweight adults. *Nutrients.* Mar 2021;13(3):966. doi:10.3390/nu13030966

215. Brown AW, Bohan Brown MM, Allison DB. Belief beyond the evidence: using the proposed effect of breakfast on obesity to show 2 practices that distort scientific evidence. *Am J Clin Nutr.* Nov 2013;98(5):1298–308. doi:10.3945/ ajcn.113.064410

216. Sievert K, Hussain SM, Page MJ, et al. Effect of breakfast on weight and energy intake: systematic review and meta-analysis of randomised controlled trials. *BMJ.* Jan 2019;364:l42. doi:10.1136/bmj.l42

217. Keim NL, Van Loan MD, Horn WF, Barbieri TF, Mayclin PL. Weight loss is greater with consumption of large morning meals and fat-free mass is preserved with large evening meals in women on a controlled weight reduction regimen. *J Nutr.* Jan 1997;127(1):75–82. doi:10.1093/ jn/127.1.75

218. Sofer S, Eliraz A, Kaplan S, et al. Greater weight loss and hormonal changes after 6 months diet with carbohydrates eaten mostly at dinner. *Obesity* (Silver Spring). Oct 2011;19(10):2006–14. doi:10.1038/oby.2011.48

219. Jakubowicz D, Barnea M, Wainstein J, Froy O. High caloric intake at breakfast vs. dinner differentially influences weight loss of overweight and obese women. *Obesity* (Silver Spring). Dec 2013;21(12):2504–12. doi:10.1002/oby.20460

220. Jakubowicz D, Froy O, Wainstein J, Boaz M. Meal timing and composition influence ghrelin levels, appetite scores and weight loss maintenance in overweight and obese adults. *Steroids*. Mar 2012;77(4):323–31. doi:10.1016/j.steroids.2011.12.006

221. Savikj M, Gabriel BM, Alm PS, et al. Afternoon exercise is more efficacious than morning exercise at improving blood glucose levels in individuals with type 2 diabetes: a randomised crossover trial. *Diabetologia*. Feb 2019;62(2):233–7. doi:10.1007/s00125-018-4767-z

222. Babraj JA, Vollaard NB, Keast C, Guppy FM, Cottrell G, Timmons JA. Extremely short duration high intensity interval training substantially improves insulin action in young healthy males. *BMC Endocr Disord*. Jan 2009;9:3. doi:10.1186/1472-6823-9-3

223. Richards JC, Johnson TK, Kuzma JN, et al. Short-term sprint interval training increases insulin sensitivity in healthy adults but does not affect the thermogenic response to beta-adrenergic stimulation. *J Physiol*. Aug 2010;588(Pt 15):2961–72. doi:10.1113/jphysiol.2010.189886

224. Murphy NE, Carrigan CT, Margolis LM. High-fat ketogenic diets and physical performance: a systematic review. *Adv Nutr*. Feb 2021;12(1):223–33. doi:10.1093/advances/nmaa101

225. Paoli A, Grimaldi K, D'Agostino D, et al. Ketogenic diet does not affect strength performance in elite artistic gymnasts. *J Int Soc Sports Nutr*. Jul 2012;9(1):34.

226. Escobar KA, VanDusseldorp TA, Kerksick CM. Carbohydrate intake and resistance-based exercise: are current recommendations reflective of actual need? *Br J Nutr*. Dec 2016;116(12):2053–65. doi:10.1017/S0007114516003949

227. McSwiney FT, Doyle L, Plews DJ, Zinn C. Impact of ketogenic diet on athletes: current insights. *Open Access J Sports Med*. Nov 2019;10:171–83. doi:10.2147/OAJSM.S180409

228. Havemann L, West S, Goedecke J, et al. Fat adaptation followed by carbohydrate loading compromises high-intensity sprint performance. *J Appl Physiol*. Jan 2006;100(1):194–202. doi:10.1152/japplphysiol.00813.2005

229. Wroble KA, Trott MN, Schweitzer GG, Rahman RS, Kelly PV, Weiss EP. Low-carbohydrate, ketogenic diet impairs anaerobic exercise performance in exercise-trained women and men: a randomized-sequence crossover trial. *J Sports Med Phys Fitness*. Apr 2019;59(4):600–7. doi:10.23736/S0022-4707.18.08318-4

230. Burke LM. Ketogenic low-CHO, high-fat diet: the future of elite endurance sport? *J Physiol*. Feb 2021;599(3):819–43. doi:10.1113/JP278928

231. Burke LM, Sharma AP, Heikura IA, et al. Crisis of confidence averted: Impairment of exercise economy and performance in elite race walkers by ketogenic low carbohydrate, high fat (LCHF) diet is reproducible. *PLoS One*. Jun 2020;15(6):e0234027. doi:10.1371/journal.pone.0234027

232. Burke LM, Whitfield J, Heikura IA, et al. Adaptation to a low carbohydrate high fat diet is rapid but impairs endurance exercise metabolism and performance despite enhanced glycogen availability. *J Physiol*. Feb 2021;599(3):771–90. doi:10.1113/JP280221

233. Cao J, Lei S, Wang X, Cheng S. The effect of a ketogenic low-carbohydrate, high-fat diet on aerobic capacity and exercise performance in endurance athletes: a systematic review and meta-analysis. *Nutrients*. Aug 2021;13(8):2896. doi:10.3390/nu13082896

234. Zajac A, Poprzecki S, Maszczyk A, Czuba M, Michalczyk M, Zydek G. The effects of a ketogenic diet on exercise metabolism and physical performance in off-road cyclists. *Nutrients*. Jul 2014;6(7):2493–508. doi: 10.3390/nu6072493

235. Bergström J, Hermansen L, Hultman E, Saltin B. Diet, muscle glycogen and physical performance. *Acta Physiol Scand*. Oct–Nov 1967;71(2):140–50. doi:10.1111/j.1748-1716.1967.tb03720.x

236. Hawley JA, Schabort EJ, Noakes TD, Dennis SC. Carbohydrate-loading and exercise performance. An update. *Sports Med*. Aug 1997;24(2):73–81. doi:10.2165/00007256-199724020-00001

237. Ormsbee MJ, Bach CW, Baur DA. Pre-exercise nutrition: the role of macronutrients, modified starches and supplements on metabolism and endurance performance. *Nutrients*. Apr 2014;6(5):1782–808. doi:10.3390/nu6051782

238. Hawley JA, Burke LM. Effect of meal frequency and timing on physical performance. *Br J Nutr*. Apr 1997;77 (Suppl 1):S91–103. doi:10.1079/bjn19970107

239. Burdon CA, Spronk I, Cheng HL, O'Connor HT. Effect of glycemic index of a pre-exercise meal on endurance exercise performance: a systematic review and meta-analysis. *Sports Med*. Jun 2017;47(6):1087–101. doi:10.1007/s40279-016-0632-8

240. Smith JW, Zachwieja JJ, Péronnet F, et al. Fuel selection and cycling endurance performance

with ingestion of [13C]glucose: evidence for a carbohydrate dose response. *J Appl Physiol* (1985). Jun 2010;108(6):1520–9. doi:10.1152/japplphysiol.91394.2008

241. Smith JW, Pascoe DD, Passe DH, et al. Curvilinear dose-response relationship of carbohydrate (0-120 g·h(-1)) and performance. *Med Sci Sports Exerc.* Feb 2013;45(2):336–41. doi:10.1249/MSS.0b013e31827205d1

242. Colombani PC, Mannhart C, Mettler S. Carbohydrates and exercise performance in non-fasted athletes: a systematic review of studies mimicking real-life. *Nutr J.* Jan 2013;12:16. doi:10.1186/1475-2891-12-16

243. Pöchmüller M, Schwingshackl L, Colombani PC, Hoffmann G. A systematic review and meta-analysis of carbohydrate benefits associated with randomized controlled competition-based performance trials. *J Int Soc Sports Nutr.* Jul 2016;13:27. doi:10.1186/s12970-016-0139-6

244. Rosset R, Egli L, Lecoultre V. Glucose-fructose ingestion and exercise performance: the gastrointestinal tract and beyond. *Eur J Sport Sci.* Aug 2017;17(7):874–84. doi:10.1080/17461391.2017.1317035

245. Rowlands DS, Houltham S, Musa-Veloso K, Brown F, Paulionis L, Bailey D. Fructose-glucose composite carbohydrates and endurance performance: critical review and future perspectives. *Sports Med.* Nov 2015;45(11):1561–76. doi:10.1007/s40279-015-0381-0

246. Brietzke C, Franco-Alvarenga PE, Coelho-Júnior HJ, Silveira R, Asano RY, Pires FO. Effects of carbohydrate mouth rinse on cycling time trial performance: a systematic review and meta-analysis. *Sports Med.* Jan 2019;49(1):57–66. doi:10.1007/s40279-018-1029-7

247. Coyle EF. Fluid and fuel intake during exercise. *J Sports Sci.* Jan 2004;22(1):39–55. doi:10.1080/0264041031000140545

248. Jeukendrup AE, Jentjens RL, Moseley L. Nutritional considerations in triathlon. *Sports Med.* 2005;35(2):163–81. doi:10.2165/00007256-200535020-00005

249. Vitale K, Getzin A. Nutrition and supplement update for the endurance athlete: review and recommendations. *Nutrients.* Jun 2019;11(6):1289. doi:10.3390/nu11061289

250. Baker LB, Barnes KA, Anderson ML, Passe DH, Stofan JR. Normative data for regional sweat sodium concentration and whole-body sweating rate in athletes. *J Sports Sci.* 2016;34(4):358–68. doi:10.1080/02640414.2015.1055291

251. Ivy JL. Glycogen resynthesis after exercise: effect of carbohydrate intake. *Int J Sports Med.* Jun 1998;19 (Suppl 2):S142–5. doi:10.1055/s-2007-971981

252. Jentjens R, Jeukendrup A. Determinants of post-exercise glycogen synthesis during short-term recovery. *Sports Med.* 2003;33(2):117–44. doi:10.2165/00007256-200333020-00004

253. Conlee RK, Lawler RM, Ross PE. Effects of glucose or fructose feeding on glycogen repletion in muscle and liver after exercise or fasting. *Ann Nutr Metab.* 1987;31(2):126–32. doi:10.1159/000177259

254. Rosset R, Lecoultre V, Egli L, et al. Postexercise repletion of muscle energy stores with fructose or glucose in mixed meals. *Am J Clin Nutr.* Mar 2017;105(3):609–17. doi:10.3945/ajcn.116.138214

255. Gonzalez JT, Fuchs CJ, Betts JA, van Loon LJ. Glucose plus fructose ingestion for post-exercise recovery—greater than the sum of its parts? *Nutrients.* Mar 2017;9(4):344. doi:10.3390/nu9040344

256. Leiper JB, Aulin KP, Söderlund K. Improved gastric emptying rate in humans of a unique glucose polymer with gel-forming properties. *Scand J Gastroenterol.* Nov 2000;35(11):1143–9. doi:10.1080/003655200750056600

257. Piehl Aulin K, Söderlund K, Hultman E. Muscle glycogen resynthesis rate in humans after supplementation of drinks containing carbohydrates with low and high molecular masses. *Eur J Appl Physiol.* Mar 2000;81(4):346–51. doi:10.1007/s004210050053

258. Stephens FB, Roig M, Armstrong G, Greenhaff PL. Post-exercise ingestion of a unique, high molecular weight glucose polymer solution improves performance during a subsequent bout of cycling exercise. *J Sports Sci.* Jan 2008;26(2):149–54. doi:10.1080/02640410701361548

259. Oliver JM, Almada AL, Van Eck LE, et al. Ingestion of high molecular weight carbohydrate enhances subsequent repeated maximal power: a randomized controlled trial. *PLoS One.* Sep 2016;11(9):e0163009. doi:10.1371/journal.pone.0163009

260. Starling RD, Trappe TA, Parcell AC, Kerr CG, Fink WJ, Costill DL. Effects of diet on muscle triglyceride and endurance performance. *J Appl Physiol* (1985). Apr 1997;82(4):1185–9. doi:10.1152/jappl.1997.82.4.1185

261. Friedman JE, Neufer PD, Dohm GL. Regulation of glycogen resynthesis following exercise. Dietary

considerations. *Sports Med.* Apr 1991;11(4):232–43. doi:10.2165/00007256-199111040-00003

262. Jeukendrup AE. Periodized nutrition for athletes. *Sports Med.* Mar 2017;47(Suppl 1):51–63. doi:10.1007/s40279-017-0694-2

263. Stellingwerff T, Spriet L, Watt M, et al. Decreased PDH activation and glycogenolysis during exercise following fat adaptation with carbohydrate restoration. *Am J Physiol Endocrinol Metab.* Feb 2006;290(2):E380–8. doi:10.1152/ajpendo.00268.2005

264. Burke L. Re-examining high-fat diets for sports performance: did we call the "nail in the coffin" too soon? *Sports Med.* Nov 2015;45 (Suppl 1): S33–49. doi: 10.1007/s40279-015-0393-9

265. Marquet LA, Brisswalter J, Louis J, et al. Enhanced endurance performance by periodization of carbohydrate intake: "sleep low" strategy. *Med Sci Sports Exerc.* Apr 2016;48(4):663–72. doi:10.1249/MSS.0000000000000823

266. Impey SG, Hearris MA, Hammond KM, et al. Fuel for the work required: a theoretical framework for carbohydrate periodization and the glycogen threshold hypothesis. *Sports Med.* May 2018;48(5):1031–48. doi:10.1007/s40279-018-0867-7

267. Gejl KD, Thams LB, Hansen M, et al. No superior adaptations to carbohydrate periodization in elite endurance athletes. *Med Sci Sports Exerc.* Dec 2017;49(12):2486–97. doi:10.1249/MSS.0000000000001377

268. National Research Council (US) Committee on Diet and Health. Diet and Health: Implications for Reducing Chronic Disease Risk. Washington (DC): National Academies Press (US); 1989. 7, Fats and Other Lipids. Available from: www.ncbi.nlm.nih.gov/books/NBK218759/

269. Le HD, Meisel JA, de Meijer VE, Gura KM, Puder M. The essentiality of arachidonic acid and docosahexaenoic acid. *Prostaglandins Leukot Essent Fatty Acids.* Aug–Sep 2009;81(2–3):165–70. doi:10.1016/j.plefa.2009.05.020

270. Richard C, Lewis ED, Field CJ. Evidence for the essentiality of arachidonic and docosahexaenoic acid in the postnatal maternal and infant diet for the development of the infant's immune system early in life. *Appl Physiol Nutr Metab.* May 2016;41(5):461–75. doi:10.1139/apnm-2015-0660

271. Siguel E. Diagnosing essential fatty acid deficiency. *Circulation.* Jun 1998;97(25):2580–3. doi:10.1161/01.cir.97.25.2580

272. Whittaker J, Wu K. Low-fat diets and testosterone in men: systematic review and meta-analysis of intervention studies. *J Steroid Biochem Mol Biol.* Jun 2021;210:105878. doi:10.1016/j.jsbmb.2021.105878

273. Iraki J, Fitschen P, Espinar S, Helms E. Nutrition recommendations for bodybuilders in the off-season: a narrative review. *Sports* (Basel). Jun 2019;7(7):154. doi:10.3390/sports7070154

274. Ruiz-Castellano C, Espinar S, Contreras C, Mata F, Aragon A, Martínez-Sanz J. Achieving an optimal fat loss phase in resistance-trained athletes: a narrative review. *Nutrients.* 2021;13(9):3255. https://doi.org/10.3390/nu13093255

275. Wohlgemuth KJ, Arieta LR, Brewer GJ, Hoselton AL, Gould LM, Smith-Ryan AE. Sex differences and considerations for female specific nutritional strategies: a narrative review. *J Int Soc Sports Nutr.* Apr 2021;18(1):27. doi:10.1186/s12970-021-00422-8

276. Childs CE, Kew S, Finnegan YE, et al. Increased dietary α-linolenic acid has sex-specific effects upon eicosapentaenoic acid status in humans: re-examination of data from a randomised, placebo-controlled, parallel study. *Nutr J.* Dec 2014;13(1):113. doi:10.1186/1475-2891-13-113

277. Mumme K, Stonehouse W. Effects of medium-chain triglycerides on weight loss and body composition: a meta-analysis of randomized controlled trials. *J Acad Nutr Diet.* Feb 2015;115(2):249–63. doi:10.1016/j.jand.2014.10.022

278. Clegg ME. Medium-chain triglycerides are advantageous in promoting weight loss although not beneficial to exercise performance. *Int J Food Sci Nutr.* Nov 2010;61(7):653–79. doi:10.3109/09637481003702114

279. Burke LM, Collier GR, Beasley SK, et al. Effect of coingestion of fat and protein with carbohydrate feedings on muscle glycogen storage. *J Appl Physiol* (1985). Jun 1995;78(6):2187–92. doi:10.1152/jappl.1995.78.6.2187

280. Fox AK, Kaufman AE, Horowitz JF. Adding fat calories to meals after exercise does not alter glucose tolerance. *J Appl Physiol* (1985). Jul 2004;97(1):11–6. doi:10.1152/japplphysiol.01398.2003

281. Elliot TA, Cree MG, Sanford AP, Wolfe RR, Tipton KD. Milk ingestion stimulates net muscle protein synthesis following resistance exercise. *Med Sci Sports Exerc.* Apr 2006;38(4):667–74. doi:10.1249/01.mss.0000210190.64458.25

282. van Vliet S, Shy EL, Abou Sawan S, et al. Consumption of whole eggs promotes greater stimulation of postexercise muscle protein synthesis than consumption of isonitrogenous amounts of egg whites in young men. *Am J Clin Nutr.* Dec 2017;106(6):1401–12. doi:10.3945/ajcn.117.159855

283. Sacks FM, Lichtenstein AH, Wu JHY, et al. Dietary fats and cardiovascular disease: a presidential advisory from the American Heart Association. *Circulation.* Jul 2017;136(3):e1–23. doi:10.1161/CIR.0000000000000510

284. US Department of Agriculture and US Department of Health and Human Services. *Dietary Guidelines for Americans, 2020–2025.* 9th Edition. December 2020. Available at DietaryGuidelines.gov.

285. Lenighan YM, McNulty BA, Roche HM. Dietary fat composition: replacement of saturated fatty acids with PUFA as a public health strategy, with an emphasis on α-linolenic acid. *Proc Nutr Soc.* May 2019;78(2):234–45. doi:10.1017/S0029665118002793

286. Hooper L, Martin N, Jimoh OF, Kirk C, Foster E, Abdelhamid AS. Reduction in saturated fat intake for cardiovascular disease. *Cochrane Database Syst Rev.* Aug 2020;8:CD011737. doi:10.1002/14651858.CD011737.pub3

287. Lawrence GD. Dietary fats and health: dietary recommendations in the context of scientific evidence. *Adv Nutr.* May 2013;4(3):294–302. doi:10.3945/an.113.003657

288. Chowdhury R, Warnakula S, Kunutsor S, et al. Association of dietary, circulating, and supplement fatty acids with coronary risk: a systematic review and meta-analysis. *Ann Intern Med.* Mar 2014;160(6):398–406. doi:10.7326/M13-1788

289. Astrup A. A changing view on saturated fatty acids and dairy: from enemy to friend. *Am J Clin Nutr.* Dec 2014;100(6):1407–8. doi:10.3945/ajcn.114.099986

290. Heileson JL. Dietary saturated fat and heart disease: a narrative review. *Nutr Rev.* Jun 2020;78(6):474–85. doi:10.1093/nutrit/nuz091

291. Shih CW, Hauser ME, Aronica L, Rigdon J, Gardner CD. Changes in blood lipid concentrations associated with changes in intake of dietary saturated fat in the context of a healthy low-carbohydrate weight-loss diet: a secondary analysis of the Diet Intervention Examining The Factors Interacting with Treatment Success (DIETFITS) trial. *Am J Clin Nutr.* Feb 2019;109(2):433–41. doi:10.1093/ajcn/nqy305

292. Gardner CD, Trepanowski JF, Del Gobbo LC, et al. Effect of low-fat vs low-carbohydrate diet on 12-month weight loss in overweight adults and the association with genotype pattern or insulin secretion: the DIETFITS randomized clinical trial. *JAMA.* Feb 2018;319(7):667–79. doi:10.1001/jama.2018.0245

293. Liu AG, Ford NA, Hu FB, Zelman KM, Mozaffarian D, Kris-Etherton PM. A healthy approach to dietary fats: understanding the science and taking action to reduce consumer confusion. *Nutr J.* Aug 2017;16(1):53. doi:10.1186/s12937-017-0271-4

294. Duarte C, Boccardi V, Amaro Andrade P, Souza Lopes AC, Jacques PF. Dairy versus other saturated fats source and cardiometabolic risk markers: systematic review of randomized controlled trials. *Crit Rev Food Sci Nutr.* 2021;61(3):450–61. doi:10.1080/10408398.2020.1736509

295. Poppitt SD. Cow's milk and dairy consumption: is there now consensus for cardiometabolic health? *Front Nutr.* 2020;7:574725. doi:10.3389/fnut.2020.574725

296. O'Sullivan TA, Hafekost K, Mitrou F, Lawrence D. Food sources of saturated fat and the association with mortality: a meta-analysis. *Am J Public Health.* Sep 2013;103(9):e31–42. doi:10.2105/AJPH.2013.301492

297. Hirahatake KM, Astrup A, Hill JO, Slavin JL, Allison DB, Maki KC. Potential cardiometabolic health benefits of full-fat dairy: the evidence base. *Adv Nutr.* May 2020;11(3):533–47. doi:10.1093/advances/nmz132

298. Chen GC, Wang Y, Tong X, et al. Cheese consumption and risk of cardiovascular disease: a meta-analysis of prospective studies. *Eur J Nutr.* Dec 2017;56(8):2565–75. doi:10.1007/s00394-016-1292-z

299. Thorning TK, Raben A, Tholstrup T, Soedamah-Muthu SS, Givens I, Astrup A. Milk and dairy products: good or bad for human health? An assessment of the totality of scientific evidence. *Food Nutr Res.* Nov 2016;60:32527. doi:10.3402/fnr.v60.32527

300. Timon CM, O'Connor A, Bhargava N, Gibney ER, Feeney EL. Dairy consumption and metabolic health. *Nutrients.* Oct 2020;12(10):3040. doi:10.3390/nu12103040

301. Rosqvist F, Smedman A, Lindmark-Månsson H, et al. Potential role of milk fat globule membrane in modulating plasma lipoproteins, gene expression, and cholesterol metabolism in humans: a randomized study. *Am J Clin Nutr.* Jul 2015;102(1):20–30. doi:10.3945/ajcn.115.107045

302. Liting P, Guoping L, Zhenyue C. Apolipoprotein B/apolipoprotein A1 ratio and non-high-density lipoprotein cholesterol. Predictive value for CHD severity and prognostic utility in CHD patients. *Herz*. Mar 2015;40 (Suppl 1):1–7. doi:10.1007/s00059-014-4147-5

303. Goswami B, Rajappa M, Mallika V, Kumar S, Shukla DK. Apo-B/apo-AI ratio: a better discriminator of coronary artery disease risk than other conventional lipid ratios in Indian patients with acute myocardial infarction. *Acta Cardiol*. Dec 2008;63(6):749–55. doi:10.2143/AC.63.6.2033393

304. Nurtazina A, Kozhakhmetova D, Dautov D, Shakhanova A, Chattu VK. Apolipoprotein B/A1 ratio as a diagnostic alternative to triglycerides and HDL-cholesterol for the prediction of metabolic syndrome among hypertensives in Kazakhstan. *Diagnostics* (Basel). Jul 2020;10(8):510. doi:10.3390/diagnostics10080510

305. Kosmerl E, Rocha-Mendoza D, Ortega-Anaya J, Jiménez-Flores R, García-Cano I. Improving human health with milk fat globule membrane, lactic acid bacteria, and Bifidobacteria. *Microorganisms*. Feb 2021;9(2):341. doi:10.3390/microorganisms9020341

306. Beals E, Kamita SG, Sacchi R, et al. Addition of milk fat globule membrane-enriched supplement to a high-fat meal attenuates insulin secretion and induction of soluble epoxide hydrolase gene expression in the postprandial state in overweight and obese subjects. *J Nutr Sci*. Apr 2019;8:e16. doi:10.1017/jns.2019.11

307. Tokede OA, Gaziano JM, Djoussé L. Effects of cocoa products/dark chocolate on serum lipids: a meta-analysis. *Eur J Clin Nutr*. Aug 2011;65(8):879–86. doi:10.1038/ejcn.2011.64

308. Ried K, Sullivan T, Fakler P, Frank OR, Stocks NP. Does chocolate reduce blood pressure? A meta-analysis. *BMC Med*. Jun 28 2010;8:39. doi:10.1186/1741-7015-8-39

309. Yuan S, Li X, Jin Y, Lu J. Chocolate consumption and risk of coronary heart disease, stroke, and diabetes: a meta-analysis of prospective studies. *Nutrients*. Jul 2017;9(7):688. doi:10.3390/nu9070688

310. de Oliveira LN, de Jesus Coelho Castro R, de Oliveira MA, de Oliveira LF. Lipid characterization of white, dark, and milk chocolates by FT-Raman spectroscopy and capillary zone electrophoresis. *J AOAC Int*. 2015 Nov–Dec 2015;98(6):1598–607. doi:10.5740/jaoacint.15-083

311. Magrone T, Russo MA, Jirillo E. Cocoa and dark chocolate polyphenols: from biology to clinical applications. *Front Immunol*. Jun 2017;8:677. doi:10.3389/fimmu.2017.00677

312. Ebaditabar M, Djafarian K, Saeidifard N, Shab-Bidar S. Effect of dark chocolate on flow-mediated dilatation: systematic review, meta-analysis, and dose-response analysis of randomized controlled trials. *Clin Nutr ESPEN*. Apr 2020;36:17–27. doi:10.1016/j.clnesp.2019.10.017

313. Neelakantan N, Seah JYH, van Dam RM. The effect of coconut oil consumption on cardiovascular risk factors: a systematic review and meta-analysis of clinical trials. *Circulation*. Mar 2020;141(10):803–14. doi:10.1161/circulationaha.119.043052

314. Wallace TC. Health effects of coconut oil—a narrative review of current evidence. *J Am Coll Nutr*. Feb 2019;38(2):97–107. doi:10.1080/07315724.2018.1497562

315. Harris M, Hutchins A, Fryda L. The impact of virgin coconut oil and high-oleic safflower oil on body composition, lipids, and inflammatory markers in postmenopausal women. *J Med Food*. Apr 2017;20(4):345–51. doi:10.1089/jmf.2016.0114

316. Khaw KT, Sharp SJ, Finikarides L, et al. Randomised trial of coconut oil, olive oil or butter on blood lipids and other cardiovascular risk factors in healthy men and women. *BMJ Open*. Mar 2018;8(3):e020167. doi:10.1136/bmjopen-2017-020167

317. Chinwong S, Chinwong D, Mangklabruks A. Daily consumption of virgin coconut oil increases high-density lipoprotein cholesterol levels in healthy volunteers: a randomized crossover trial. *Evid Based Complement Alternat Med*. 2017;2017:7251562. doi:10.1155/2017/7251562

318. Cardoso DA, Moreira AS, de Oliveira GM, Raggio Luiz R, Rosa G. A coconut extra virgin oil-rich diet increases HDL cholesterol and decreases waist circumference and body mass in coronary artery disease patients. *Nutr Hosp*. Nov 2015;32(5):2144–52. doi:10.3305/nh.2015.32.5.9642

319. Assunção ML, Ferreira HS, dos Santos AF, Cabral CR, Florêncio TM. Effects of dietary coconut oil on the biochemical and anthropometric profiles of women presenting abdominal obesity. *Lipids*. Jul 2009;44(7):593–601. doi:10.1007/s11745-009-3306-6

320. Valente FX, Cândido FG, Lopes LL, et al. Effects of coconut oil consumption on energy metabolism,

cardiometabolic risk markers, and appetitive responses in women with excess body fat. *Eur J Nutr.* Jun 2018;57(4):1627–37. doi:10.1007/s00394-017-1448-5

321. Marina AM, Man YB, Nazimah SA, Amin I. Antioxidant capacity and phenolic acids of virgin coconut oil. *Int J Food Sci Nutr.* 2009;60 (Suppl 2):114–23. doi:10.1080/09637480802549127

322. World Cancer Research Fund, American Institute for Cancer Research. Limit red and processed meat. Accessed Oct 2021. www.wcrf.org/dietandcancer/limit-red-and-processed-meat/.

323. National Health Service (UK). Red meat and the risk of bowel cancer. Accessed October 2021. www.nhs.uk/live-well/eat-well/red-meat-and-the-risk-of-bowel-cancer/

324. O'Connor LE, Kim JE, Campbell WW. Total red meat intake of ≥0.5 servings/d does not negatively influence cardiovascular disease risk factors: a systemically searched meta-analysis of randomized controlled trials. *Am J Clin Nutr.* Jan 2017;105(1):57–69. doi:10.3945/ajcn.116.142521

325. Kruger C, Zhou Y. Red meat and colon cancer: a review of mechanistic evidence for heme in the context of risk assessment methodology. *Food Chem Toxicol.* Aug 2018;118:131–53. doi:10.1016/j.fct.2018.04.048

326. Maximova K, Khodayari Moez E, Dabravolskaj J, et al. Co-consumption of vegetables and fruit, whole grains, and fiber reduces the cancer risk of red and processed meat in a large prospective cohort of adults from Alberta's Tomorrow Project. *Nutrients.* Jul 2020;12(8):2265. doi:10.3390/nu12082265

327. McNeill SH. Inclusion of red meat in healthful dietary patterns. *Meat Sci.* Nov 2014;98(3):452–60. doi:10.1016/j.meatsci.2014.06.028

328. O'Connor LE, Paddon-Jones D, Wright AJ, Campbell WW. A Mediterranean-style eating pattern with lean, unprocessed red meat has cardiometabolic benefits for adults who are overweight or obese in a randomized, crossover, controlled feeding trial. *Am J Clin Nutr.* Jul 2018;108(1):33–40. doi:10.1093/ajcn/nqy075

329. Roussell MA, Hill AM, Gaugler TL, et al. Beef in an optimal lean diet study: effects on lipids, lipoproteins, and apolipoproteins. *Am J Clin Nutr.* Jan 2012;95(1):9–16. doi:10.3945/ajcn.111.016261

330. Beauchesne-Rondeau E, Gascon A, Bergeron J, Jacques H. Plasma lipids and lipoproteins in hypercholesterolemic men fed a lipid-lowering diet containing lean beef, lean fish, or poultry. *Am J Clin Nutr.* Mar 2003;77(3):587–93. doi:10.1093/ajcn/77.3.587

331. Maki KC, Van Elswyk ME, Alexander DD, Rains TM, Sohn EL, McNeill S. A meta-analysis of randomized controlled trials that compare the lipid effects of beef versus poultry and/or fish consumption. *J Clin Lipidol.* Jul–Aug 2012;6(4):352–61. doi:10.1016/j.jacl.2012.01.001

332. Mah E, Chen CO, Liska DJ. The effect of egg consumption on cardiometabolic health outcomes: an umbrella review. *Public Health Nutr.* Apr 2020;23(5):935–55. doi:10.1017/S1368980019002441

333. Drouin-Chartier JP, Chen S, Li Y, et al. Egg consumption and risk of cardiovascular disease: three large prospective US cohort studies, systematic review, and updated meta-analysis. *BMJ.* Mar 2020;368:m513. doi:10.1136/bmj.m513

334. Krittanawong C, Narasimhan B, Wang Z, et al. Association between egg consumption and risk of cardiovascular outcomes: a systematic review and meta-analysis. *Am J Med.* Jan 2021;134(1):76–83.e2. doi:10.1016/j.amjmed.2020.05.046

335. Fuller NR, Sainsbury A, Caterson ID, et al. Effect of a high-egg diet on cardiometabolic risk factors in people with type 2 diabetes: the Diabetes and Egg (DIABEGG) Study—randomized weight-loss and follow-up phase. *Am J Clin Nutr.* Jun 2018;107(6):921–31. doi:10.1093/ajcn/nqy048

336. Sugano M, Matsuoka R. Nutritional viewpoints on eggs and cholesterol. *Foods.* Feb 2021;10(3):494. doi:10.3390/foods10030494

337. Zhang X, Lv M, Luo X, et al. Egg consumption and health outcomes: a global evidence mapping based on an overview of systematic reviews. *Ann Transl Med.* Nov 2020;8(21):1343. doi:10.21037/atm-20-4243

338. Khalighi Sikaroudi M, Soltani S, Kolahdouz-Mohammadi R, et al. The responses of different dosages of egg consumption on blood lipid profile: an updated systematic review and meta-analysis of randomized clinical trials. *J Food Biochem.* Aug 2020;44(8):e13263. doi:10.1111/jfbc.13263

339. DiMarco DM, Missimer A, Murillo AG, et al. Intake of up to 3 eggs/day increases HDL cholesterol and plasma choline while plasma trimethylamine-N-oxide is unchanged in a healthy population. *Lipids.* Mar 2017;52(3):255–63. doi:10.1007/s11745-017-4230-9

340. DiMarco DM, Norris GH, Millar CL, Blesso CN, Fernandez ML. Intake of up to 3 eggs per day is associated with changes in HDL function

and increased plasma antioxidants in healthy, young adults. *J Nutr.* Mar 2017;147(3):323–9. doi:10.3945/jn.116.241877

341. Lemos BS, Medina-Vera I, Blesso CN, Fernandez ML. Intake of 3 eggs per day when compared to a choline bitartrate supplement, downregulates cholesterol synthesis without changing the LDL/HDL ratio. *Nutrients.* Feb 2018;10(2):258. doi:10.3390/nu10020258

342. Buzzard IM, McRoberts MR, Driscoll DL, Bowering J. Effect of dietary eggs and ascorbic acid on plasma lipid and lipoprotein cholesterol levels in healthy young men. *Am J Clin Nutr.* Jul 1982;36(1):94–105. doi:10.1093/ajcn/36.1.94

343. Flynn MA, Nolph GB, Osio Y, et al. Serum lipids and eggs. *J Am Diet Assoc.* Nov 1986;86(11): 1541–8.

344. Clark RM, Herron KL, Waters D, Fernandez ML. Hypo- and hyperresponse to egg cholesterol predicts plasma lutein and beta-carotene concentrations in men and women. *J Nutr.* Mar 2006;136(3):601–7. doi:10.1093/jn/136.3.601

345. Mutungi G, Ratliff J, Puglisi M, et al. Dietary cholesterol from eggs increases plasma HDL cholesterol in overweight men consuming a carbohydrate-restricted diet. *J Nutr.* Feb 2008;138(2):272–6. doi:10.1093/jn/138.2.272

346. Mutungi G, Waters D, Ratliff J, et al. Eggs distinctly modulate plasma carotenoid and lipoprotein subclasses in adult men following a carbohydrate-restricted diet. *J Nutr Biochem.* Apr 2010;21(4):261–7. doi:10.1016/j.jnutbio.2008.12.011

347. Blesso CN, Andersen CJ, Barona J, Volek JS, Fernandez ML. Whole egg consumption improves lipoprotein profiles and insulin sensitivity to a greater extent than yolk-free egg substitute in individuals with metabolic syndrome. *Metabolism.* Mar 2013;62(3):400–10. doi:10.1016/j.metabol.2012.08.014

348. Wright CS, Zhou J, Sayer RD, Kim JE, Campbell WW. Effects of a high-protein diet including whole eggs on muscle composition and indices of cardiometabolic health and systemic inflammation in older adults with overweight or obesity: a randomized controlled trial. *Nutrients.* Jul 2018;10(7):946. doi:10.3390/nu10070946

349. Wallace SK, Mozaffarian D. Trans-fatty acids and nonlipid risk factors. *Curr Atheroscler Rep.* Nov 2009;11(6):423–33. doi:10.1007/s11883-009-0064-0

350. Gayet-Boyer C, Tenenhaus-Aziza F, Prunet C, et al. Is there a linear relationship between the dose of ruminant trans-fatty acids and cardiovascular risk markers in healthy subjects: results from a systematic review and meta-regression of randomised clinical trials. *Br J Nutr.* Dec 2014;112(12):1914–22. doi:10.1017/S0007114514002578

351. Allen BC, Vincent MJ, Liska D, Haber LT. Meta-regression analysis of the effect of trans fatty acids on low-density lipoprotein cholesterol. *Food Chem Toxicol.* Dec 2016;98(Pt B):295–307. doi:10.1016/j.fct.2016.10.014

352. Hu Y, Hu FB, Manson JE. Marine omega-3 supplementation and cardiovascular disease: an updated meta-analysis of 13 randomized controlled trials involving 127,477 participants. *J Am Heart Assoc.* Oct 2019;8(19):e013543. doi:10.1161/JAHA.119.013543

353. Bowman L, Mafham M, Wallendszus K, et al. Effects of n-3 fatty acid supplements in diabetes mellitus. *N Engl J Med.* Oct 2018;379(16):1540–50. doi:10.1056/NEJMoa1804989

354. Manson JE, Cook NR, Lee IM, et al. Marine n-3 fatty acids and prevention of cardiovascular disease and cancer. *N Engl J Med.* Jan 2019;380(1):23–32. doi:10.1056/NEJMoa1811403

355. Bhatt DL, Steg PG, Miller M, et al. Cardiovascular risk reduction with icosapent ethyl for hypertriglyceridemia. *N Engl J Med.* Jan 2019;380(1):11–22. doi:10.1056/NEJMoa1812792

356. Kris-Etherton PM, Harris WS, Appel LJ, Committee AHAN. Fish consumption, fish oil, omega-3 fatty acids, and cardiovascular disease. *Circulation.* Nov 19 2002;106(21):2747–57. doi:10.1161/01.cir.0000038493.65177.94

357. Kris-Etherton PM, Richter CK, Bowen KJ, et al. Recent clinical trials shed new light on the cardiovascular benefits of omega-3 fatty acids. *Methodist Debakey Cardiovasc J.* 2019 Jul–Sep 2019;15(3):171–8. doi:10.14797/mdcj-15-3-171

358. Baker EJ, Miles EA, Burdge GC, Yaqoob P, Calder PC. Metabolism and functional effects of plant-derived omega-3 fatty acids in humans. *Prog Lipid Res.* Oct 2016;64:30–56. doi:10.1016/j.plipres.2016.07.002

359. Lane K, Derbyshire E, Li W, Brennan C. Bioavailability and potential uses of vegetarian sources of omega-3 fatty acids: a review of the literature. *Crit Rev Food Sci Nutr.* 2014;54(5):572–9. doi:10.1080/10408398.2011.596292

360. Craddock JC, Neale EP, Probst YC, Peoples GE. Algal supplementation of vegetarian eating patterns improves plasma and serum

docosahexaenoic acid concentrations and omega-3 indices: a systematic literature review. *J Hum Nutr Diet.* Dec 2017;30(6):693–9. doi:10.1111/jhn.12474

361. Simopoulos AP. The importance of the ratio of omega-6/omega-3 essential fatty acids. *Biomed Pharmacother.* Oct 2002;56(8):365–79. doi:10.1016/s0753-3322(02)00253-6

362. Simopoulos AP. The omega-6/omega-3 fatty acid ratio, genetic variation, and cardiovascular disease. *Asia Pac J Clin Nutr.* 2008;17 (Suppl 1):131–4.

363. Johnson GH, Fritsche K. Effect of dietary linoleic acid on markers of inflammation in healthy persons: a systematic review of randomized controlled trials. *J Acad Nutr Diet.* Jul 2012; 112(7):1029–41, 1041.e1–15. doi:10.1016/j. jand.2012.03.029

364. Ramsden CE, Hibbeln JR, Majchrzak SF, Davis JM. n-6 fatty acid-specific and mixed polyunsaturate dietary interventions have different effects on CHD risk: a meta-analysis of randomised controlled trials. *Br J Nutr.* Dec 2010;104(11):1586–600. doi:10.1017/ S0007114510004010

365. Ramsden CE, Zamora D, Leelarthaepin B, et al. Use of dietary linoleic acid for secondary prevention of coronary heart disease and death: evaluation of recovered data from the Sydney Diet Heart Study and updated meta-analysis. *BMJ.* Feb 2013;346:e8707. doi:10.1136/bmj.e8707

366. Ramsden CE, Zamora D, Majchrzak-Hong S, et al. Re-evaluation of the traditional diet-heart hypothesis: analysis of recovered data from Minnesota Coronary Experiment (1968–73). *BMJ.* Apr 2016;353:i1246. doi:10.1136/bmj.i1246

367. Hooper L, Al-Khudairy L, Abdelhamid AS, et al. Omega-6 fats for the primary and secondary prevention of cardiovascular disease. *Cochrane Database Syst Rev.* Nov 2018;11:CD011094. doi:10.1002/14651858.CD011094.pub4

368. Farvid MS, Ding M, Pan A, et al. Dietary linoleic acid and risk of coronary heart disease: a systematic review and meta-analysis of prospective cohort studies. *Circulation.* Oct 2014;130(18):1568–78. doi:10.1161/ CIRCULATIONAHA.114.010236

369. Li J, Guasch-Ferré M, Li Y, Hu FB. Dietary intake and biomarkers of linoleic acid and mortality: systematic review and meta-analysis of prospective cohort studies. *Am J Clin Nutr.* Jul 2020;112(1):150–67. doi:10.1093/ajcn/nqz349

370. Marangoni F, Agostoni C, Borghi C, et al. Dietary linoleic acid and human health: focus on cardiovascular and cardiometabolic effects. *Atherosclerosis.* Jan 2020;292:90–8. doi:10.1016/j. atherosclerosis.2019.11.018

371. Schwingshackl L, Bogensberger B, Benčič A, Knüppel S, Boeing H, Hoffmann G. Effects of oils and solid fats on blood lipids: a systematic review and network meta-analysis. *J Lipid Res.* Sept 2018;59(9):1771–82. doi:10.1194/jlr.P085522

372. Kamil A, Chen CY. Health benefits of almonds beyond cholesterol reduction. *J Agric Food Chem.* Jul 2012;60(27):6694–702. doi:10.1021/ jf2044795

373. Alexiadou K, Katsilambros N. Nuts: anti-atherogenic food? *Eur J Intern Med.* Apr 2011; 22(2):141–6. doi:10.1016/j.ejim.2010.11.008

374. Vadivel V, Kunyanga CN, Biesalski HK. Health benefits of nut consumption with special reference to body weight control. *Nutrition.* Nov–Dec 2012;28(11–12):1089–97. doi:10.1016/j. nut.2012.01.004

375. Ros E. Nuts and CVD. *Br J Nutr.* Apr 2015; 113 (Suppl 2):S111–20. doi:10.1017/ S0007114514003924

376. de Souza RGM, Schincaglia RM, Pimentel GD, Mota JF. Nuts and human health outcomes: a systematic review. *Nutrients.* Dec 2017; 9(12):1311. doi:10.3390/nu9121311

377. Harris WS. The omega-6:omega-3 ratio: a critical appraisal and possible successor. *Prostaglandins Leukot Essent Fatty Acids.* May 2018;132:34–40. doi:10.1016/j.plefa.2018.03.003

378. Forouhi NG, Krauss RM, Taubes G, Willett W. Dietary fat and cardiometabolic health: evidence, controversies, and consensus for guidance. *BMJ.* Jun 2018;361:k2139. doi:10.1136/bmj.k2139

379. Swann JP. The history of efforts to regulate dietary supplements in the USA. *Drug Test Anal.* Mar–Apr 2016;8(3–4):271–82. doi:10.1002/ dta.1919

380. Dickinson A. History and overview of DSHEA. *Fitoterapia.* Jan 2011;82(1):5–10. doi:10.1016/j. fitote.2010.09.001

381. Lordan R. Dietary supplements and nutraceuticals market growth during the coronavirus pandemic—implications for consumers and regulatory oversight. *PharmaNutrition.* Dec 2021;18:100282. doi:10.1016/j.phanu.2021.100282

382. Benito PJ, Cupeiro R, Ramos-Campo DJ, Alcaraz PE, Rubio-Arias J. A systematic review with meta-analysis of the effect of resistance training

on whole-body muscle growth in healthy adult males. *Int J Environ Res Public Health.* Feb 2020;17(4):1285. doi:10.3390/ijerph17041285

383. Aguiar AF, Grala AP, da Silva RA, et al. Free leucine supplementation during an 8-week resistance training program does not increase muscle mass and strength in untrained young adult subjects. *Amino Acids.* Jul 2017;49(7):1255–62. doi:10.1007/s00726-017-2427-0

384. Marcon M, Zanella PB. The effect of branched-chain amino acids supplementation in physical exercise: a systematic review of human randomized controlled trials. *Science & Sports.* 2022;(January [in press]) https://doi.org/10.1016/j.scispo.2021.05.006

385. Manore MM. Dietary supplements for improving body composition and reducing body weight: where is the evidence? *Int J Sport Nutr Exerc Metab.* Apr 2012;22(2):139–54. doi:10.1123/ijsnem.22.2.139

386. Stohs SJ, Badmaev V. A review of natural stimulant and non-stimulant thermogenic agents. *Phytother Res.* May 2016;30(5):732–40. doi:10.1002/ptr.5583

387. Watanabe M, Risi R, Masi D, et al. Current evidence to propose different food supplements for weight loss: a comprehensive review. *Nutrients.* Sep 2020;12(9):2873. doi:10.3390/nu12092873

388. Clark JE, Welch S. Comparing effectiveness of fat burners and thermogenic supplements to diet and exercise for weight loss and cardiometabolic health: systematic review and meta-analysis. *Nutr Health.* Dec 2021;27(4):445–59. doi:10.1177/0260106020982362

389. Tabrizi R, Saneei P, Lankarani KB, et al. The effects of caffeine intake on weight loss: a systematic review and dose-response meta-analysis of randomized controlled trials. *Crit Rev Food Sci Nutr.* 2019;59(16):2688–96. doi:10.1080/10408398.2018.1507996

390. Kamangar F, Emadi A. Vitamin and mineral supplements: do we really need them? *Int J Prev Med.* Mar 2012;3(3):221–6.

391. Kim J, Choi J, Kwon SY, et al. Association of multivitamin and mineral supplementation and risk of cardiovascular disease: a systematic review and meta-analysis. *Circ Cardiovasc Qual Outcomes.* Jul 2018;11(7):e004224. doi:10.1161/CIRCOUTCOMES.117.004224

392. Sesso HD, Christen WG, Bubes V, et al. Multivitamins in the prevention of cardiovascular disease in men: the Physicians' Health Study II randomized controlled trial. *JAMA.* Nov 2012;308(17):1751–60. doi:10.1001/jama.2012.14805

393. Hercberg S, Galan P, Preziosi P, et al. The SU.VI. MAX study: a randomized, placebo-controlled trial of the health effects of antioxidant vitamins and minerals. *Arch Intern Med.* Nov 2004;164(21):2335–42. doi:10.1001/archinte.164.21.2335

394. USDA, USDHHS. *2015–2020 Dietary Guidelines for Americans,* 8th Edition. US Government Printing Office. https://health.gov/dietaryguidelines/2015/resources/2015-2020_Dietary_Guidelines.pdf

395. Huang HY, Caballero B, Chang S, et al. Multivitamin/mineral supplements and prevention of chronic disease. *Evid Rep Technol Assess (Full Rep).* May 2006;(139):1–117.

396. Bird JK, Murphy RA, Ciappio ED, McBurney MI. Risk of deficiency in multiple concurrent micronutrients in children and adults in the United States. *Nutrients.* Jun 2017;9(7):655. doi:10.3390/nu9070655

397. Calton JB. Prevalence of micronutrient deficiency in popular diet plans. *J Int Soc Sports Nutr.* Jun 2010;7:24. doi:10.1186/1550-2783-7-24

398. G Engel M, J Kern H, Brenna JT, H Mitmesser S. Micronutrient gaps in three commercial weight-loss diet plans. *Nutrients.* Jan 2018;10(1):108. doi:10.3390/nu10010108

399. Kleiner SM, Bazzarre TL, Litchford MD. Metabolic profiles, diet, and health practices of championship male and female bodybuilders. *J Am Diet Assoc.* Jul 1990;90(7):962–7.

400. Kleiner SM, Bazzarre TL, Ainsworth BE. Nutritional status of nationally ranked elite bodybuilders. *Int J Sport Nutr.* Mar 1994;4(1):54–69. doi:10.1123/ijsn.4.1.54

401. Misner B. Food alone may not provide sufficient micronutrients for preventing deficiency. *J Int Soc Sports Nutr.* Jun 2006;3:51–5. doi:10.1186/1550-2783-3-1-51

402. Ward E. Addressing nutritional gaps with multivitamin and mineral supplements. *Nutr J.* Jul 15 2014;13:72. doi:10.1186/1475-2891-13-72

403. Joncquel-Chevalier Curt M, Voicu PM, Fontaine M, et al. Creatine biosynthesis and transport in health and disease. *Biochimie.* Dec 2015;119:146–65. doi:10.1016/j.biochi.2015.10.022

404. Kreider RB. Effects of creatine supplementation on performance and training adaptations. *Mol Cell Biochem.* Feb 2003;244(1-2):89–94.

405. Persky AM, Brazeau GA. Clinical pharmacology of the dietary supplement creatine monohydrate. *Pharmacol Rev.* Jun 2001;53(2):161–76.

406. Cooper R, Naclerio F, Allgrove J, Jimenez A. Creatine supplementation with specific view to exercise/sports performance: an update. *J Int Soc Sports Nutr.* Jul 2012;9(1):33. doi:10.1186/1550-2783-9-33

407. Brosnan ME, Brosnan JT. The role of dietary creatine. *Amino Acids.* Aug 2016;48(8):1785–91. doi:10.1007/s00726-016-2188-1

408. Riesberg LA, Weed SA, McDonald TL, Eckerson JM, Drescher KM. Beyond muscles: The untapped potential of creatine. *Int Immunopharmacol.* Aug 2016;37:31–42. doi:10.1016/j.intimp.2015.12.034

409. Roschel H, Gualano B, Ostojic SM, Rawson ES. Creatine supplementation and brain health. *Nutrients.* Feb 2021;13(2):586. doi:10.3390/nu13020586

410. Naderi A, de Oliveira EP, Ziegenfuss TN, Willems MT. Timing, optimal dose and intake duration of dietary supplements with evidence-based use in sports nutrition. *J Exerc Nutrition Biochem.* Dec 2016;20(4):1–12. doi:10.20463/jenb.2016.0031

411. Antonio J, Ciccone V. The effects of pre versus post workout supplementation of creatine monohydrate on body composition and strength. *J Int Soc Sports Nutr.* Aug 2013;10:36. doi:10.1186/1550-2783-10-36

412. Candow DG, Vogt E, Johannsmeyer S, Forbes SC, Farthing JP. Strategic creatine supplementation and resistance training in healthy older adults. *Appl Physiol Nutr Metab.* Jul 2015;40(7):689–94. doi:10.1139/apnm-2014-0498

413. Candow DG, Zello GA, Ling B, et al. Comparison of creatine supplementation before versus after supervised resistance training in healthy older adults. *Res Sports Med.* 2014;22(1):61–74. doi:10.1080/15438627.2013.852088

414. Ribeiro F, Longobardi I, Perim P, et al. Timing of creatine supplementation around exercise: a real concern? *Nutrients.* Aug 2021;13(8):2844. doi:10.3390/nu13082844

415. Buford TW, Kreider RB, Stout JR, et al. International Society of Sports Nutrition position stand: creatine supplementation and exercise. *J Int Soc Sports Nutr.* Aug 2007;4:6. doi:10.1186/1550-2783-4-6

416. Rawson ES, Persky AM, Price TB, Clarkson PM. Effects of repeated creatine supplementation on muscle, plasma, and urine creatine levels. *J Strength Cond Res.* Feb 2004;18(1):162–7. doi:10.1519/1533-4287(2004)0182.0.co;2

417. Jäger R, Purpura M, Shao A, Inoue T, Kreider RB. Analysis of the efficacy, safety, and regulatory status of novel forms of creatine. *Amino Acids.* May 2011;40(5):1369–83. doi:10.1007/s00726-011-0874-6

418. Antonio J, Candow DG, Forbes SC, et al. Common questions and misconceptions about creatine supplementation: what does the scientific evidence really show? *J Int Soc Sports Nutr.* Feb 2021;18(1):13. doi:10.1186/s12970-021-00412-w

419. Trexler ET, Smith-Ryan AE. Creatine and caffeine: considerations for concurrent supplementation. *Int J Sport Nutr Exerc Metab.* Dec 2015;25(6):607–23. doi:10.1123/ijsnem.2014-0193

420. Marinho AH, Gonçalves JS, Araújo PK, Lima-Silva AE, Ataide-Silva T, de Araujo GG. Effects of creatine and caffeine ingestion in combination on exercise performance: a systematic review. *Crit Rev Food Sci Nutr.* Nov 2021:1–14. doi:10.1080/10408398.2021.2007470

421. van der Merwe J, Brooks NE, Myburgh KH. Three weeks of creatine monohydrate supplementation affects dihydrotestosterone to testosterone ratio in college-aged rugby players. *Clin J Sport Med.* Sep 2009;19(5):399–404. doi:10.1097/JSM.0b013e3181b8b52f

422. Kaufman KD. Androgens and alopecia. *Mol Cell Endocrinol.* Dec 2002;198(1-2):89–95. doi:10.1016/s0303-7207(02)00372-6

423. Artioli GG, Gualano B, Smith A, Stout J, Lancha AH. Role of beta-alanine supplementation on muscle carnosine and exercise performance. *Med Sci Sports Exerc.* Jun 2010;42(6):1162–73. doi:10.1249/MSS.0b013e3181c74e38

424. Everaert I, Mooyaart A, Baguet A, et al. Vegetarianism, female gender and increasing age, but not CNDP1 genotype, are associated with reduced muscle carnosine levels in humans. *Amino Acids.* Apr 2011;40(4):1221–9. doi:10.1007/s00726-010-0749-2

425. Hobson RM, Saunders B, Ball G, Harris RC, Sale C. Effects of β-alanine supplementation on exercise performance: a meta-analysis. *Amino Acids.* Jul 2012;43(1):25–37. doi:10.1007/s00726-011-1200-z

426. Saunders B, Elliott-Sale K, Artioli GG, et al. β-alanine supplementation to improve exercise capacity and performance: a systematic review and meta-analysis. *Br J Sports Med.* Apr 2017;51(8):658–69. doi:10.1136/bjsports-2016-096396

427. Brisola GMP, Zagatto AM. Ergogenic effects of β-alanine supplementation on different sports modalities: strong evidence or only incipient findings? *J Strength Cond Res.* Jan 2019;33(1):253–82. doi:10.1519/JSC.0000000000002925

428. Harris RC, Tallon MJ, Dunnett M, et al. The absorption of orally supplied beta-alanine and its effect on muscle carnosine synthesis in human vastus lateralis. *Amino Acids.* May 2006;30(3):279–89. doi:10.1007/s00726-006-0299-9

429. Saunders B, DE Salles Painelli V, DE Oliveira LF, et al. Twenty-four weeks of β-alanine supplementation on carnosine content, related genes, and exercise. *Med Sci Sports Exerc.* May 2017;49(5):896–906. doi:10.1249/MSS.0000000000001173

430. Stegen S, Bex T, Vervaet C, Vanhee L, Achten E, Derave W. β-alanine dose for maintaining moderately elevated muscle carnosine levels. *Med Sci Sports Exerc.* Jul 2014;46(7):1426–32. doi:10.1249/MSS.0000000000000248

431. Dolan E, Swinton PA, Painelli VS, et al. A systematic risk assessment and meta-analysis on the use of oral β-alanine supplementation. *Adv Nutr.* May 2019;10(3):452–63. doi:10.1093/advances/nmy115

432. Sale C, Saunders B, Harris RC. Effect of beta-alanine supplementation on muscle carnosine concentrations and exercise performance. *Amino Acids.* Jul 2010;39(2):321–33. doi:10.1007/s00726-009-0443-4

433. Décombaz J, Beaumont M, Vuichoud J, Bouisset F, Stellingwerff T. Effect of slow-release β-alanine tablets on absorption kinetics and paresthesia. *Amino Acids.* Jul 2012;43(1):67–76. doi:10.1007/s00726-011-1169-7

434. de Salazar L, Segarra I, López-Román FJ, Torregrosa-García A, Pérez-Piñero S, Ávila-Gandía V. Increased bioavailability of β-alanine by a novel controlled-release powder blend compared to a slow-release tablet. *Pharmaceutics.* Sep 2021;13(9):1517. doi:10.3390/pharmaceutics13091517

435. Blancquaert L, Everaert I, Missinne M, et al. Effects of histidine and β-alanine supplementation on human muscle carnosine storage. *Med Sci Sports Exerc.* Mar 2017;49(3):602–9. doi:10.1249/MSS.0000000000001213

436. Grgic J, Rodriguez RF, Garofolini A, et al. Effects of sodium bicarbonate supplementation on muscular strength and endurance: a systematic review and meta-analysis. *Sports Med.* Jul 2020;50(7):1361–75. doi:10.1007/s40279-020-01275-y

437. Calvo JL, Xu H, Mon-López D, Pareja-Galeano H, Jiménez SL. Effect of sodium bicarbonate contribution on energy metabolism during exercise: a systematic review and meta-analysis. *J Int Soc Sports Nutr.* Feb 2021;18(1):11. doi:10.1186/s12970-021-00410-y

438. Peart DJ, Siegler JC, Vince RV. Practical recommendations for coaches and athletes: a meta-analysis of sodium bicarbonate use for athletic performance. *J Strength Cond Res.* Jul 2012;26(7):1975–83. doi:10.1519/JSC.0b013e3182576f3d

439. Carr AJ, Hopkins WG, Gore CJ. Effects of acute alkalosis and acidosis on performance: a meta-analysis. *Sports Med.* Oct 2011;41(10):801–14. doi:10.2165/11591440-000000000-00000

440. Matson LG, Tran ZV. Effects of sodium bicarbonate ingestion on anaerobic performance: a meta-analytic review. *Int J Sport Nutr.* Mar 1993;3(1):2–28. doi:10.1123/ijsn.3.1.2

441. Grgic J, Pedisic Z, Saunders B, et al. International Society of Sports Nutrition position stand: sodium bicarbonate and exercise performance. *J Int Soc Sports Nutr.* Sep 2021;18(1):61. doi:10.1186/s12970-021-00458-w

442. Ducker KJ, Dawson B, Wallman KE. Effect of beta alanine and sodium bicarbonate supplementation on repeated-sprint performance. *J Strength Cond Res.* Dec 2013;27(12):3450–60. doi:10.1519/JSC.0b013e31828fd310

443. Hadzic M, Eckstein ML, Schugardt M. The impact of sodium bicarbonate on performance in response to exercise duration in athletes: a systematic review. *J Sports Sci Med.* Jun 2019;18(2):271–81.

444. Maughan RJ, Burke LM, Dvorak J, et al. IOC consensus statement: dietary supplements and the high-performance athlete. *Br J Sports Med.* Apr 2018;52(7):439–55. doi:10.1136/bjsports-2018-099027

445. McMahon NF, Leveritt MD, Pavey TG. The effect of dietary nitrate supplementation on endurance exercise performance in healthy adults: a systematic review and meta-analysis. *Sports Med.* Apr 2017;47(4):735–56. doi:10.1007/s40279-016-0617-7

446. Gao C, Gupta S, Adli T, et al. The effects of dietary nitrate supplementation on endurance exercise performance and cardiorespiratory measures in

healthy adults: a systematic review and meta-analysis. *J Int Soc Sports Nutr.* Jul 2021;18(1):55. doi:10.1186/s12970-021-00450-4

447. Gallardo EJ, Coggan AR. What's in your beet juice? Nitrate and nitrite content of beet juice products marketed to athletes. *Int J Sport Nutr Exerc Metab.* Jul 2019;29(4):345–9. doi:10.1123/ijsnem.2018-0223

448. Clements WT, Lee SR, Bloomer RJ. Nitrate ingestion: a review of the health and physical performance effects. *Nutrients.* Nov 2014; 6(11):5224–64. doi:10.3390/nu6115224

449. Hord NG, Tang Y, Bryan NS. Food sources of nitrates and nitrites: the physiologic context for potential health benefits. *Am J Clin Nutr.* Jul 2009;90(1):1–10. doi:10.3945/ajcn.2008.27131

450. Larsen FJ, Schiffer TA, Ekblom B, et al. Dietary nitrate reduces resting metabolic rate: a randomized, crossover study in humans. *Am J Clin Nutr.* Apr 2014;99(4):843–50. doi:10.3945/ajcn.113.079491

451. Pawlak-Chaouch M, Boissière J, Gamelin FX, Cuvelier G, Berthoin S, Aucouturier J. Effect of dietary nitrate supplementation on metabolic rate during rest and exercise in human: a systematic review and a meta-analysis. *Nitric Oxide.* Feb 2016;53:65–76. doi:10.1016/j.niox.2016.01.001

452. Cappelletti S, Piacentino D, Daria P, Sani G, Aromatario M. Caffeine: cognitive and physical performance enhancer or psychoactive drug? *Curr Neuropharmacol.* Jan 2015;13(1):71–88. doi:10.2174/1570159X13666141210215655

453. Meredith SE, Juliano LM, Hughes JR, Griffiths RR. Caffeine use disorder: a comprehensive review and research agenda. *J Caffeine Res.* Sep 2013;3(3):114–30. doi:10.1089/jcr.2013.0016

454. Martins GL, Guilherme JPLF, Ferreira LHB, de Souza-Junior TP, Lancha AH. Caffeine and exercise performance: possible directions for definitive findings. *Front Sports Act Living.* Dec 2020;2:574854. doi:10.3389/fspor.2020.574854

455. Goldstein ER, Ziegenfuss T, Kalman D, et al. International Society of Sports Nutrition position stand: caffeine and performance. *J Int Soc Sports Nutr.* Jan 2010;7(1):5. doi:10.1186/1550-2783-7-5

456. Grgic J, Trexler ET, Lazinica B, Pedisic Z. Effects of caffeine intake on muscle strength and power: a systematic review and meta-analysis. *J Int Soc Sports Nutr.* Mar 2018;15:11. doi:10.1186/s12970-018-0216-0

457. Grgic J, Grgic I, Pickering C, Schoenfeld BJ, Bishop DJ, Pedisic Z. Wake up and smell the coffee: caffeine supplementation and exercise performance—an umbrella review of 21 published meta-analyses. *Br J Sports Med.* Jun 2020;54(11):681–8. doi:10.1136/bjsports-2018-100278

458. Guest NS, VanDusseldorp TA, Nelson MT, et al. International Society of Sports Nutrition position stand: caffeine and exercise performance. *J Int Soc Sports Nutr.* Jan 2021;18(1):1. doi:10.1186/s12970-020-00383-4

459. Campbell B, Wilborn C, La Bounty P, et al. International Society of Sports Nutrition position stand: energy drinks. *J Int Soc Sports Nutr.* Jan 2013;10(1):1. doi:10.1186/1550-2783-10-1

460. Generali JA. Energy drinks: food, dietary supplement, or drug? *Hosp Pharm.* Jan 2013;48(1):5–9. doi:10.1310/hpj4801-5.test

461. Al-Shaar L, Vercammen K, Lu C, Richardson S, Tamez M, Mattei J. Health effects and public health concerns of energy drink consumption in the United States: a mini-review. *Front Public Health.* Aug 2017;5:225. doi:10.3389/fpubh.2017.00225

462. Satel S. Is caffeine addictive? A review of the literature. *Am J Drug Alcohol Abuse.* 2006;32(4): 493–502. doi:10.1080/00952990600918965

463. Kim Y, Je Y, Giovannucci E. Coffee consumption and all-cause and cause-specific mortality: a meta-analysis by potential modifiers. *Eur J Epidemiol.* Aug 2019;34(8):731–52. doi:10.1007/s10654-019-00524-3

464. Ruiz LD, Scherr RE. Risk of energy drink consumption to adolescent health. *Am J Lifestyle Med.* Jan–Feb 2019;13(1):22–5. doi:10.1177/1559827618803069

465. Poole R, Kennedy OJ, Roderick P, Fallowfield JA, Hayes PC, Parkes J. Coffee consumption and health: umbrella review of meta-analyses of multiple health outcomes. *BMJ.* Nov 2017; 359:j5024. doi:10.1136/bmj.j5024

466. Doepker C, Franke K, Myers E, et al. Key findings and implications of a recent systematic review of the potential adverse effects of caffeine consumption in healthy adults, pregnant women, adolescents, and children. *Nutrients.* Oct 2018; 10(10):1536. doi:10.3390/nu10101536

467. Higgins S, Straight CR, Lewis RD. The effects of preexercise caffeinated coffee ingestion on endurance performance: an evidence-based review. *Int J Sport Nutr Exerc Metab.* Jun 2016; 26(3):221–39. doi:10.1123/ijsnem.2015-0147

468. Grgic J, Pickering C, Del Coso J, Schoenfeld BJ, Mikulic P. CYP1A2 genotype and acute

ergogenic effects of caffeine intake on exercise performance: a systematic review. *Eur J Nutr.* Apr 2021;60(3):1181–95. doi:10.1007/s00394-020-02427-6

469. Kouri EM, Pope HG, Katz DL, Oliva P. Fat-free mass index in users and nonusers of anabolic-androgenic steroids. *Clin J Sport Med.* Oct 1995;5(4):223–8. doi:10.1097/00042752-199510000-00003

470. Trexler ET, Smith-Ryan AE, Blue MNM, et al. Fat-free mass index in NCAA Division I and II collegiate American football players. *J Strength Cond Res.* Oct 2017;31(10):2719–27. doi:10.1519/JSC.0000000000001737

471. Hattori K, Kondo M, Abe T, Tanaka S, Fukunaga T. Hierarchical differences in body composition of professional sumo wrestlers. *Ann Hum Biol.* Mar–Apr 1999;26(2):179–84. doi:10.1080/030144699282886

472. Wilson JM, Lowery RP, Joy JM, et al. The effects of 12 weeks of beta-hydroxy-beta-methylbutyrate free acid supplementation on muscle mass, strength, and power in resistance-trained individuals: a randomized, double-blind, placebo-controlled study. *Eur J Appl Physiol.* Jun 2014;114(6):1217–27. doi:10.1007/s00421-014-2854-5

473. Kyle UG, Schutz Y, Dupertuis YM, Pichard C. Body composition interpretation. Contributions of the fat-free mass index and the body fat mass index. *Nutrition.* Jul–Aug 2003;19(7–8):597–604. doi:10.1016/s0899-9007(03)00061-3

474. van der Ploeg GE, Brooks AG, Withers RT, Dollman J, Leaney F, Chatterton BE. Body composition changes in female bodybuilders during preparation for competition. *Eur J Clin Nutr.* Apr 2001;55(4):268–77. doi:10.1038/sj.ejcn.1601154

475. Cureton KJ, Collins MA, Hill DW, McElhannon FM. Muscle hypertrophy in men and women. *Med Sci Sports Exerc.* Aug 1988;20(4):338–44. doi:10.1249/00005768-198808000-00003

476. Levine JA, Eberhardt NL, Jensen MD. Role of nonexercise activity thermogenesis in resistance to fat gain in humans. *Science.* Jan 1999;8;283(5399):212–4. doi: 10.1126/science.283.5399.212

477. Gentil P, Steele J, Pereira MC, Castanheira RP, Paoli A, Bottaro M. Comparison of upper body strength gains between men and women after 10 weeks of resistance training. *PeerJ.* Feb 2016;4:e1627. doi:10.7717/peerj.1627

478. Janssen I, Heymsfield SB, Wang ZM, Ross R. Skeletal muscle mass and distribution in 468 men and women aged 18–88 yr. *J Appl Physiol* (1985). Jul 2000;89(1):81–8. doi:10.1152/jappl.2000.89.1.81

479. Abe T, Bell ZW, Wong V, et al. Skeletal muscle size distribution in large-sized male and female athletes. *Am J Hum Biol.* Mar 2021;33(2):e23473. doi:10.1002/ajhb.23473

480. Norgan NG. The beneficial effects of body fat and adipose tissue in humans. *Int J Obes Relat Metab Disord.* Sep 1997;21(9):738–46. doi:10.1038/sj.ijo.0800473

481. El Ghoch M, Milanese C, Calugi S, Pellegrini M, Battistini NC, Dalle Grave R. Body composition, eating disorder psychopathology, and psychological distress in anorexia nervosa: a longitudinal study. *Am J Clin Nutr.* Apr 2014;99(4):771–8. doi:10.3945/ajcn.113.078816

482. Manuelli M, Blundell JE, Biino G, Cena H. Body composition and resting energy expenditure in women with anorexia nervosa: is hyperactivity a protecting factor? *Clin Nutr ESPEN.* Feb 2019;29:160–4. doi:10.1016/j.clnesp.2018.10.015

483. Abernathy RP, Black DR. Healthy body weights: an alternative perspective. *Am J Clin Nutr.* Mar 1996;63(3 Suppl):448S–51S. doi:10.1093/ajcn/63.3.448

484. Fleck SJ. Body composition of elite American athletes. *Am J Sports Med.* Nov–Dec 1983; 11(6):398–403. doi:10.1177/036354658301100604

485. Hulmi JJ, Isola V, Suonpää M, et al. The effects of intensive weight reduction on body composition and serum hormones in female fitness competitors. *Front Physiol.* Jan 2016;7:689. doi:10.3389/fphys.2016.00689

486. Rossow LM, Fukuda DH, Fahs CA, Loenneke JP, Stout JR. Natural bodybuilding competition preparation and recovery: a 12-month case study. *Int J Sports Physiol Perform.* Sep 2013;8(5):582–92. doi:10.1123/ijspp.8.5.582

487. Nackers L, Ross K, Perri M. The association between rate of initial weight loss and long-term success in obesity treatment: does slow and steady win the race? *Int J Behav Med.* Sep 2010;17(3):161–7. doi: 10.1007/s12529-010-9092-y

488. Garthe I, Raastad T, Refsnes P, Koivisto A, Sundgot-Borgen J. Effect of two different weight-loss rates on body composition and strength and power-related performance in elite athletes. *Int J Sport Nutr Exerc Metab.* Apr 2011;21(2):97–104. doi: 10.1123/ijsnem.21.2.97

489. Helms E, Aragon A, Fitschen P. Evidence-based recommendations for natural bodybuilding contest preparation: nutrition and supplementation. *J Int Soc Sports Nutr.* May 2014 12;11:20.

490. von Loeffelholz C, Birkenfeld A. The role of non-exercise activity thermogenesis in human obesity. 2018 Apr 9. In: Feingold KR, Anawalt B, Boyce A, Chrousos G, de Herder WW, Dhatariya K, Dungan K, Hershman JM, Hofland J, Kalra S, Kaltsas G, Koch C, Kopp P, Korbonits M, Kovacs CS, Kuohung W, Laferrère B, Levy M, McGee EA, McLachlan R, Morley JE, New M, Purnell J, Sahay R, Singer F, Sperling MA, Stratakis CA, Trence DL, Wilson DP, editors. Endotext [Internet]. South Dartmouth (MA): MDText.com, Inc.; 2000–. PMID: 25905303.

491. Wing RR, Phelan S. Long-term weight loss maintenance. *Am J Clin Nutr.* Jul 2005;82(1 Suppl):222S–5S. doi:10.1093/ajcn/82.1.222S

492. Keesey RE, Boyle PC. Effects of quinine adulteration upon body weight of LH-lesioned and intact male rats. *J Comp Physiol Psychol.* Jul 1973;84(1):38–46. doi:10.1037/h0035016

493. Wirtshafter D, Davis JD. Set points, settling points, and the control of body weight. *Physiol Behav.* Jul 1977;19(1):75–8. doi:10.1016/0031-9384(77)90162-7

494. Fazzino TL, Rohde K, Sullivan DK. Hyper-palatable foods: development of a quantitative definition and application to the US Food System Database. *Obesity* (Silver Spring). Nov 2019;27(11):1761–8. doi:10.1002/oby.22639

495. Johnson F, Wardle J. Variety, palatability, and obesity. *Adv Nutr.* Nov 2014;5(6):851–9. doi:10.3945/an.114.007120

496. Hall KD. Did the food environment cause the obesity epidemic? *Obesity* (Silver Spring). Jan 2018;26(1):11–3. doi:10.1002/oby.22073

497. Müller MJ, Geisler C, Heymsfield SB, Bosy-Westphal A. Recent advances in understanding body weight homeostasis in humans. *F1000Res.* 2018;7. doi:10.12688/f1000research.14151.1

498. Sherman AM, Bowen DJ, Vitolins M, et al. Dietary adherence: characteristics and interventions. *Control Clin Trials.* Oct 2000;21(5 Suppl):206S–11S. doi:10.1016/s0197-2456(00)00080-5

499. Lemstra M, Bird Y, Nwankwo C, Rogers M, Moraros J. Weight loss intervention adherence and factors promoting adherence: a meta-analysis. *Patient Prefer Adherence.* Aug 2016;10:1547–59. doi:10.2147/PPA.S103649

500. Cruwys T, Norwood R, Chachay VS, Ntontis E, Sheffield J. "An important part of who I am": the predictors of dietary adherence among weight-loss, vegetarian, vegan, Paleo, and gluten-free dietary groups. *Nutrients.* Apr 2020;12(4):970. doi:10.3390/nu12040970

501. Spreckley M, Seidell J, Halberstadt J. Perspectives into the experience of successful, substantial long-term weight-loss maintenance: a systematic review. *Int J Qual Stud Health Well-being.* Dec 2021;16(1):1862481. doi:10.1080/17482631.2020.1862481

502. Resnicow K, Page SE. Embracing chaos and complexity: a quantum change for public health. *Am J Public Health.* Aug 2008;98(8):1382–9. doi:10.2105/AJPH.2007.129460

503. Hall K. A review of the carbohydrate-insulin model of obesity. *Eur J Clin Nutr.* Mar 2017;71(3):323–6. doi: 10.1038/ejcn.2016.260

504. Hall KD, Guyenet SJ, Leibel RL. The carbohydrate-insulin model of obesity is difficult to reconcile with current evidence. *JAMA Intern Med.* Aug 2018;178(8):1103–5. doi:10.1001/jamainternmed.2018.2920

505. Patrick H, Williams GC. Self-determination theory: its application to health behavior and complementarity with motivational interviewing. *Int J Behav Nutr Phys Act.* Mar 2012;9:18. doi:10.1186/1479-5868-9-18

506. Yancy WS, Mayer SB, Coffman CJ, et al. Effect of allowing choice of diet on weight loss: a randomized trial. *Ann Intern Med.* Jun 2015;162(12):805–14. doi:10.7326/M14-2358

507. McClain AD, Otten JJ, Hekler EB, Gardner CD. Adherence to a low-fat vs. low-carbohydrate diet differs by insulin resistance status. *Diabetes Obes Metab.* Jan 2013;15(1):87–90. doi:10.1111/j.1463-1326.2012.01668.x

508. Rosanoff A, Weaver CM, Rude RK. Suboptimal magnesium status in the United States: are the health consequences underestimated? *Nutr Rev.* Mar 2012;70(3):153–64. doi:10.1111/j.1753-4887.2011.00465.x

509. Cogswell ME, Zhang Z, Carriquiry AL, et al. Sodium and potassium intakes among US adults: NHANES 2003–2008. *Am J Clin Nutr.* Sep 2012;96(3):647–57. doi:10.3945/ajcn.112.034413

510. Vadiveloo M, Sacks FM, Champagne CM, Bray GA, Mattei J. Greater healthful dietary variety is associated with greater 2-year changes in weight and adiposity in the preventing overweight using novel dietary strategies (POUNDS lost) trial. *J Nutr.* Aug 2016;146(8):1552–9. doi:10.3945/jn.115.224683

511. Loria-Kohen V, Gómez-Candela C, Fernández-Fernández C, Pérez-Torres A, García-Puig J, Bermejo LM. Evaluation of the usefulness of a low-calorie diet with or without bread in the treatment of overweight/obesity. *Clin Nutr.* Aug 2012;31(4):455–61. doi:10.1016/j.clnu.2011.12.002

512. Farhangi MA, Jahangiry L. Dietary diversity score is associated with cardiovascular risk factors and serum adiponectin concentrations in patients with metabolic syndrome. *BMC Cardiovasc Disord.* Apr 2018;18(1):68. doi:10.1186/s12872-018-0807-3

513. Steinberg DM, Bennett GG, Askew S, Tate DF. Weighing every day matters: daily weighing improves weight loss and adoption of weight control behaviors. *J Acad Nutr Diet.* Apr 2015;115(4):511–8. doi:10.1016/j.jand.2014.12.011

514. Peterson ND, Middleton KR, Nackers LM, Medina KE, Milsom VA, Perri MG. Dietary self-monitoring and long-term success with weight management. *Obesity* (Silver Spring). Sep 2014;22(9):1962–7. doi:10.1002/oby.20807

515. Klos LA, Esser VE, Kessler MM. To weigh or not to weigh: the relationship between self-weighing behavior and body image among adults. *Body Image.* Sep 2012;9(4):551–4. doi:10.1016/j.bodyim.2012.07.004

516. Rohde P, Arigo D, Shaw H, Stice E. Relation of self-weighing to future weight gain and onset of disordered eating symptoms. *J Consult Clin Psychol.* Aug 2018;86(8):677–87. doi:10.1037/ccp0000325

517. Aragon A. How can we track body composition changes with minimal technology and resources? *AARR,* May 2020.

518. Macdiarmid J, Blundell J. Assessing dietary intake: who, what and why of under-reporting. *Nutr Res Rev.* Dec 1998;11(2):231–53. doi:10.1079/NRR19980017

519. Schwingshackl L, Zähringer J, Nitschke K, et al. Impact of intermittent energy restriction on anthropometric outcomes and intermediate disease markers in patients with overweight and obesity: systematic review and meta-analyses. *Crit Rev Food Sci Nutr.* 2021;61(8):1293–304. doi:10.1080/10408398.2020.1757616

520. Cui Y, Cai T, Zhou Z, et al. Health effects of alternate-day fasting in adults: a systematic review and meta-analysis. *Front Nutr.* Nov 2020;7:586036. doi:10.3389/fnut.2020.586036

521. Gabel K, Hoddy KK, Haggerty N, et al. Effects of 8-hour time restricted feeding on body weight and metabolic disease risk factors in obese adults: a pilot study. *Nutr Healthy Aging.* Jun 2018;4(4):345–53. doi:10.3233/NHA-170036

522. Lowe DA, Wu N, Rohdin-Bibby L, et al. Effects of time-restricted eating on weight loss and other metabolic parameters in women and men with overweight and obesity: the TREAT randomized clinical trial. *JAMA Intern Med.* Nov 2020;180(11):1491–9. doi:10.1001/jamainternmed.2020.4153

523. Headland ML, Clifton PM, Keogh JB. Effect of intermittent compared to continuous energy restriction on weight loss and weight maintenance after 12 months in healthy overweight or obese adults. *Int J Obes* (Lond). Oct 2019;43(10):2028–36. doi:10.1038/s41366-018-0247-2

524. Conley M, Le Fevre L, Haywood C, Proietto J. Is two days of intermittent energy restriction per week a feasible weight loss approach in obese males? A randomised pilot study. *Nutr Diet.* Feb 2018;75(1):65–72. doi:10.1111/1747-0080.12372

525. Cioffi I, Evangelista A, Ponzo V, et al. Intermittent versus continuous energy restriction on weight loss and cardiometabolic outcomes: a systematic review and meta-analysis of randomized controlled trials. *J Transl Med.* Dec 2018;16(1):371. doi:10.1186/s12967-018-1748-4

526. Harris L, Hamilton S, Azevedo LB, et al. Intermittent fasting interventions for treatment of overweight and obesity in adults: a systematic review and meta-analysis. *JBI Database System Rev Implement Rep.* Feb 2018;16(2):507–47. doi:10.11124/JBISRIR-2016-003248

527. Meng H, Zhu L, Kord-Varkaneh H, O Santos H, Tinsley GM, Fu P. Effects of intermittent fasting and energy-restricted diets on lipid profile: a systematic review and meta-analysis. *Nutrition.* Sept 2020;77:110801. doi:10.1016/j.nut.2020.110801

528. Headland M, Clifton PM, Carter S, Keogh JB. Weight-loss outcomes: a systematic review and meta-analysis of intermittent energy restriction trials lasting a minimum of 6 months. *Nutrients.* Jun 2016;8(6):354. doi:10.3390/nu8060354

529. Keenan S, Cooke MB, Belski R. The effects of intermittent fasting combined with resistance training on lean body mass: a systematic review of human studies. *Nutrients.* Aug 2020;12(8):2349. doi:10.3390/nu12082349

530. Seimon R, Roekenes J, Zibellini J, et al. Do intermittent diets provide physiological benefits over continuous diets for weight loss?

A systematic review of clinical trials. *Mol Cell Endocrinol.* 2015;418(Pt 2):153–72. doi: 10.1016/j.mce.2015.09.014

531. Welton S, Minty R, O'Driscoll T, et al. Intermittent fasting and weight loss: systematic review. *Can Fam Physician.* Feb 2020;66(2):117–25.

532. Adafer R, Messaadi W, Meddahi M, et al. Food timing, circadian rhythm and chrononutrition: a systematic review of time-restricted eating's effects on human health. *Nutrients.* Dec 2020;12(12):3770. doi:10.3390/nu12123770

533. O'Connor SG, Boyd P, Bailey CP, et al. Perspective: time-restricted eating compared with caloric restriction: potential facilitators and barriers of long-term weight loss maintenance. *Adv Nutr.* Mar 2021;12(2):325–33. doi:10.1093/advances/nmaa168

534. Headland ML, Clifton PM, Keogh JB. Impact of intermittent vs. continuous energy restriction on weight and cardiometabolic factors: a 12-month follow-up. *Int J Obes* (Lond). Jun 2020;44(6):1236–42. doi:10.1038/s41366-020-0525-7

535. Campbell BI, Aguilar D, Colenso-Semple LM, et al. Intermittent energy restriction attenuates the loss of fat free mass in resistance trained individuals. a randomized controlled trial. *J Funct Morphol Kinesiol.* Mar 2020;5(1):19. doi:10.3390/jfmk5010019

536. Peos JJ, Helms ER, Fournier PA, et al. Continuous versus intermittent dieting for fat loss and fat-free mass retention in resistance-trained adults: the ICECAP trial. *Med Sci Sports Exerc.* Aug 2021;53(8):1685–98. doi:10.1249/MSS.0000000000002636

537. Kysel P, Haluzíková D, Doležalová RP, et al. The influence of cyclical ketogenic reduction diet vs. nutritionally balanced reduction diet on body composition, strength, and endurance performance in healthy young males: a randomized controlled trial. *Nutrients.* Sep 2020;12(9):2832. doi:10.3390/nu12092832

538. Byrne NM, Sainsbury A, King NA, Hills AP, Wood RE. Intermittent energy restriction improves weight loss efficiency in obese men: the MATADOR study. *Int J Obes* (Lond). Feb 2018;42(2):129–38. doi:10.1038/ijo.2017.206

539. Antonio J, Peacock C, Ellerbroek A, Fromhoff B, Silver T. The effects of consuming a high protein diet (4.4 g/kg/d) on body composition in resistance-trained individuals. *J Int Soc Sports Nutr.* May 2014;11:19. doi:10.1186/1550-2783-11-19

540. Wing RR, Jeffery RW. Prescribed "breaks" as a means to disrupt weight control efforts. *Obes Res.* Feb 2003;11(2):287–91. doi:10.1038/oby.2003.43

541. Peos JJ, Helms ER, Fournier PA, Krieger J, Sainsbury A. A 1-week diet break improves muscle endurance during an intermittent dieting regime in adult athletes: a pre-specified secondary analysis of the ICECAP trial. *PLoS One.* Feb 2021;16(2):e0247292. doi:10.1371/journal.pone.0247292

542. do Vale R, Pieters R, Zeelenberg M. The benefits of behaving badly on occasion: successful regulation by planned hedonic deviations. *Journal of Consumer Psychology.* Jan 2016;26(1):17–28. https://doi.org/10.1016/j.jcps.2015.05.001

543. Corney RA, Sunderland C, James LJ. Immediate pre-meal water ingestion decreases voluntary food intake in lean young males. *Eur J Nutr.* Mar 2016;55(2):815–9. doi:10.1007/s00394-015-0903-4

544. Dennis EA, Dengo AL, Comber DL, et al. Water consumption increases weight loss during a hypocaloric diet intervention in middle-aged and older adults. *Obesity* (Silver Spring). Feb 2010;18(2):300–7. doi:10.1038/oby.2009.235

545. Daniels MC, Popkin BM. Impact of water intake on energy intake and weight status: a systematic review. *Nutr Rev.* Sep 2010;68(9):505–21. doi:10.1111/j.1753-4887.2010.00311.x

546. National Institute on Alcohol Abuse and Alcoholism, National Institutes of Health. Drinking patterns and their definitions. *Alcohol Research: Current Reviews.* Jan 2018, Vol 39, Issue 1.

547. Golan R, Gepner Y, Shai I. Wine and health—new evidence. *Eur J Clin Nutr.* Jul 2019;72(Suppl 1):55–59. doi:10.1038/s41430-018-0309-5

548. Chiva-Blanch G, Badimon L. Benefits and risks of moderate alcohol consumption on cardiovascular disease: current findings and controversies. *Nutrients.* Dec 2019;12(1):108. doi:10.3390/nu12010108

549. Castaldo L, Narváez A, Izzo L, et al. Red wine consumption and cardiovascular health. *Molecules.* Oct 2019;24(19):3626. doi:10.3390/molecules24193626

550. Estruch R, Hendriks HFJ. Associations between low to moderate consumption of alcoholic beverage types and health outcomes: a systematic review. *Alcohol Alcohol.* Mar 2022;57(2):176–84. doi:10.1093/alcalc/agab082

551. Pavlidou E, Mantzorou M, Fasoulas A, Tryfonos C, Petridis D, Giaginis C. Wine: An aspiring agent in promoting longevity and preventing chronic diseases. *Diseases.* Aug 2018;6(3):73. doi:10.3390/diseases6030073

552. Rehm J. The risks associated with alcohol use and alcoholism. *Alcohol Res Health.* 2011;34(2):135–43.

553. Dirlewanger M, di Vetta V, Guenat E, et al. Effects of short-term carbohydrate or fat overfeeding on energy expenditure and plasma leptin concentrations in healthy female subjects. *Int J Obes Relat Metab Disord.* Nov 2000;24(11):1413–8. doi:10.1038/sj.ijo.0801395

554. Soeliman FA, Azadbakht L. Weight loss maintenance: a review on dietary related strategies. *J Res Med Sci.* Mar 2014;19(3):268–75.

555. Jensen MD, Ryan DH, Apovian CM, et al. 2013 AHA/ACC/TOS guideline for the management of overweight and obesity in adults: a report of the American College of Cardiology/American Heart Association Task Force on Practice Guidelines and the Obesity Society. *Circulation.* Jun 2014;129(25 Suppl 2):S102–38. doi:10.1161/01.cir.0000437739.71477.ee

556. Wing RR, Hill JO. Successful weight loss maintenance. *Annu Rev Nutr.* 2001;21:323–41. doi:10.1146/annurev.nutr.21.1.323

557. Ribeiro AS, Nunes JP, Schoenfeld BJ, Aguiar AF, Cyrino ES. Effects of different dietary energy intake following resistance training on muscle mass and body fat in bodybuilders: a pilot study. *J Hum Kinet.* Nov 2019;70:125–34. doi:10.2478/hukin-2019-0038

558. Lichtman S, Pisarska K, Berman E, et al. Discrepancy between self-reported and actual caloric intake and exercise in obese subjects. *N Engl J Med.* Dec 1992;327(27):1893–8. doi:10.1056/NEJM199212313272701

559. Thomas DM, Martin CK, Redman LM, et al. Effect of dietary adherence on the body weight plateau: a mathematical model incorporating intermittent compliance with energy intake prescription. *Am J Clin Nutr.* Sep 2014;100(3):787–95. doi:10.3945/ajcn.113.079822

560. Townshend T, Lake A. Obesogenic environments: current evidence of the built and food environments. *Perspect Public Health.* Jan 2017;137(1):38–44. doi:10.1177/1757913916679860

561. Rosenbaum M, Leibel RL. Adaptive thermogenesis in humans. *Int J Obes* (Lond). Oct 2010;34 Suppl 1:S47–55. doi:10.1038/ijo.2010.184

562. Clark J. Periodization of exercise induces long-term weight loss while focusing strictly on improvements in cardiovascular and musculoskeletal fitness for individuals who are overfat. *Sport Sciences for Health.* Apr 2018;14:517–30. https://doi.org/10.1007/s11332-018-0450-5

563. Aragon A. *The Cycle of Progress* (evolved version of what originally appeared in *Girth Control,* 2007). 2021.

564. Hahn SL, Kaciroti N, Eisenberg D, Weeks HM, Bauer KW, Sonneville KR. Introducing dietary self-monitoring to undergraduate women via a calorie counting app has no effect on mental health or health behaviors: results from a randomized controlled trial. *J Acad Nutr Diet.* Dec 2021;121(12):2377–88. doi:10.1016/j.jand.2021.06.311

565. Levinson CA, Fewell L, Brosof LC. My Fitness Pal calorie tracker usage in the eating disorders. *Eat Behav.* Dec 2017;27:14–6. doi:10.1016/j.eatbeh.2017.08.003

566. Simpson CC, Mazzeo SE. Calorie counting and fitness tracking technology: associations with eating disorder symptomatology. *Eat Behav.* Aug 2017;26:89–92. doi:10.1016/j.eatbeh.2017.02.002

567. Eikey E. Effects of diet and fitness apps on eating disorder behaviours: qualitative study. *BJPsych Open.* Sept 2021;7(5):e176. doi:10.1192/bjo.2021.1011

568. Griffiths C, Harnack L, Pereira MA. Assessment of the accuracy of nutrient calculations of five popular nutrition tracking applications. *Public Health Nutr.* Jun 2018;21(8):1495–502. doi:10.1017/S1368980018000393

569. Passler S, Bohrer J, Blöchinger L, Senner V. Validity of wrist-worn activity trackers for estimating VO. *Int J Environ Res Public Health.* Aug 2019;16(17):3037. doi:10.3390/ijerph16173037

INDEX

A

abbreviations, 12–13

Abe, T., 206

Academy of Nutrition and Dietetics (AND), 20, 50, 95–96, 124

acceptable macronutrient distribution range (AMDR), 64, 142–143

accountability, individualizing, 247–253

ADA Courier (newsletter), 20

adaptive thermogenesis, 282

added sugars, 171

adenosine, 188

adenosine triphosphate (ATP), 35, 106, 111, 138

adherence. *See* dietary adherence

age-related anabolic resistance, 69

alcohol, 268–270

Allen, B. C., 161

alpha-linolenic acid (ALA), 141, 147, 163

alternate-day fasting (ADF), 255

American College of Sports Medicine (ACSM), 50, 95–96, 124

American Diabetes Association, 51

American Dietetic Association (ADA), 20

American Heart Association (AHA), 145, 152, 157, 162

American Institute for Cancer Research, 158

amino acids. *See* protein

anabolic response, 71, 101

anabolic window concept, 81

anaerobic exercise, 35

analysis of results, in scientific method, 36

androgen, 142

anecdotes, 47–48

animal-derived proteins

about, 99

compared with plant protein, 70–72

anthropometry, 199

anti-carb campaign, 240

anticatabolism, 116

Antonio, J., 65, 261–262

apolipoproteins, 155

arachidonic acid (AA), 141

Aragon, Alan

Girth Control, 9, 250

The Lean Muscle Diet, 243

online calculator, 304

Areta, Jose, 125

Arnal, M. A., 91

The Art and Science of Low Carbohydrate Performance (Volek and Phinney), 89

Ashtary-Larky, D., 112

athletes, protein requirements for fat loss in, 85

athletic performance

role of carbohydrates in, 122–137, 139

role of exercise performance–enhancing supplements for, 178–191

role of protein in, 94–99

timing of carbohydrates relative to, 126–137

medium-chain triglycerides (MCTs), 148–149

MEDLINE database, 51

men

    metabolism of fat by, 146–147

    muscle gain in, 233

    protein metabolism for, 76–77

Merwe, J., 181–182

Messina, M., 72

meta-analyses, 49–50

metabolic slowing, 258

metabolism

    of fat, 146–147

    of protein based on sex, 76–77

    sex-based differences in carbohydrate, 110–111

micromanagement, 234

micronutrients, 23

Mifflin St. Jeor online calculator, 212

milk, 151

milk fat globule membrane (MFGM), 155

mini-cuts, 275

Minnesota Coronary Experiment, 165

misinformation, prevalence of, 30–31, 41

Misner, B., 177

mitochondrial remodeling, 87

mmol/L, 89

mnemonic, 145

monohydrate form, 181

monosaccharides, 103

Moore, D. R., 80–81

Morton, R. W., 116

motivation, as a strategy to breach barriers to dietary change, 237

Müller, M. J., 236

multiple transportable carbohydrate model, 129

multivitamin-mineral (MVM) supplements, 174–178, 193, 302

muscle anabolism. *See* muscle gain

muscle gain

    distribution of protein throughout the day for, 77–79

    fasting and, 80–81

    maximizing, 77, 101

    in men, 233

    potential over long term, 201–203

    protein and, 100

    role of carbohydrates in, 111–117, 139

    role of protein in, 67–84

    time frame determined by rate of, 203–205

    timing of carbohydrates relative to training session for, 113–117

    timing of protein relative to training session for, 81–84

    total daily carbohydrate requirements for, 111–112

    total daily protein requirements for, 68–70

    in women, 206, 233

muscle glycogen synthesis, 131

muscle hypertrophy. *See* muscle gain

muscle protein breakdown (MPB), 67, 82, 101

muscle protein synthesis (MPS), 54, 56, 67, 71, 76, 78, 99, 116

muscle protein turnover, 68

myonuclei, 87

myristic acid, 156

N

O

P

ABOUT THE AUTHOR

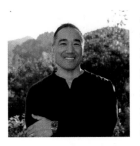 Alan Aragon is a nutrition researcher and educator with over 25 years of success in the field. He is known as one of the most influential figures in the fitness industry's movement toward evidence-based information. Notable clients Alan has worked with include "Stone Cold" Steve Austin, Derek Fisher, and Pete Sampras.

Alan writes a monthly research review, AARR, providing cutting-edge theoretical and practical information. His work has been published in popular magazines as well as the peer-reviewed scientific literature. He is the lead author of the International Society of Sports Nutrition Position Stand on Diets & Body Composition. Alan also maintains a private practice designing programs for athletes and regular people striving to be their best.